T0205228

METHODS IN MOLECULAR BIOLOGY

Series Editor
John M. Walker
School of Life and Medical Sciences
University of Hertfordshire
Hatfield, Hertfordshire, AL10 9AB, UK

For further volumes:
http://www.springer.com/series/7651

MicroRNA Profiling

Methods and Protocols

Edited by

Sweta Rani

Department of Science, Waterford Institute of Technology, Waterford, Ireland

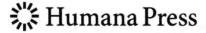 Humana Press

Editor
Sweta Rani
Department of Science
Waterford Institute of Technology
Waterford, Ireland

ISSN 1064-3745   ISSN 1940-6029   (electronic)
Methods in Molecular Biology
ISBN 978-1-4939-8225-7   ISBN 978-1-4939-6524-3   (eBook)
DOI 10.1007/978-1-4939-6524-3

This Humana Press imprint is published by Springer Nature
The registered company is Springer Science+Business Media LLC

Preface

MicroRNAs (miRNAs) are a small non-coding, single-stranded RNA molecule consisting of 20–24 nucleotides. It is found in animals and plants as well as some viruses and is involved in the regulation of gene expression. The primary function of miRNA is, at the post-transcriptional level, downregulating gene expression by regulating translational repression, mRNA cleavage, and deadenylation. Since the discovery of miRNAs in 1993, this field has garnered major interests among the scientists worldwide.

This volume of *Methods in Molecular Biology* book collates chapters by the experts in their respective field. This book not only provides classical techniques to profile miRNA but also includes newer approaches. The chapters include step-by-step easy-to-follow protocol and troubleshooting tips to ensure successful experiment.

To summarize, this book includes comprehensive descriptions of miRNA biogenesis and their role in the development and progression of various human diseases. The first few chapters describe the effect of overexpressing and repressing of a target miRNA and their effect on cell viability and proliferation. Applications and limitations of several RNA isolation kit have been outlined. A hands-on, optimized protocol for total RNA isolation using formalin-fixed paraffin-embedded (FFPE) tissue and plants tissues is described in this book.

Extracellular miRNAs are found to be resistant to nucleases. Some of these extracellular miRNAs are found to be encapsulated in exosomes or extracellular vesicles. Isolation and characterization of exosomes from medium conditioned by cell lines, serum, and plasma specimens are also outlined in few chapters.

Induced pluripotent stem (iPS) cells are gaining importance to be used in cell replacement therapies. To generate the iPS cells one has to understand the molecular mechanism controlling differentiation. miRNA expression associated with the pluripotent state of the iPS cells has important functional significance and is described in an easy-to-follow protocol in this book. Diverse miRNA detection methods are available and newer ones are continuously being developed and are described in this book. This book also includes novel method of miRNA profiling, like Ligo-miR, to identify unique miRNA.

Modern technologies such as TLDA, Microarrays, and Next Generation Sequencing generate a huge amount of data. Managing and analyzing the miRNA expression data requires the understanding of several software and tools. Bioinformatics analysis allows extraction of biologically useful results from large amounts of raw data. There are several software tools available including miRandola, PicTar, DIANA, and miRWalk, which are described in this book.

Waterford, Ireland *Sweta Rani*

Contents

Preface. . . . . *v*
Contributors. . . . . *ix*

1 MiRNA Biogenesis and Regulation of Diseases: An Overview 1
   Anchal Vishnoi and Sweta Rani

2 Assessment of Basic Biological Functions Exerted by miRNAs. 11
   John Nolan, Raymond L. Stallings, and Olga Piskareva

3 Extraction of miRNAs from Formalin-Fixed Paraffin-Embedded
   (FFPE) Tissues 17
   Karen Howe

4 MiRNA Isolation from Plants Rich in Polysaccharides and Polyphenols 25
   K.K. Sabu, Fasiludeen Nadiya, and Narayanannair Anjali

5 MicroRNA Profiling of Exosomes. 37
   Melissa Daly and Lorraine O'Driscoll

6 MiRNA Profiling in Human Induced Pluripotent Stem Cells. 47
   Erica Hennessy

7 MiRNA Expression in Cystic Fibrosis Bronchial Epithelial Cells 57
   Irene K. Oglesby and Paul J. McKiernan

8 TaqMan Low Density Array: MicroRNA Profiling for Biomarker
   and Oncosuppressor Discovery 71
   Keith O'Brien

9 Detection of MicroRNAs in Brain Slices Using In Situ Hybridization 85
   **Sean Quinlan, Christine Henke, Gary P. Brennan, David C. Henshall,
   and Eva M. Jimenez-Mateos**

10 Exosomal MicroRNA Discovery in Age-Related Macular Degeneration. 93
   Hanan Elshelmani and Sweta Rani

11 Profiling the MicroRNA Payload of Exosomes Derived
   from Ex Vivo Primary Colorectal Fibroblasts. 115
   **Rahul Bhome, Rebecca Goh, Karen Pickard, Massimiliano Mellone,
   A. Emre Sayan, and Alex Mirnezami**

12 Circulating MicroRNAs in Cancer. 123
   **Killian P. O'Brien, Eimear Ramphul, Linda Howard,
   William M. Gallagher, Carmel Malone, Michael J. Kerin,
   and Róisín M. Dwyer**

13 Profiling Circulating MiRNAs from the Plasma of Individuals
   with Metabolic Syndrome 141
   Sadhbh O'Neill and Lorraine O'Driscoll

14   Manipulating MiRNA Expression to Uncover Hidden Functions 151
     Sinéad T. Aherne and Nga T. Lao

15   Analysis of the Distribution Profiles of Circulating MicroRNAs
     by Asymmetrical Flow Field Flow Fractionation. 161
     Kenneth Flack, Luis A. Jimenez, and Wenwan Zhong

16   MicroRNA Expression Profiling Using Agilent One-Color Microarray 169
     Carmela Dell'Aversana, Cristina Giorgio, and Lucia Altucci

17   A Multiplex Ligation Assay for MiRNA Copy Number Profiling 185
     Duncan Kilburn, Yunke Song, Tza-Huei Wang, and Kelvin J. Liu

18   Practical Bioinformatics Analysis of MiRNA Data Using Online Tools. 195
     James A.L. Brown and Emer Bourke

19   Visualization and Analysis of MiRNA–Targets Interactions Networks 209
     Luis E. León and Sebastián D. Calligaris

20   Guidelines on Designing MicroRNA Sponges: From Construction
     to Stable Cell Line 221
     Manoela Marques Ortega and Hakim Bouamar

21   Customization of Artificial MicroRNA Design 235
     Tien Van Vu and Vinh Nang Do

Index 245

Contributors

SINÉAD T. AHERNE • *Department of Tumor Biology, H. Lee Moffitt Cancer Center and Research Institute, Tampa, FL, USA*

National Institute for Cellular Biotechnology, Dublin City University, Dublin, Ireland

LUCIA ALTUCCI • *Institute of Genetics and Biophysics, CNR, Naples, Italy; Department of Biochemistry, Biophysics and General Pathology, Second University of Naples, Naples, Italy*

NARAYANANNAIR ANJALI • *Biotechnology and Bioinformatics Division, Jawaharlal Nehru Tropical Botanic Garden and Research Institute (JNTBGRI), Thiruvananthapuram, India*

RAHUL BHOME • *Cancer Sciences, University of Southampton, Southampton, UK; University Surgical Unit, Southampton General Hospital, Southampton, UK*

HAKIM BOUAMAR • *Department of Cellular and Structural Biology, University of Texas Health Science Center at San Antonio, San Antonio, TX, USA*

EMER BOURKE • *Discipline of Pathology, College of Medicine, Lambe Institute for Translational Research, National University of Ireland Galway, Galway, Ireland*

GARY P. BRENNAN • *Department of Physiology and Medical Physics, Royal College of Surgeons in Ireland, Dublin, Ireland*

JAMES A.L. BROWN • *Discipline of Surgery, College of Medicine, Lambe Institute for Translational Research, National University of Ireland Galway, Galway, Ireland*

SEBASTIÁN D. CALLIGARIS • *Centro de Medicina Regenerativa, Facultad de Medicina, Clínica Alemana-Universidad del Desarrollo, Santiago, Chile*

MELISSA DALY • *School of Pharmacy and Pharmaceutical Science and Trinity Biomedical Sciences Institute, Trinity College Dublin, Dublin, Ireland*

CARMELA DELL'AVERSANA • *Institute of Genetics and Biophysics, CNR, Naples, Italy; Department of Biochemistry, Biophysics and General Pathology, Second University of Naples, Naples, Italy*

VINH NANG DO • *National Key Laboratory for Plant Cell Biotechnology, Agricultural Genetics Institute, Ha Noi, Vietnam*

RÓISÍN M. DWYER • *Discipline of Surgery, Lambe Institute for Translational Research, National University of Ireland Galway, Galway, Ireland*

HANAN ELSHELMANI • *Zoology Department, School of Natural Sciences, Trinity College Dublin, Dublin, Ireland*

KENNETH FLACK • *Department of Chemistry, University of California, Riverside, CA, USA*

WILLIAM M. GALLAGHER • *Cancer Biology and Therapeutics Laboratory, UCD School of Biomolecular and Biomedical Science, UCD Conway Institute, University College Dublin, Dublin, Ireland*

CRISTINA GIORGIO • *Department of Biochemistry, Biophysics and General Pathology, Second University of Naples, Naples, Italy*

REBECCA GOH • *Cancer Sciences, University of Southampton, Southampton, UK*

CHRISTINE HENKE • *Department of Physiology and Medical Physics, Royal College of Surgeons in Ireland, Dublin, Ireland*

ERICA HENNESSY • *National Institute for Cellular Biotechnology, Dublin City University, Dublin, Ireland*

DAVID C. HENSHALL • *Department of Physiology and Medical Physics, Royal College of Surgeons in Ireland, Dublin, Ireland*

LINDA HOWARD • *Regenerative Medicine Institute, National University of Ireland Galway, Galway, Ireland*

KAREN HOWE • *National institute for Cellular Biotechnology, Dublin City University, Dublin, Ireland*

LUIS A. JIMENEZ • *Program in Biomedical Sciences, University of California, Riverside, CA, USA*

EVA M. JIMENEZ-MATEOS • *Department of Physiology and Medical Physics, Royal College of Surgeons in Ireland, Dublin, Ireland*

MICHAEL J. KERIN • *Discipline of Surgery, Lambe Institute for Translational Research, National University of Ireland Galway, Galway, Ireland*

DUNCAN KILBURN • *Circulomics Inc., Baltimore, MD, USA*

NGA T. LAO • *National Institute for Cellular Biotechnology, Dublin City University, Dublin, Ireland*

LUIS E. LEÓN • *Centro de Genética y Genómica, Facultad de Medicina, Clínica Alemana-Universidad del Desarrollo, Santiago, Chile*

KELVIN J. LIU • *Circulomics Inc., Baltimore, MD, USA*

CARMEL MALONE • *Discipline of Surgery, Lambe Institute for Translational Research, National University of Ireland Galway, Galway, Ireland*

PAUL J. MCKIERNAN • *Royal College of Surgeons in Ireland, Education and Research Centre, Beaumont Hospital, Dublin, Ireland*

MASSIMILIANO MELLONE • *Cancer Sciences, University of Southampton, Southampton, UK*

ALEX MIRNEZAMI • *Cancer Sciences, University of Southampton, Southampton, UK; University Surgical Unit, Southampton General Hospital, Southampton, UK*

FASILUDEEN NADIYA • *Biotechnology and Bioinformatics Division, Jawaharlal Nehru Tropical Botanic Garden and Research Institute (JNTBGRI), Thiruvananthapuram, India*

JOHN NOLAN • *Molecular and Cellular Therapeutics, Royal College of Surgeons in Ireland, Dublin, Ireland; National Children's Research Centre Our Lady's Children's Hospital, Crumlin, Dublin, Ireland*

KEITH O'BRIEN • *School of Pharmacy and Pharmaceutical Sciences & Trinity Biomedical Sciences Institute, Trinity College, Dublin, Ireland*

KILLIAN P. O'BRIEN • *Discipline of Surgery, Lambe Institute for Translational Research, National University of Ireland Galway, Galway, Ireland*

LORRAINE O'DRISCOLL • *School of Pharmacy and Pharmaceutical Sciences and Trinity Biomedical Sciences Institute, Trinity College Dublin, Dublin, Ireland*

SADHBH O'NEILL • *School of Pharmacy and Pharmaceutical Sciences and Trinity Biomedical Sciences Institute, Trinity College Dublin, Dublin, Ireland*

IRENE K. OGLESBY • *Royal College of Surgeons in Ireland, Education and Research Centre, Beaumont Hospital, Dublin, Ireland*

MANOELA MARQUES ORTEGA • *Post Graduate Program in Health Sciences, São Francisco University, Bragança Paulista, São Paulo, Brazil*

KAREN PICKARD • *Cancer Sciences Unit, University of Southampton, Southampton, UK*

OLGA PISKAREVA • *Molecular and Cellular Therapeutics, Royal College of Surgeons in Ireland, Dublin, Ireland; National Children's Research Centre Our Lady's Children's Hospital, Crumlin, Dublin, Ireland*

SEAN QUINLAN • *Department of Physiology and Medical Physics, Royal College of Surgeons in Ireland, Dublin, Ireland*

EIMEAR RAMPHUL • *Discipline of Surgery, Lambe Institute for Translational Research, National University of Ireland Galway, Galway, Ireland*

SWETA RANI • *Department of Science, Waterford Institute of Technology, Waterford, Ireland*

K.K. SABU • *Biotechnology and Bioinformatics Division, Jawaharlal Nehru Tropical Botanic garden & Research Institute (JNTBGRI), Thiruvananthapuram, India*

A. EMRE SAYAN • *Cancer Sciences, University of Southampton, Southampton, UK*

YUNKE SONG • *Biomedical Engineering Department, Johns Hopkins University, Baltimore, MD, USA*

RAYMOND L. STALLINGS • *Molecular and Cellular Therapeutics, Royal College of Surgeons in Ireland, Dublin, Ireland; National Children's Research Centre Our Lady's Children's Hospital, Crumlin, Dublin, Ireland*

ANCHAL VISHNOI • *SEQOME Ltd., Waterford, Ireland*

TIEN VAN VU • *National Key Laboratory for Plant Cell Biotechnology, Agricultural Genetics Institute, Ha Noi, Vietnam*

TZA-HUEI WANG • *Biomedical Engineering Department, Johns Hopkins University, Baltimore, MD, USA; Mechanical Engineering Department, Johns Hopkins University, Baltimore, MD, USA; Sidney Kimmel Comprehensive Cancer Center, Johns Hopkins University, Baltimore, MD, USA; Center of Cancer Nanotechnology Excellence, Johns Hopkins University, Baltimore, MD, USA*

WENWAN ZHONG • *Department of Chemistry, University of California, Riverside, CA, USA*

Chapter 1

MiRNA Biogenesis and Regulation of Diseases: An Overview

Anchal Vishnoi and Sweta Rani

Abstract

MicroRNAs (miRNAs) are small RNA molecules, with their role in gene silencing and translational repression by binding to target mRNAs. Since it was discovered in 1993, miRNA are found in all eukaryotic cells conserved across the species. In recent years, regulation of miRNAs are extensively studied for their role in biological processes as well as in development and progression of various human diseases including retinal disorder, neurodegenerative diseases, cardiovascular disease and cancer. This chapter summarises miRNA biogenesis and explores their potential roles in a variety of diseases. miRNAs holds huge potential for diagnostic and prognostic biomarkers, and as predictors of drug response.

Key words miRNA, Retinal disorder, Neurodegenerative diseases, Cardiovascular disease, Cancer

1 Introduction

1.1 microRNAs (miRNA)

microRNA (miRNA) was first observed in *Caenorhabditis elegans* [1] and is the most abundant small RNA [2]. It has now been detected in nearly all animal model systems and their numbers largely correlate with the complexity of the organism [3]. Humans have approximately 2000 annotated miRNA genes and total number of microRNA loci annotated is 24, 521 loci in 206 species [4]. Human genome consist of large number of miRNA genes accounting for 1–5 % of all predicted human genes [5] and mammalian miRNAs are known to regulate approximately 30 % of all protein-coding genes [6]. As multiple miRNAs target the same mRNA there is no linear correlation between miRNA and mRNA expression [7].

Ambros and Ruvkun were the first to discover miRNA in 1993. Lin-4 was the first miRNA to be discovered in *C. elegans* [1, 8]. In 2000 a second miRNA was discovered called let-7 and found to be conserved across the species [9]. This finding boosted the miRNA discovery studies and soon many more miRNAs were found in *C. elegans*, *Drosophila melanogaster* and human genomes [10–12].

Sweta Rani (ed.), *MicroRNA Profiling: Methods and Protocols*, Methods in Molecular Biology, vol. 1509, DOI 10.1007/978-1-4939-6524-3_1, © Springer Science+Business Media New York 2017

miRNA are small non-coding RNAs, single-stranded RNA molecules of approximately 21–23 nucleotides in length. miRNA has a uridine at their 5′-end and partially complementary to the 3′-end untranslated regions of the messenger RNA (mRNA). miRNA recruits Argonaute (AGO) protein complex to a complementary target mRNA, which results in translation repression or degradation or deadenylation of the mRNA [13].

2   miRNA Biogenesis

2.1   Transcription of miRNA

The miRNA biogenesis in human follows a two step process with nuclear and cytoplasmic cleavage event. In the nucleus the miR-NAs are transcribed as a long transcript called pri-miRNA, either by their own promoters or by sharing promoters of their host gene [14]. For the majority of miRNA among the two RNA polymerase RNA pol II and RNA pol III, RNA pol II is thought to be responsible for the pri-miRNA transcription (Fig. 1a). The preference for RNA pol II is evident by the length of pri-miRNA, which is more than 1 kb longer than the pol III transcript. Also pri-miRNA contains sequences of uridine residues, which terminates pol III transcription. These all, support the preference of pol II for transcription of pri-miRNA though there is exception, transcription of miR-142 by RNA pol III [15]. In addition to the above-mentioned features, the transcriptional start sites are located far away from the genes and promoters contain features typical of RNA pol II [16]. The transcriptional regulation of miRNA sometimes follow feedback loop where positive or negative regulation of miRNA down-regulates or amplify their own expression [17].

miRNAs which resides in introns are known as mirtrons. Mirtrons presence is widespread in Drosophila, *C. elegans*, vertebrates and plants [18]. The transcription, primarily for mirtrons, take place independent of the host gene (Fig. 1a).

2.2   Formation of pre-miRNA

The nuclear cleavage of the pri-miRNA, is carried out by Drosha RNase III endonuclease (Fig. 1a 2). Drosha RNase III endonuclease cleaves both strands of the stem at sites near the base of the primary stem loop releasing ~60–70 nt stem loop intermediate, called miRNA precursor, or the pre-miRNA. Only that, pri-miRNA matures into functional miRNA that has a flexible terminal loop (≥10 bp) and 5′ phosphate and ~2 nt 3′ single-stranded RNA overhangs. It is mediated via RNase III endonuclease Drosha and the double-stranded RNA-binding protein DiGeorge syndrome critical region gene 8 (DGCR8) also known as pasha [14]. The pre-miRNA has a staggered cut with 5′ phosphate and 3′ 2 nucleotide overhang [19]. The mirtrons are exception, and bypass the Drosha pathway releasing the precursor splicing [20] (Fig. 1a).

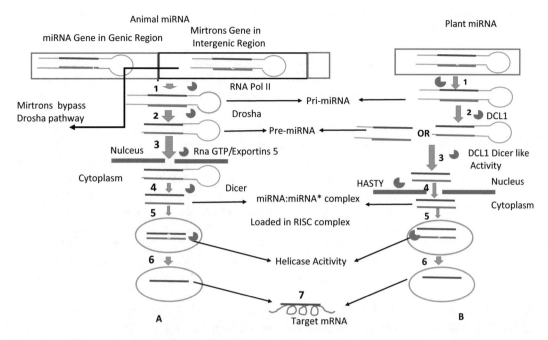

Fig. 1 miRNA biogenesis in (**a**) animal and (**b**) plant. (1). RNA pol II responsible for the pri-miRNA transcription (2). Drosha RNase III endonuclease cleavs pri-miRNA near the base of the primary stem loop. In plant DCL1 has a siilar function as drosha. (3). The pre-miRNA transported into the cytoplasm (4). pre-miRNA maturation in the cytoplasm is carried out by RNase III endonuclease Dicer (5). The helicase domain recognises the loop region and cleaves both the strands (6). Short RNA fragment called miRNA (7). MiRNA bind to their target mRNA and negatively regulate its expression

This pre-miRNA is transported into the cytoplasm through the interaction of exportin-5 and Ran-GTP [21] (Fig. 1a 3).

2.3 Maturation of Pre-miRNA in Cytoplasm

The pre-miRNA maturation in the cytoplasm is further carried out by RNase III endonuclease Dicer (Fig. 1a 4). It recognize the 5′ phosphate and 3′ overhang approximately at the two helical turn away from the base, and cut the double strand. The cleavage separate the loop structure and the imperfect double strand is known as miRNA:miRNA* complex. miRNA is a mature miRNA whereas miRNA* is the opposing arm of the miRNA, this complex and miRNA* is short lived as revealed by cloning of the miRNA [22, 23]. The Dicer is characterized by the presence of helicase, a PAZ domain, double stranded RNA binding domain and a RNAIII domain. The PAZ domain recognizes the 3′ overhang [24]. The helicase domain recognized the loop region and the two RNAIII domain cleaves both the strands, the whole procedure occurs only when the miRNA complex is loaded in the Dicer [24, 25]. In plants, Dicer-like 1 (DCL1) protein has similar function as Drosha and perhaps functions as Dicer (which is not clear yet) in processing the miRNA-miRNA* complex in the nucleus [26]. This complex is then transported nucleus by HASTY the Arabidopsis homolog of exportin 5 [27] (Fig. 1b).

3   Regulation of Dicer

Different pathways regulate Dicer, which in turn regulates the amount of miRNA in the cell. In human sometimes, the Dicer is regulated by its miRNA through the binding sites, as present in the let-7 miRNA [28]. In addition to miRNA regulation of Dicer activity, the helicase domain has an auto-inhibitory effect on Dicer [29]. Many protein interactions also affect the efficiency of the Dicer. The HIV-1 TAR RNA-binding protein (TRBP) and protein activator of PKR (PACT) a dsRNA binding protein increase the cleavage efficiency of Dicer through helicase binding [29, 30]. On the other hand, the monocyte chemoattractant protein 1-induced protein 1 (MCPIP1), also known as Zinc-finger CCCH-type containing 12A (Zc3h12a) degrades the miRNA precursor. The MCPIP1 is a nuclease, which works opposite to Dicer cleaving the loop region of miRNA precursor resulting in its rapid degradation [31].

3.1   Maturation of miRNA in RISC

Both in plants and animals, the miRNA from the miRNA–miRNA* complex are loaded into RNA induced silencing complex (RISC). Further, maturation of miRNAs are carried out by the RISC-loading complex (RLC) [32].

The Argonaute protein, a catalytic component of RISC helps in uptake of miRNA and freeing of Dicer. In some case, as in mammalian cells, Ago2, a Argonaute protein have endonuclease activity and cleave the 3′ arm of the miRNA before being processed by Dicer, this in turn may help in determining the mature miRNA strand [32, 33]. The structure of the miRNA is likely to determine the specificity of Ago2 [33, 34]. There are three categories of Argonaute, (1) Ago, which works in miRNA and siRNA pathways; (2) piwi, which regulates the piRNAs; and (3) worm specific subfamilies [35]. It then directs RISC to down-regulate the target gene. The miRNA either cleave the target mRNA if it has the sufficient complementarity to the miRNA or miRNA repress the translation of mRNA [36]. The target recognition of mRNA by miRNA is done by conserved region of miRNA, as in case of invertebrate miRNA where 2–8 residues are perfectly complementary to 3′UTR motifs is shown to mediate posttranscriptional repression [37].

The Argonaute proteins in addition to targeting the mRNA also regulate the stability of the miRNAs. In *C. elegans* by unknown mechanism the ALG-1 (Argonautes) play a role in miRNA stability and precursor processing [38]. Association of miRNA with the Argonaute protein protects them from exonuclease (XRN-1 and XRN-2) degradation [38]. The base pairing of miRNA with its target also determines miRNA stability. In Drosophila a strong base pairing between the target and miRNA leads to addition of nucleotide at 3′ end, which further trim the miRNA [39]. Similarly, in human a uridine is added to miR-223 when there is perfect match with target, which leads to its degradation [40].

The addition of nucleotide at 3′ end of miRNA does not always lead to its degradation. In mice, poly(A) polymerase GLD-2 determines the addition of single adenosine at the 3′ end of the miR-122, which in turn protect it from the exonuclease activity and thus increasing its life [41]. In another example, RNA binding protein Quaking (QKI) stabilizes the structure of miR-20a in human cells [42]. The QKI is a tumour suppressor, regulating glioblastoma multiforme (GBM) pathogenesis, by its effect on miR-20a. The level of miR-20a levels decrease in absence of QKI, which in turn, increases the level of TGFβ~ R2 involved in onco-genesis [42].

The miRNA biogenesis pathway is also regulated by other miRNA. For example, in mouse the miR-709 binds to the compli-mentary sites of primary miR-15a/16-1 and repress it's Drosha processing [43]. Therefore, it can be said that there are different pathways, which degrade or stabilize the structure of miRNA alter-ing its level in the cell.

4 Extracellular Vesicles (EVs)

Extracellular vesicles (EVs) are nano-sized (40–100 nm in diame-ter) vesicles of endosomal origin [44]. Pan and Johnstone were the first to isolate small vesicles secreted by sheep reticulocytes in 1980 [45]. The cargo is driven into the EVs from the cytoplasm of the host cell. EVs cargo includes proteins, microRNA (miRNA), mRNA and lipids [46, 47]. EVs are subsequently internalised by other cells via direct membrane fusion, endocytosis or cell-type specific phagocytosis [48–50].

4.1 Role of EVs and miRNA in Diseases

With the discovery of miRNAs, it has garnered huge interest in determining their role in various diseases. Dysregulation of miRNA expression plays an important role in disease progression and their expression profiling is likely to become important diagnostic and prognostic tools. miRNA therapeutics is not only challenging but also promising for several diseases.

4.2 Retinal Disorder

miRNAs has been found to play essential roles in not only retinal development and survival, but also in their normal functioning. It is still not clear if every cell type has their own miRNA phenotype but studies have confirmed the presence of differentially expressed miRNA in neural retina and their expression patterns can be used to distinguish retinal cell types [51]. Reduced expression of miR-NAs in the retina is observed in the absence of Dicer [52], a prin-cipal enzyme in miRNA biogenesis, leading to altered function and survival of retinal neurons and ultimately impaired vision [53].

miR-183/96/182 cluster provide a protective role in retinal neurons and inactivation of this cluster in transgenic mice resulted in gradual synaptic connectivity defects of the photoreceptors causing extreme sensitivity to light and severe retinal degeneration [54]. In an attempt to identify biomarker, specifically circulating biomarker for ocular disorder, Ragusa et al. analysed vitreous humor (VH) and found more than 100-fold difference in miRNA expression when compared to serum from patients affected by various ocular diseases [55].

4.3 Neurodegenerative Diseases

Cause of central nervous system diseases could be attributed to the altered expression of miRNAs. Study of miRNA expression could lead to novel molecular information and therapeutic option including enhancing or inhibiting specific miRNAs to improve the disease treatment.

Earlier in 2012, Xin et al. demonstrated that MSCs communicate via exosomes with brain parenchymal cells and regulate neurite outgrowth by horizontal transfer of miR-133b to neural cells in vitro [56]. MSCs are known to contribute to neurological recovery after stroke, and with the discovery of exosomes as a carrier of miR-133b to astrocytes and neurons after cerebral ischemia, a theory has emerged that these exosomes shuttles miR-133b stimulating neurite outgrowth and thereby improving recovery after stroke [56].

4.4 Cardiovascular Disease

miRNAs plays an important role in the development of cardiac tissue at all stages [57]. Various miRNA and in particular, miR-143 regulates myocardial cell morphology and is also essential for the functioning and formation of cardiac chamber. Vascular smooth muscle cell (VSMC) differentiation is also regulated via miR-143 and miR-145 [58]. In recent years, it has been reported that deregulation of miRNA is associated with several cardiovascular diseases. Decreased expression of miR-143/145 was reported by acute and chronic vascular stresses [58].

miRNAs associated with MSC-EVs also play an important role in cardio-protection and was found that miR-22-loaded EVs targeted methyl CpG binding protein 2 (Mecp2) promoting cardiac remodelling following myocardial infarction [59]. Similarly, miR-221 level was found to be significantly higher in MSC-EVs compared to their parent MSCs, enhancing cardio-protection by reducing the expression of p53 up-regulated modulator of apoptosis (PUMA) [60].

4.5 Cancer

miRNAs are known as critical regulator of gene expression, and in cancer, miRNA play a role in oncogenesis, metastasis, and resistance to various therapies. miRNAs can be classified as oncogenes (oncomirs), tumor-suppressor genes, pro-metastatic ('metastamiRs') and metastasis-suppressor [61].

Number of studies suggests that miRNAs exist in sera that are associated with non-small cell lung cancer. A group of 6 miRNAs (miR-30c-1*, miR-616*, miR-146b-3p, miR-566, miR-550, and miR-939) was found to exist at substantially higher levels in the ADC compared to control sera [62]. Loss of miR-486 expression in stage 1 NSCLC tumors, compared to adjacent non-cancerous lung tissues, suggest that its downregulation may be important in lung cancer development. miR-486 is reported to be potent tumor suppressor of lung cancer, regulating components of insulin growth factor (IGF) signaling, including insulin-like growth factor 1 (IGF1), IGF1 receptor (IGF1R), and phosphoinositide-3-kinase, regulatory subunit 1 (alpha) (PIK3R1, or p85a) both in vitro and in vivo [63].

miRNAs has the potential as breast cancer biomarkers. A tsudy analysing the 54 Luminal A-like breast cancer blood samples and 56 normal blood samples has reported that the expression of 3 miRNAs (miR-29a, miR-181a, and miR-652), has the potential to facilitate accurate subtype-specific breast tumor diagnosis in combination with mammography [64]. miR-10b overexpression not only initiates invasion and metastasis in breast cancer models but its expression in primary breast carcinomas also correlates with clinical progression [65].

5   Conclusion

As summarised in this chapter, miRNAs and EVs have potential therapeutic and prognostic application in range of disease models. Therapeutic effects of EVs are mediated via it's ability to transfer biological information in the form of proteins, mRNA and miRNA from one cell to another. EVs also hold immense potential for precision medicine where, EVs can be used as targeted drug (or RNAi) delivery system for cell-specific disease treatment.

References

1. Lee RC, Feinbaum RL, Ambros V (1993) The C. elegans heterochronic gene lin-4 encodes small RNAs with antisense complementarity to lin-14. Cell 75(5):843–854

2. Felekkis K, Touvana E, Stefanou C et al (2010) microRNAs: a newly described class of encoded molecules that play a role in health and disease. Hippokratia 14(4):236–240

3. Friedlander MR, Lizano E, Houben AJ et al (2014) Evidence for the biogenesis of more than 1,000 novel human microRNAs. Genome Biol 15(4):R57. doi:10.1186/gb-2014-15-4-r57

4. Kozomara A, Griffiths-Jones S (2011) miR-Base: integrating microRNA annotation and deep-sequencing data. Nucleic Acids Res 39(Database issue):D152–D157. doi:10.1093/nar/gkq1027

5. Bentwich I, Avniel A, Karov Y et al (2005) Identification of hundreds of conserved and nonconserved human microRNAs. Nat Genet 37(7):766–770. doi:10.1038/ng1590

6. Filipowicz W, Bhattacharyya SN, Sonenberg N (2008) Mechanisms of post-transcriptional regulation by microRNAs: are the answers in sight? Nat Rev Genet 9(2):102–114. doi:10.1038/nrg2290

7. Saetrom P, Heale BS, Snove O Jr et al (2007) Distance constraints between microRNA target sites dictate efficacy and cooperativity. Nucleic Acids Res 35(7):2333–2342. doi:10.1093/nar/gkm133

8. Bartel DP (2004) MicroRNAs: genomics, biogenesis, mechanism, and function. Cell 116(2):281–297

9. Reinhart BJ, Slack FJ, Basson M et al (2000) The 21-nucleotide let-7 RNA regulates developmental timing in Caenorhabditis elegans. Nature 403(6772):901–906. doi:10.1038/35002607

10. Lagos-Quintana M, Rauhut R, Lendeckel W et al (2001) Identification of novel genes coding for small expressed RNAs. Science (New York, NY) 294(5543):853–858. doi:10.1126/science.1064921

11. Lau NC, Lim LP, Weinstein EG et al (2001) An abundant class of tiny RNAs with probable regulatory roles in Caenorhabditis elegans. Science (New York, NY) 294(5543):858–862. doi:10.1126/science.1065062

12. Lee RC, Ambros V (2001) An extensive class of small RNAs in Caenorhabditis elegans. Science (New York, NY) 294(5543):862–864. doi:10.1126/science.1065329

13. Wu L, Fan J, Belasco JG (2006) MicroRNAs direct rapid deadenylation of mRNA. Proc Natl Acad Sci U S A 103(11):4034–4039. doi:10.1073/pnas.0510928103

14. Lee Y, Jeon K, Lee JT et al (2002) MicroRNA maturation: stepwise processing and subcellular localization. EMBO J 21(17):4663–4670

15. Chen CZ, Li L, Lodish HF et al (2004) MicroRNAs modulate hematopoietic lineage differentiation. Science (New York, NY) 303(5654):83–86. doi:10.1126/science.1091903

16. Monteys AM, Spengler RM, Wan J et al (2010) Structure and activity of putative intronic miRNA promoters. RNA 16(3):495–505. doi:10.1261/rna.1731910

17. Martinez NJ, Ow MC, Barrasa MI et al (2008) A C. elegans genome-scale microRNA network contains composite feedback motifs with high flux capacity. Genes Dev 22(18):2535–2549. doi:10.1101/gad.1678608

18. Okamura K, Hagen JW, Duan H et al (2007) The mirtron pathway generates microRNA-class regulatory RNAs in Drosophila. Cell 130(1):89–100. doi:10.1016/j.cell.2007.06.028

19. Lee Y, Ahn C, Han J et al (2003) The nuclear RNase III Drosha initiates microRNA processing. Nature 425(6956):415–419. doi:10.1038/nature01957

20. Westholm JO, Lai EC (2011) Mirtrons: microRNA biogenesis via splicing. Biochimie 93(11):1897–1904. doi:10.1016/j.biochi.2011.06.017

21. Yi R, Qin Y, Macara IG et al (2003) Exportin-5 mediates the nuclear export of pre-microRNAs and short hairpin RNAs. Genes Dev 17(24):3011–3016. doi:10.1101/gad.1158803

22. Aravin AA, Lagos-Quintana M, Yalcin A et al (2003) The small RNA profile during Drosophila melanogaster development. Dev Cell 5(2):337–350

23. Lagos-Quintana M, Rauhut R, Yalcin A et al (2002) Identification of tissue-specific microRNAs from mouse. Curr Biol 12(9):735–739

24. MacRae IJ, Doudna JA (2007) Ribonuclease revisited: structural insights into ribonuclease III family enzymes. Curr Opin Struct Biol 17(1):138–145. doi:10.1016/j.sbi.2006.12.002

25. Lau PW, Guiley KZ, De N et al (2012) The molecular architecture of human Dicer. Nat Struct Mol Biol 19(4):436–440. doi:10.1038/nsmb.2268

26. Papp I, Mette MF, Aufsatz W et al (2003) Evidence for nuclear processing of plant micro RNA and short interfering RNA precursors. Plant Physiol 132(3):1382–1390

27. Bollman KM, Aukerman MJ, Park MY et al (2003) HASTY, the Arabidopsis ortholog of exportin 5/MSN5, regulates phase change and morphogenesis. Development 130(8):1493–1504

28. Forman JJ, Legesse-Miller A, Coller HA (2008) A search for conserved sequences in coding regions reveals that the let-7 microRNA targets Dicer within its coding sequence. Proc Natl Acad Sci U S A 105(39):14879–14884. doi:10.1073/pnas.0803230105

29. Ma E, MacRae IJ, Kirsch JF et al (2008) Autoinhibition of human dicer by its internal helicase domain. J Mol Biol 380(1):237–243. doi:10.1016/j.jmb.2008.05.005

30. Lee Y, Hur I, Park SY et al (2006) The role of PACT in the RNA silencing pathway. EMBO J 25(3):522–532. doi:10.1038/sj.emboj.7600942

31. Suzuki HI, Arase M, Matsuyama H et al (2011) MCPIP1 ribonuclease antagonizes dicer and terminates microRNA biogenesis through precursor microRNA degradation. Mol Cell 44(3):424–436. doi:10.1016/j.molcel.2011.09.012

32. Sanghvi VR, Steel LF (2011) The cellular TAR RNA binding protein, TRBP, promotes HIV-1 replication primarily by inhibiting the activation of double-stranded RNA-dependent kinase PKR. J Virol 85(23):12614–12621. doi:10.1128/JVI.05240-11

33. Diederichs S, Haber DA (2007) Dual role for argonautes in microRNA processing and post-transcriptional regulation of microRNA expression. Cell 131(6):1097–1108. doi:10.1016/j.cell.2007.10.032

34. Yang N, Cao Y, Han P et al (2012) Tools for investigation of the RNA endonuclease activity of mammalian Argonaute2 protein. Anal Chem 84(5):2492–2497. doi:10.1021/ac2032854

35. Tolia NH, Joshua-Tor L (2007) Slicer and the argonautes. Nat Chem Biol 3(1):36–43. doi:10.1038/nchembio848

36. Hutvagner G, Zamore PD (2002) A microRNA in a multiple-turnover RNAi enzyme complex. Science (New York, NY) 297(5589):2056–2060. doi:10.1126/science.1073827

37. Lai EC (2002) Micro RNAs are complementary to 3′ UTR sequence motifs that mediate negative post-transcriptional regulation. Nat Genet 30(4):363–364. doi:10.1038/ng865

38. Grishok A, Pasquinelli AE, Conte D et al (2001) Genes and mechanisms related to RNA interference regulate expression of the small temporal RNAs that control C. elegans developmental timing. Cell 106(1):23–34

39. Ameres SL, Horwich MD, Hung JH et al (2010) Target RNA-directed trimming and tailing of small silencing RNAs. Science (New York, NY) 328(5985):1534–1539. doi:10.1126/science.1187058

40. Baccarini A, Chauhan H, Gardner TJ et al (2011) Kinetic analysis reveals the fate of a microRNA following target regulation in mammalian cells. Curr Biol 21(5):369–376. doi:10.1016/j.cub.2011.01.067

41. Katoh T, Sakaguchi Y, Miyauchi K et al (2009) Selective stabilization of mammalian microRNAs by 3′ adenylation mediated by the cytoplasmic poly(A) polymerase GLD-2. Genes Dev 23(4):433–438. doi:10.1101/gad.1761509

42. Chen AJ, Paik JH, Zhang H et al (2012) STAR RNA-binding protein Quaking suppresses cancer via stabilization of specific miRNA. Genes Dev 26(13):1459–1472. doi:10.1101/gad.189001.112

43. Tang R, Li L, Zhu D et al (2012) Mouse miRNA-709 directly regulates miRNA-15a/16-1 biogenesis at the posttranscriptional level in the nucleus: evidence for a microRNA hierarchy system. Cell Res 22(3):504–515. doi:10.1038/cr.2011.137

44. Colombo M, Moita C, van Niel G et al (2013) Analysis of ESCRT functions in exosome biogenesis, composition and secretion highlights the heterogeneity of extracellular vesicles. J Cell Sci 126(Pt 24):5553–5565. doi:10.1242/jcs.128868

45. Pan BT, Johnstone RM (1983) Fate of the transferrin receptor during maturation of sheep reticulocytes in vitro: selective externalization of the receptor. Cell 33(3):967–978

46. Rani S, Ryan AE, Griffin MD et al (2015) Mesenchymal stem cell-derived extracellular vesicles: toward cell-free therapeutic applications. Mol Ther 23(5):812–823. doi:10.1038/mt.2015.44

47. Rani S, Ritter T (2015) The Exosome—a naturally secreted nanoparticle and its application to wound healing. Adv Mater. doi:10.1002/adma.201504009

48. Feng D, Zhao WL, Ye YY et al (2010) Cellular internalization of exosomes occurs through phagocytosis. Traffic (Copenhagen, Denmark) 11(5):675–687. doi:10.1111/j.1600-0854.2010.01041.x

49. Morelli AE, Larregina AT, Shufesky WJ et al (2004) Endocytosis, intracellular sorting, and processing of exosomes by dendritic cells. Blood 104(10):3257–3266. doi:10.1182/blood-2004-03-0824

50. Svensson KJ, Christianson HC, Wittrup A et al (2013) Exosome uptake depends on ERK1/2-heat shock protein 27 signaling and lipid Raft-mediated endocytosis negatively regulated by caveolin-1. J Biol Chem 288(24):17713–17724. doi:10.1074/jbc.M112.445403

51. Andreeva K, Cooper NG (2014) MicroRNAs in the neural retina. Int J Genomics 2014:165897. doi:10.1155/2014/165897

52. Damiani D, Alexander JJ, O'Rourke JR et al (2008) Dicer inactivation leads to progressive functional and structural degeneration of the mouse retina. J Neurosci 28(19):4878–4887. doi:10.1523/jneurosci.0828-08.2008

53. Pinter R, Hindges R (2010) Perturbations of microRNA function in mouse dicer mutants produce retinal defects and lead to aberrant axon pathfinding at the optic chiasm. PLoS One 5(4), e10021. doi:10.1371/journal.pone.0010021

54. Lumayag S, Haldin CE, Corbett NJ et al (2013) Inactivation of the microRNA-183/96/182 cluster results in syndromic retinal degeneration. Proc Natl Acad Sci U S A 110(6):E507–E516. doi:10.1073/pnas.1212655110

55. Ragusa M, Caltabiano R, Russo A et al (2013) MicroRNAs in vitreus humor from patients with ocular diseases. Mol Vis 19:430–440

56. Xin H, Li Y, Buller B et al (2012) Exosome-mediated transfer of miR-133b from multipotent mesenchymal stromal cells to neural cells contributes to neurite outgrowth. Stem Cells (Dayton, Ohio) 30(7):1556–1564. doi:10.1002/stem.1129

57. Romaine SP, Tomaszewski M, Condorelli G et al (2015) MicroRNAs in cardiovascular disease: an introduction for clinicians. Heart 101(12):921–928. doi:10.1136/heartjnl-2013-305402

58. Zhao W, Zhao SP, Zhao YH (2015) MicroRNA-143/-145 in cardiovascular diseases. BioMed Res Int 2015:531740. doi:10.1155/2015/531740

59. Feng Y, Huang W, Wani M et al (2014) Ischemic preconditioning potentiates the protective effect of stem cells through secretion of exosomes by targeting Mecp2 via miR-22. PLoS One 9(2), e88685. doi:10.1371/journal.pone.0088685

60. Yu B, Gong M, Wang Y et al (2013) Cardiomyocyte protection by GATA-4 gene engineered mesenchymal stem cells is partially mediated by translocation of miR-221 in microvesicles. PLoS One 8(8), e73304. doi:10.1371/journal.pone.0073304

61. van Schooneveld E, Wildiers H, Vergote I et al (2015) Dysregulation of microRNAs in breast cancer and their potential role as prognostic and predictive biomarkers in patient management. Breast Cancer Res 17:21. doi:10.1186/s13058-015-0526-y

62. Rani S, Gately K, Crown J et al (2013) Global analysis of serum microRNAs as potential biomarkers for lung adenocarcinoma. Cancer Biol Ther 14(12):1104–1112. doi:10.4161/cbt.26370

63. Peng Y, Dai Y, Hitchcock C et al (2013) Insulin growth factor signaling is regulated by microRNA-486, an underexpressed microRNA in lung cancer. Proc Natl Acad Sci U S A 110(37):15043–15048. doi:10.1073/pnas.1307107110

64. Zhu J, Zheng Z, Wang J et al (2014) Different miRNA expression profiles between human breast cancer tumors and serum. Front Genet 5:149. doi:10.3389/fgene.2014.00149

65. Gee HE, Camps C, Buffa FM et al (2008) MicroRNA-10b and breast cancer metastasis. Nature 455(7216):E8–E9. doi:10.1038/nature07362, author reply E9

Chapter 2

Assessment of Basic Biological Functions Exerted by miRNAs

John Nolan, Raymond L. Stallings, and Olga Piskareva

Abstract

Assessment of cell viability and proliferation under different miRNA expression levels is an important step in the evaluation of basic miRNA functional effects within the cell. Here, we describe the overexpression of miRNA in question in cells achieved by transfection with subsequent examination of cell viability and proliferation over a period of time using the acid phosphatase assay.

Key words miRNA, Cell viability, Proliferation, Transfection

1 Introduction

The discovery of microRNAs (miRNAs), a new class of gene expression regulator at translational level, has revolutionized our understanding of gene regulatory networks. MiRNAs are short sequences of non-coding RNAs, which in mature form are approximately 22 nucleotides in length. They can regulate cellular processes by binding to a 3′-UTR seed region on corresponding mRNA sequences and inhibiting translation of the gene or inducing cleavage of the mRNA depending on the degree of complementarity. There are more than one thousand miRNAs encoded in the human genome [1], which are estimated to regulate one-third of human mRNAs [2]. Many major cellular pathways are regulated by miRNAs including cell development, differentiation, proliferation, death, and metabolism [3]. They have been shown to be broadly involved in a diverse range of pathological conditions, such as cancer, cardiovascular and autoimmune diseases, mental disorders, and many more [2–6].

Investigation of the impact of miRNAs on target gene expression and on cell viability in vitro is essential in elucidating the role of miRNA in various diseases and cellular processes. This can be achieved by ectopically expressing miRNA of interest in cells by

Sweta Rani (ed.), *MicroRNA Profiling: Methods and Protocols*, Methods in Molecular Biology, vol. 1509,
DOI 10.1007/978-1-4939-6524-3_2, © Springer Science+Business Media New York 2017

lipofection. Lipofection is a method of lipid-mediated transfection, which depends on cationic lipid molecules. These molecules have dual roles, forming a complex with negatively charged miRNA to form unilamellar liposomes and subsequently mediating the fusion of these miRNA containing liposomes with the negatively charged plasma membrane. Fusion of the liposome is further facilitated by a helper lipid, which allows the release of miRNA into the cytosol. Generally, miRNA concentration of 10 nM is recommended for transfection; however, the efficiency of the chosen miRNA sequence, the target genes rate of transcription, and the stability of the resulting protein all affect the extent of target gene knockdown. It may therefore be necessary to titrate the miRNA concentration and assay time to obtain desired gene silencing. A positive control for uptake efficiency and negative control for background toxic effect of transfection are necessary. For this purpose, siRNA targeting KIFF11, a molecular motor protein involved in spindle dynamics [7], is used as a positive control to induce mitotic arrest and "rounding-up" in transfected cell leading to cell death. A scrambled oligonucleotide, which does not target any genes, is used as a negative control to evaluate baseline toxicity of the transfection method. The effect of the miRNA of interest can therefore be determined relative to these controls.

Following transfection with miRNA, it is important to assess its influence on cell behavior such as cell viability and proliferation. There are various assays available for the determination of cell viability based on numerous cellular processes including cell membrane permeability, enzyme activity, ATP production, nucleotide uptake activity, and coenzyme production. The acid phosphatase assay described in this study is based on the conversion of p-nitrophenol phosphate (pNPP) to p-nitrophenol by cytosolic acid phosphatase. This assay has similar sensitivity and a wider linear response range than the commonly used MTS and [^{3}H] thymidine incorporation assay [8]. It also has the added advantage of not requiring radioactive isotopes, negating the need for special protective precautions and the production of hazardous waste. It is also a relatively fast and simple method for accurate cell quantification.

2   Materials

2.1   Cell Line

The adherent neuroblastoma cell line SK-N-AS used in this study was obtained from the American Type Culture Collection (ATCC).

2.2   Growth Media

1. Minimum essential media, store at 4 °C.

2. 1 % non-essential amino acids, store at 4 °C.

3. 200 mM L-glutamine, store at 4 °C.

4. 10 % fetal bovine serum, store at 4 °C.

5. 1% pen/strep, store at 4 °C.

2.3 Transfection Reagents

1. Plain minimum essential media, store at 4 °C.

2. OptiMEM (Gibco), store at 4 °C.

3. Lipofectamine™ RNAiMAX (Invitrogen, #13775-150), store at 4 °C.

4. Negative Control #1 (Ambion), Silencer select siRNA KIFF11 (Ambion) and *mir*Vana™ miRNA Mimic (Ambion), store at −20 °C.

2.4 Acid Phosphatase Reagents

1. Phosphatase substrate, store at −20 °C.

2. 0.1 M sodium acetate, 0.1% Triton X-100, (pH 5.5), store at 4 °C.

3. 1 M NaOH, store at room temperature.

2.5 Equipment

1. Class II down-flow recirculating laminar flow cabinet.

2. Forma™ Steri-Cycle™ CO_2 Incubator, 5% CO_2 at 37 °C.

3. Perkin Elmer Victor™X3 plate reader.

4. 96 well microplates.

5. Pipettes 0.001–1 mL, single channel and 0.01–0.3 mL, multi-channel.

3 Methods

3.1 MiRNA Forward Transfection

1. SK-N-AS cells were seeded at 3000 cells/well of a 96-well plate in 100 μL growth media 24 h prior to transfection. Cell density at the time of transfection should be 30–50% confluent. The full growth media is removed from wells and replaced with 100 μL growth media without serum and antibiotics. Empty wells are used for detection of background signal (*see* **Notes 1** and **2**).

2. *For each well to be transfected*, prepare miRNA duplex-Lipofectamine™ RNAiMAX complexes as follows.

    (a) Dilute 1.2 pmol miRNA duplex in 10 μL Opti-MEM® Reduced serum medium and mix gently.

    (b) Mix Lipofectamine™ RNAiMAX gently and dilute 0.2 μL in 10 μL Opti-MEM® Reduced serum medium and mix gently.

    (c) Mix the diluted Lipofectamine™ RNAiMAX with the diluted miRNA duplex and incubate at room temperature for 10–20 min to allow complexes to form.

3. Add the miRNA duplex-Lipofectamine™ RNAiMAX to appropriate wells giving a final volume of 120 μL and a final RNA concentration of 10 nM. Rock plate back and forth to mix.

4. Incubate cells at 37 °C with 5 % CO_2 for 4–6 h, before replacing the transfection media with 200 μL complete media. Cells are then maintained at 37 °C with 5 % CO_2 until they are assessed by acid phosphatase assay at 0, 24, 48, 72, 96, and 120 h.

3.2 Acid Phosphatase Assay

1. *For each selected time point:* remove all media from wells using a multi-channel pipette, being careful not to disturb cell monolayer (*see* **Note 3**).

2. Wash wells once with 200 μL phosphate-buffered saline at 37 °C (*see* **Note 4**).

3. Add 100 μL freshly prepared acid phosphatase substrate to each well (10 mM *p*-nitrophenol phosphate in 0.1 M sodium acetate, 0.1 % Triton X-100, pH 5.5).

4. Incubate the plate in 5 % CO_2 at 37 °C away from light for 2 h to allow reaction to occur.

5. Add 50 μL of 1 M NaOH to each well to increase pH and stop the reaction following incubation.

6. Read plate on microplate reader at 405 nm to assess color change and relative cell number (*see* **Note 5**).

3.3 Example Result

1. *Linearity of viable cell number with OD level:* Cells were plated in 6 technical repeats at increasing concentration from 0.25×10^3 to 32×10^3 cells/well (*see* **Note 6**). Following acid phosphatase assay the relationship between cell number and OD was graphed demonstrating a linear relationship between color change and cell number across a broad range (Fig. 1).

2. *Cell viability of transfected cells:* The mean absorbance for empty wells represents the background OD of the phosphatase substrate. This value was subtracted from all other samples (*see* **Note 7**). The mean absorbance values were calculated and plotted for each treatment groups shown (Fig. 2a). The cell viability can be also calculated and plotted as a percentage of the negative control at the final time point using the equation in Fig. 2b.

3. *Proliferation of transfected cells:* The proliferative rate of transfected cells was determined by calculating cell viability as above every 24 h over a 120 h period. All values were then plotted (Fig. 3).

4 Notes

1. The protocol was optimised for the use of neuroblastoma cell line SK-N-AS, however it is widely applicable to other cell lines. Please refer to RNAiMAX guidelines for recommended initial concentrations to be used with different cell lines.

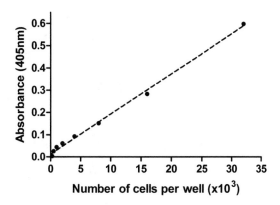

Fig. 1 Demonstration of linear relationship between acid phosphatase activity and number of viable cells

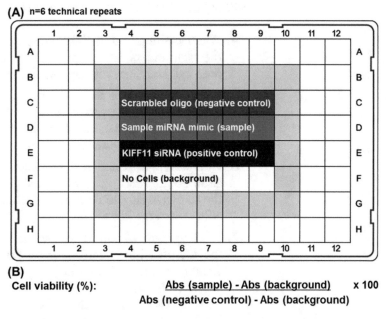

(B)
Cell viability (%): $\dfrac{\text{Abs (sample) - Abs (background)}}{\text{Abs (negative control) - Abs (background)}}$ x 100

Fig. 2 (**a**) Example of treatment arrangement using a 96-well plate for transfection. Cells are plated in 6 wells for each treatment and 6 wells are left empty to determine background absorbance. (**b**) Equation for determination of viable cells as a percentage of negative control (representing maximal viability)

2. Cell concentration plated varies dependent on cell line. When running acid phosphatase assay on a cell line for the first time, increasing cell concentrations should be plated before commencing transfection. This allows for the determination of optimum cell number for different time points and the relation of absorbance to viable cell number.

3. When removing media and PBS from wells, tilt the 96-well plate and aspirate gently from the edge of the well avoiding touching cell.

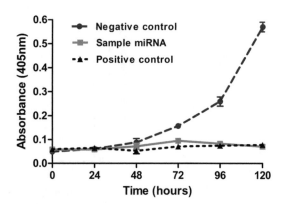

Fig. 3 Growth curve of SK-N-AS cell line. Combination of cell viability assays taken every 24 h, representing number of viable cells in each treatment group and proliferation over 120 h following transfection. All values are represented as corresponding absorbance value mean without background absorbance

4. When washing wells with PBS dispense slowly down the side of the well and gently rock by hand. Dispensing PBS directly onto cell layer may dislodge weakly adherent cells.

5. The upper limit for the microplate reader may be surpassed if too many cells are present. The number of cells plated should therefore be adjusted based on whether the cells are promoted or inhibited by transfected miRNA.

6. Cells should be plated in at least triplicate for each treatment to allow for inherent variation in cell plating. Wells surrounding the test wells should be filled with 200 μL PBS to reduce edge effect on outer test wells.

7. Plotting a growth curve from sequential time points allows for the identification of optimum time points for assessment of cell viability as cell growth will plateau at a certain point due to contact inhibition, exhaustion of media, and surpassing of the maximal OD value which can be accurately measured.

References

1. microRNA.org - Targets and Expression (2010). http://www.microrna.org/microrna/getMirnaForm.do. Accessed 4 Jan 2016

2. Urbich C, Kuehbacher A, Dimmeler S (2008) Role of microRNAs in vascular diseases, inflammation, and angiogenesis. Cardiovasc Res 79:581–588. doi:10.1093/cvr/cvn156

3. Lin S, Gregory R (2015) MicroRNA biogenesis pathways in cancer. Nat Rev Cancer 15:321–333. doi:10.1038/nrc3932

4. Romaine SP, Tomaszewski M, Condorelli G, Samani NJ (2015) MicroRNAs in cardiovascular disease: an introduction for clinicians. Heart 101:921–928. doi:10.1136/heartjnl-2013-305402

5. Pua HH, Ansel KM (2015) MicroRNA regulation of allergic inflammation and asthma. Curr Opin Immunol 36:101–108. doi:10.1016/j.coi.2015.07.006

6. Issler O, Chen A (2015) Determining the role of microRNAs in psychiatric disorders. Nat Rev Neurosci 16:201–212. doi:10.1038/nrn3879

7. Rath O, Kozielski F (2012) Kinesins and cancer. Nat Rev Cancer 12: 527–39. doi:10.1038/nrc3310. PMID 22825217

8. Yang TT, Sinai P, Kain SR (1996) An acid phosphatase assay for quantifying the growth of adherent and nonadherent cells. Anal Biochem 241:103–108

Chapter 3

Extraction of miRNAs from Formalin-Fixed Paraffin-Embedded (FFPE) Tissues

Karen Howe

Abstract

miRNAs are small non-coding RNAs that regulate gene expression and are involved in numerous diseases ranging from osteoporosis, cardiovascular disease, and numerous cancer indications. Most of the clinical material that is accessible for study is archival FFPE blocks. Due to the harsh nature of fixation and embedding procedures involved in preserving clinical material, these samples are heavily fragmented and chemically cross-linked by formalin. miRNAs, due to their small size and increased stability, are easier to retrieve and study in these precious tissues. Therefore, miRNAs have become useful tools in the diagnosis, prognosis, and prediction of diseases. Due to their increased importance, isolation of miRNAs from FFPE material is extremely clinically relevant. Here, we describe the best method for miRNA extraction from FFPE tissue blocks and determine the Qiagen miRNeasy FFPE kit to be the best kit for this task.

Key words microRNA (miRNA), Formalin-fixed paraffin-embedded (FFPE), RNA extraction, miR-Neasy, Cell culture donor block (CCDB)

1   Introduction

miRNAs are a family of 21–25-nucleotide-long RNAs expressed in a wide variety of organisms ranging from plants to worms and humans [1]. miRNAs account for greater than 3% of all human genes [2]. miRNA levels are known to have significant bearing on the development of tumors and the progression of cancers [3, 4]. miRNAs function in gene expression repression carried out by mRNA cleavage, mRNA degradation and translational repression [5]. miRNAs have many physiological functions such as developmental timing, cell proliferation and differentiation, apoptosis, disease and antiviral defense [6]. Due to their importance in regulation of physiological processes, it has been shown that their deficiencies or excesses are linked to numerous disease types including cancer, cardiovascular disease, inflammatory disease, and neuro-developmental disease [7]. In 2005, it was reported that miRNA expression profiles may classify cancer types [4]. Recently, miR-21 has

Sweta Rani (ed.), *MicroRNA Profiling: Methods and Protocols*, Methods in Molecular Biology, vol. 1509,
DOI 10.1007/978-1-4939-6524-3_3, © Springer Science+Business Media New York 2017

been identified as an oncomiR along with other miRNAs in glioblastoma multiforme (GBM) [8]. More recently, Ganepola *et al.* discovered a panel of three miRNAs that could be used as diagnostic markers for early pancreatic cancer [9]. In September 2010, the American Association for Cancer Research (AACR) released a press release for a miRNA-based screening tool that can be used to detect early-stage colorectal cancer [10]. As miRNAs may play functional and diagnostic roles in disease, they hold invaluable information and need to be explored fully. Formalin fixation is the standard method of preserving patient tissue samples. However upon formalin fixation, cross-linking of DNA and degradation occur which can cause difficulties in extracting intact DNA. miRNAs are more stable than DNA and mRNA, and therefore are ideal candidates for investigating biomarkers in archival patient samples [11]. Previously, microRNAs have successfully been extracted from FFPE material [12]. These eluates have also been successfully analyzed by miRNA expression analysis and small RNA sequencing [13, 14]. In this chapter, we explore three different miRNA extraction kits that are suitable for formalin-fixed paraffin-embedded material and determine the best starting material for optimum analysis.

2   Materials

1. Three miRNA/Total RNA isolation kits specific for FFPE tissues were tested to identify the optimal kit for the extraction of miRNA (detailed in Table 1).

    (a) RecoverAll™ Total Nucleic Acid Isolation Kit (Ambion), which extracts total RNA.

    (b) High Pure miRNA Isolation kit (Roche) which extracts miRNAs and total RNA.

    (c) miRNeasy FFPE Kit (Qiagen) which extracts miRNA and total RNA.

2. Cell culture donor blocks (CCDB) or archival FFPE blocks.

3. Different sources of starting material; full-face sections (10 μM) and cores (1.0 mm and 1.5 mm).

4. Microtome.

5. 100% Xylene stored at room temperature.

6. 100% Ethanol stored at room temperature.

7. Nuclease-free 1.5 mL microcentrifuge tubes.

8. Nuclease-free water stored at room temperature.

9. RNase Zap.

Table 1
Summary of RNA extraction protocols for the three commercially available kits tested in this study

	Roche High Pure miRNA Isolation Kit	Ambion RecoverAll Total Nucleic Acid Isolation Kit	Qiagen miRNeasy FFPE kit
Sample input	One 10 μM FFPE section or 1.0 mm/1.5 mm Core		
Deparaffinization	Xylene & 2 Ethanol Steps with a drying step of 55 °C for 10 mins	Xylene & 2 Ethanol steps with a melting step of 50 °C for 3 mins and an air-dry step of 45 mins	Xylene & Ethanol step with a drying incubation at RT
Lysis conditions	55 °C overnight	50 °C for 15 mins and 80 °C for 15 mins	56 °C for 15 mins and 80 °C for 15 mins
Proteinase K step	Included in Lysis step	N/A	Included in Lysis Step
DNase digest step	Optional	Included in protocol	Included in protocol
Elution volume	50 μL	60 μL	14–30 μL

10. RNase-free filter tips.

11. Nanodrop 1000 Spectrophotometer—RNA quantity (μg) and $A_{260/280}$ (~1.8–2.2) were determined.

12. Agilent 2100 BioAnalyzer—RNA integrity is determined by RNA integrity number (RIN).

3 Methods

3.1 Identification of Best Optimal miRNA FFPE Extraction Kit

All three kits used a column-based approach for isolating miRNAs. The differences in the kits were minimal. Each kit had a slightly different deparaffinization step but included both xylene and ethanol steps. The Roche kit included an overnight lysis step at 55 °C compared to two 15 min incubation step at 55 °C and 80 °C. There are Proteinase K steps in the Roche and Qiagen kits, however none in the Ambion kit. Proteinase K is widely used to inactivate DNase and RNAse that may degrade the DNA or RNA during purification protocols. A DNase digestion step is included in both the Ambion and Qiagen kit but is an optional step in the Roche kit. The elution volumes vary between the kits (14–60 μL).

Initial testing was carried out using CCDB which were prepared using the HER2-positive SKBR3 breast cancer cell line as follows:

Preparation of cell culture donor blocks

1. Cells were grown to 75–80 % confluency, trypsinized and resuspended in 10 mL of media.

2. Cells were pelleted by centrifugation at $75 \times g$ for 3 min and the supernatant was removed, washed once in PBS, re-pelleted and the supernatant was removed.

3. Cell pellet was fixed in 5 mL of a 10 % (v/v) neutral-buffered formalin solution and incubated overnight at room temperature.

4. Cells were pelleted by centrifugation at $75 \times g$ for 3 min, washed with PBS and re-pelleted.

5. Cells were resuspended in 200 μL of a 0.8 % agarose solution and transferred to the lid of a 1.5 mL microcentrifuge tube, from which the tapered end had been removed.

6. The agarose plug was left to solidify within the tube, removed via the cap end and transferred to an embedding cassette.

7. The cassettes were placed in a slide bath and were washed for 1 h each in the following solutions:

    (a) Ultra-high purity (UHP) water,

    (b) 50 % ethanol

    (c) 70 % ethanol

    (d) 90 % ethanol

    (e) 100 % ethanol.

    (f) 100 % xylene for 2×1 h washes

    (g) Melted Paraffin for 2 h.

8. Using the Leica EG1150H machine the cassettes were placed in plastic moulds, embedded with paraffin and left to cool.

9. Once the paraffin was set the cell culture blocks were stored at 4 °C with desiccant prior to sectioning.

Sections and cores were isolated and processed using the three extraction kits in triplicate. RNA yield and purity were analyzed by spectrophotometry using the NanoDrop ND1000 spectrophotometer. NanoDrop analysis of all elutes determined all kits had successful extraction of miRNA/RNA (Table 2). The $A_{260/280}$ values ranged from 2.0 to 2.2 and the $A_{260/230}$ from 1.3 to 2. To further assess the RNA integrity and determine if small RNAs were present, Bioanalyser analysis was carried out and the resulting electropherograms can be seen in Fig. 1. The RNA interference values (RIN) ranged from 1.0 to 2.1 (Table 3). Overall, we determined the Qiagen miRNeasy kit achieved successful miRNA elutes with small RNA peaks visible in the Bioanalyser analysis. This kit allows for 50 reactions, is cheaper and has a greater ease of handling overall.

Table 2
Average total RNA (µg), $A_{260/280}$, and $A_{260/230}$ ratios from three individual extractions analyzed using the NanoDrop spectrophotometer (ND1000, Thermo Scientific) extracted from sections (10 µM), cores; 1.0 mm and 1.5 mm using three commercially available kits

	RecoverAll™ Total Nucleic Acid Isolation Kit			High Pure miRNA Isolation Kit			miRNeasy FFPE Kit		
	µg	$A_{260/280}$	$A_{260/230}$	µg	$A_{260/280}$	$A_{260/230}$	µg	$A_{260/280}$	$A_{260/230}$
Section (10 µM)	2.3	2.2	1.5	3.7	2.2	1.5	4.4	2.0	2.0
Core (1 mm)	2.4	2.0	1.3	2.4	2.1	1.3	1.2	2.1	2.0
Core (1.5 mm)	3.7	2.1	1.4	6.0	2.0	1.4	2.6	2.0	2.1

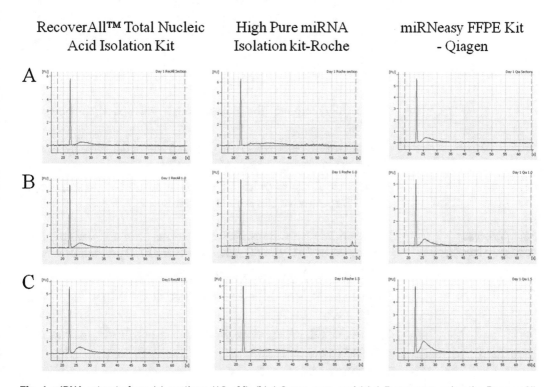

Fig. 1 miRNA extracts from (**a**) sections (10 µM), (**b**) 1.0 mm core, and (**c**) 1.5 mm core using the RecoverAll, High Pure and Qiagen kit were analyzed using the Agilent Bioanalyzer. Electropherograms shown are representative of triplicate RNA extractions

3.2 Deparaffinization Using Xylene

1. Cut and trim section (10 µM) (*see* **Note 1**) and place directly into a nuclease-free 1.5 mL microcentrifuge tube.

2. Add 1 mL of Xylene (*see* **Note 2**). Vortex vigorously for 10 s and centrifuge at room temperature on a table top centrifuge at full speed for 2 min.

Table 3
Average RNA interference values (RIN) from Bioanalyser analysis of the RNA eluates from the three FFPE extraction kits

		RIN
RecoverAll™ Total Nucleic Acid Isolation Kit	Section (10 µM)	1.8 ± 0.6
	Core (1 mm)	1.2 ± 0.1
	Core (1.5 mm)	2.1 ± 0.7
High Pure miRNA Isolation Kit	Section (10 µM)	1.4 ± 0.2
	Core (1 mm)	1.2 ± 0.1
	Core (1.5 mm)	1.4 ± 0.3
miRNeasy FFPE Kit	Section (10 µM)	1.0 ± 0.0
	Core (1 mm)	1.1 ± 0.6
	Core (1.5 mm)	1.8 ± 0.4

3. Carefully remove the supernatant without disturbing the pellet.

4. Add 1 mL of ethanol (96–100%) to the pellet, mix by vortexing and centrifuge at full speed for 2 min.

5. Incubate samples (with lid open) at room temperature or at 37 °C to remove all residual ethanol.

3.3 Proteinase and DNase Digestion

1. Depending on the number of sections used add 150 µL (*1–2 sections*) or 240 µL (*>2 sections*) Buffer PKD, vortex briefly.

2. Add 10 µL Proteinase K, mix by pipetting.

3. Incubate at 56 °C for 15 min, then at 80 °C for 15 min (*see* **Note 3**).

4. Transfer the lower, clear phase into a new 2 mL microcentrifuge tube.

5. Incubate on ice for 3 min.

6. Centrifuge for 15 min at $20,000 \times g$ and transfer supernatant to a new 2 mL microcentrifuge tube. Do not disturb the pellet.

7. Add DNase booster equivalent to a tenth of the total sample volume (approximately 16 µL (*1–2 sections*) or 25 µL (*>2 sections*)) and 10 µL DNase I stock solution.

8. Mix by inversion and centrifuge briefly to collect residual liquid from the sides of the tube.

9. Incubate at room temperature for 15 min.

3.4 RNA Isolation

1. Add 320 μL (*1–2 sections*) or 500 μL (*>2 sections*) Buffer RBC and mix lysate thoroughly.

2. Add 1120 μL (*1–2 sections*) or 1750 μL (*>2 sections*) ethanol (96–100%) and mix by pipetting. Do not centrifuge.

3. Transfer 700 μL of samples (including any precipitate that may have formed) to an RNeasy MinElute spin column placed in a 2 mL collection tube (stored at 2–8 °C). Centrifuge for 15 s at $8000 \times g$. Discard flow through.

4. Repeat **step 3** until entire sample has been passed through the spin column.

5. Add 500 μL Buffer RPE to the spin column and centrifuge for 15 s at $8000 \times g$. Discard flow through.

6. Add a further 500 μL Buffer RPE to the spin column. Centrifuge for 2 min at $8000 \times g$ to wash the spin column membrane. Discard the collection tube with flow through.

3.5 RNA Elution

1. Place the RNeasy MinElute spin column in a new 2 mL collection tube. Open the lid of the spin column and centrifuge at full speed for 5 min. Discard flow through (*see* **Note 4**).

2. Place the RNeasy MinElute spin column in a new 1.5 mL collection tube (supplied with kit).

3. Add 14–30 μL pre-heated (37–42 °C) Nuclease-free water directly to the centre of the spin column membrane. Incubate at room temperature for 1–5 min to improve RNA recovery. Centrifuge for 1 min at full speed to elute the RNA (*see* **Note 5**).

4 Notes

1. Increased number of sections can be added up to 80 μM (8×10 μM or 4×20 μM).

2. Xylene is a toxic chemical and all work should be carried out in a fume hood and waste should be disposed of correctly.

3. If using one heat block, leave sample at room temperature until the heating block reaches 80 °C.

4. To avoid damage to lids, place spin columns in centrifuge with at least one empty position between columns. Ensure the lids are orientated toward the centre of centrifuge.

5. Elution with smaller volumes of RNase water leads to higher total RNA concentration but lower RNA yields. The dead volume of the spin column is 2 μL, therefore 14 μL nuclease-free water yields 12 μL eluate.

References

1. Pillai RS (2005) MicroRNA function: multiple mechanisms for a tiny RNA? RNA 11(12):1753–1761. doi:10.1261/rna.2248605

2. Bentwich I, Avniel A, Karov Y et al (2005) Identification of hundreds of conserved and nonconserved human microRNAs. Nat Genet 37(7):766–770

3. He L, Thomson JM, Hemann MT et al (2005) A microRNA polycistron as a potential human oncogene. Nature 435(7043): 828–833

4. Lu J, Getz G, Miska EA et al (2005) MicroRNA expression profiles classify human cancers. Nature 435(7043):834–838

5. Gu S, Kay MA (2010) How do miRNAs mediate translational repression? Silence 1(1):11. doi:10.1186/1758-907X-1-11

6. Wang Y, Stricker HM, Gou D et al (2007) MicroRNA: past and present. Front Biosci 12:2316–2329, doi:2234 [pii]

7. Ardekani AM, Naeini MM (2010) The role of MicroRNAs in human diseases. Avicenna J Med Biotechnol 2(4):161–179

8. Moller HG, Rasmussen AP, Andersen HH et al (2013) A systematic review of microRNA in glioblastoma multiforme: micro-modulators in the mesenchymal mode of migration and invasion. Mol Neurobiol 47(1):131–144. doi:10.1007/s12035-012-8349-7

9. Ganepola GA, Rutledge JR, Suman P et al (2014) Novel blood-based microRNA biomarker panel for early diagnosis of pancreatic cancer. World J Gastrointest Oncol 6(1):22–33. doi:10.4251/wjgo.v6.i1.22

10. Søren Jensby Nielsen PD (2010) Screening Tool Can Detect Colorectal Cancer from a Small Blood Sample. American Association for Cancer Research. http://www.aacr.org/home/public--media/aacr-press-releases.aspx?d=2068. Accessed 22 Dec 2010

11. Liu A, Tetzlaff MT, Vanbelle P et al (2009) MicroRNA expression profiling outperforms mRNA expression profiling in formalin-fixed paraffin-embedded tissues. Int J Clin Exp Pathol 2(6):519–527

12. Liu A, Xu X (2011) MicroRNA isolation from formalin-fixed paraffin-embedded tissues. Methods Mol Biol 724:259–267. doi:10.1007/978-1-61779-055-3_16

13. Tanić M, Yanowski K, Andrés E et al (2015) miRNA expression profiling of formalin-fixed paraffin-embedded (FFPE) hereditary breast tumors. Genomics Data 3:75–79. doi:10.1016/j.gdata.2014.11.008

14. Peng J, Feng Y, Rinaldi G et al (2014) Profiling miRNAs in nasopharyngeal carcinoma FFPE tissue by microarray and Next Generation Sequencing. Genomics Data 2:285–289. doi:10.1016/j.gdata.2014.08.005

Chapter 4

MiRNA Isolation from Plants Rich in Polysaccharides and Polyphenols

K.K. Sabu, Fasiludeen Nadiya, and Narayanannair Anjali

Abstract

MicroRNAs (miRNAs) are a group of 18–22-nucleotide-long noncoding RNAs, which show wide array of roles in various biological and metabolic processes in both animals and plants. They are formed endogenously and have evolutionary conserved sequences. RNA quality is extremely important for sequencing miRNAs using next-generation sequencing platforms. However, isolation and quantification of miRNAs from plant samples are often technically difficult and recovery of miRNAs from total RNA might be problematic. Degradation of RNA weakens the true miRNAs present in the sample, hence it is crucial to use a protocol that effectively retains good integrity miRNAs. In this chapter, we outline few protocols that can be used to maximize the retrieval of good-quality miRNA and total RNA to be used in miRNA analysis for plants rich in polysaccharides and polyphenols.

Key words RNA, miRNA, Plant, miRNA isolation, Secondary metabolite, Polysaccharide, Polyphenol, NGS, Next-generation sequencing

1 Introduction

Plants possessing diverse level of polysaccharides and polyphenols make the RNA isolation protocol more tedious. The hydroxyl group attached to the 2′ position of the pentose ring makes the RNA less stable than DNA because it is more susceptible to hydrolysis. Most of the RNA isolation protocols reported are species-specific due to the varying concentration of polysaccharides, low nucleic acid, and different types of phenolics (tannins) and fibrous tissues such as lignin (wood), which will be more strenuous to remove [1]. The existence of bountiful secondary metabolites and formation of insoluble complexes between protein and RNA cause degradation and low yield of functional mRNA and small RNA through polyphenolic oxidation and polysaccharide co-precipitation which compromises the purity of RNA resulted in the modification of extraction protocols while moving from one plant species to another [2]. Although there are numerous total RNA isolation

Sweta Rani (ed.), *MicroRNA Profiling: Methods and Protocols*, Methods in Molecular Biology, vol. 1509,
DOI 10.1007/978-1-4939-6524-3_4, © Springer Science+Business Media New York 2017

protocols, most of them cannot be applied for small RNA or miRNA isolation. The choice and optimization of RNA purification methods are vital for successful isolation of good-quality RNA for employing to stable downstream applications.

Multiple factors may get interfered into the RNA isolation process and should be examined separately. As a safeguard for preserving the integrity of RNA, it is critical to keep going with an RNase (ribonuclease)-free environment beginning with tissue sampling to RNA purification. Unlike DNase, RNase does not need metal ion cofactors and can continue its activity even after autoclaving, hence RNA is exceedingly vulnerable to degradation through endogenous or exogenous RNase, both are omnipresent and tough to inactivate. Therefore, caution must be taken to protect RNA from all sources of RNase. Wearing gloves is essential while handling the chemicals and reagents for RNA isolation. Avoid touching surfaces, equipment or skin, when wearing gloves, to keep away RNase from the sterilized material. Designate a special area exclusively for RNA work. Clean workbenches, pipettes, and instruments, with commercially available RNase inactivating agents like RNase AWAY or RNase Zap. Glassware should be immersed overnight in 0.01% diethyl pyrocarbonate (DEPC) and baked at 160 °C for 5 h. Utensils that would not resist this temperature can be cleaned with 1% hydrogen peroxide followed by rinsing with DEPC-water. All the reagents used should be prepared using DEPC-treated autoclaved distilled water. Electrophoresis gel tank, gel comb, and gel tray should be immersed in a soaking buffer (0.1 M NaOH and 100 mM EDTA) for 2 h and rinsed well with DEPC-treated water. Make sure all the components used for agarose gel electrophoresis are RNase-free.

Plant tissue harvesting for RNA isolation should be expeditious, snap freeze in liquid nitrogen, and should not be thawed until processing. Uninterrupted homogenization of cells or tissues is another vital step in RNA isolation that blocks both RNA dropping and RNA degradation. The choice of homogenization should be customized to the cell or tissue type.

It has been reported that the presence of polysaccharides and polyphenols interferes with the total RNA isolation in most of the plants [3–6]. miRNA analysis through next-generation technology demands high-integrity miRNA but the practice of extracting small RNAs in recalcitrant plant tissues with diverse secondary metabolites is not proficiently demonstrated, mostly for tropical and subtropical plant species with abundant polysaccharides and polyphenols [7]. Recently, Yockteng et al. [8] published a high-quality RNA extraction method for diverse types of plants for gene expression analysis and next-generation sequencing. Several RNA extraction methods were reported in various plant species; most of them are plant-specific and are particularly established for model organisms. The success of these protocols for other non-model plant species should be checked [8]. Besides these methods there are many commercially available RNA isolation kits that efficiently precipitate RNA, but in most cases the secondary metabolites may co-precipitate with the RNA and compromise the purity.

2 Materials

The material required and precautions to be taken during the miRNA isolation are listed below:

1. Workbench should be cleaned twice with ethanol and RNase AWAY reagent.

2. Prepare RNase-free mortars, pestles, spatulas, and scissors: immerse all in DEPC overnight, dry and wrap in aluminum foil and bake at 160 °C at least for 5 h (*see* **Note 1**).

3. Use commercially available RNase-free tips and microcentrifuge tubes.

4. DEPC-water: Add 0.1% DEPC to distilled water, stir overnight and autoclave (121 °C for 15 min). RNase-free water is also available commercially.

5. Reagents: All reagents and solutions should be made with DEPC-treated distilled water.

6. Instruments: Centrifuge with rotor ($30,000 \times g$), Microcentrifuge and Spectrophotometer should be wiped with RNase Zap reagent before using for analysis (*see* **Note 2**).

7. Gloves: Use powder-free, RNase-free sterile gloves and keep the gloves clean entire time while handling RNA solutions (*see* **Note 3**).

8. Liquid nitrogen.

2.1 Isolation of Small RNAs from Recalcitrant Plant Tissues Rich in Polyphenols and Polysaccharides

1. CTAB buffer-PVPP lysis buffer: 2% (w/v) CTAB, 4 M guanidinium thiocyanate, 100 mM Tris–HCl (pH 8.5), 25 mM EDTA, 2 M NaCl, 2% (w/v) PVPP, and 2% (v/v) β-mercaptoethanol (add just before use).

2. Precipitation buffer—PEG 8000 (Polyethylene glycol 8000), 20% (w/v) PEG 8000, 1 M NaCl, 4 M LiCl.

3. 3 M sodium acetate.

2.2 High-Quality Small RNA Isolation Using Combined CTAB and Qiagen miRNeasy Mini Kit [9]

1. CTAB extraction buffer: 1 M Tris, 2% CTAB, 0.5 M EDTA, 2 M NaCl, 2% PVP.

2. Chloroform isoamyl alcohol.

3. 8 M lithium chloride.

4. 70% ethanol.

5. Isopropanol.

6. Qiagen miRNeasy Mini Kit.

2.3 Isolation of LMW RNA Using Low Salt Concentration Buffer (LSC) [10]

1. LSC extraction buffer: 2% CTAB, 2% PVP, 0.4 M NaAc (pH 5.2), 20 mM EDTA, 2% β-ME (add just before use).

2. Washing buffer (pH 7.4): 25 mM Tris–Cl, 10 mM EDTA, 80% ethanol.

3. TE buffer (pH 8.0): 10 mM Tris, 1 mM EDTA.

4. PCI (Phenol–chloroform–isoamylalcohol, 25:24:1): 50 mL water saturated phenol, 48 mL chloroform, 2 mL isoamylalcohol (total volume 100 mL).

5. CI (chloroform–isoamylalcohol, 24:1): 96 mL chloroform, 4 mL isoamylalcohol (total volume 100 mL).

2.4 An Economical Method for Low Molecular Weight RNA Isolation [11]

1. Extraction buffer; 2% CTAB, 25 mM EDTA, 2 M NaCl, 4% PVP-40 (w/v), 100 mM Tris–HCl (pH-8), 0.5 g/L spermidine.

2. β-Mercaptoethanol.

3. Acid-saturated phenol.

4. Chloroform:isoamyl alcohol.

5. PEG 8000.

6. Ethanol.

7. Formaldehyde.

8. Urea.

2.5 Small RNA Analysis Using 17% PAGE

1. Polyacrylamide stock solution: 12.5% polyacrylamide (acrylamide:bisacrylamide 19:1), 0.5× TBE buffer, pH 8.0, 7 M Urea, Gel tank soaking buffer; 0.1 M NaOH, 100 mM EDTA.

2. Denaturing polyacrylamide gel (for one gel 20 mL): 5 mL of polyacrylamide stock, 25 μL of 20% APS (ammonium persulfate), 5 μL TEMED (N,N,N,N'-tetramethylethylenediamine).

3. Staining solution: 0.001% SYBR Gold (Invitrogen), 0.5× TBE buffer, pH 8.0.

2.6 Total RNA Analysis Using AGE

1. 1.4% Agarose in 1× TBE (pH 8), Ethidium bromide or any safe DNA stain, Bromophenol blue.

3 Methods

Before describing details of various miRNA isolation procedures, some of the steps shared in all methods are given below:

Homogenization of plant samples. The homogenization method is similar in all RNA isolation methods described in this chapter.

1. The plant tissues from RNA to be isolated should be collected fresh and immediately frozen in liquid nitrogen (*see* **Note 4**).

2. Chill the sterile mortar and pestle with liquid nitrogen before placing the sample for grinding.

3. Place the tissues to the mortar and carefully start grinding gently to break the bigger pieces. Apply force to speed grinding till samples became fine powder. Continue adding liquid nitrogen and grind until no tissue particles are visible, sufficiently ground till green tissue appears almost white.

4. Use a chilled RNase-free spatula for transferring the powder to an RNase-free chilled tube (*see* **Note 5**) and allow the liquid nitrogen to evaporate, close the tube and detach the tube cap immediately to liberate any pressure which may have emerged due to the evaporation of leftover liquid nitrogen. This step is exceptionally significant if the transferred powder looks wet, designating that the liquid nitrogen has not entirely volatized.

5. Add the extraction buffer of choice (must contain suitable RNase deactivation chemicals (*see* **Note 6**) after the complete evaporation of liquid nitrogen and before tissue thawing.

6. Proceed to specific RNA isolation protocols as soon as possible (*see* **Note 7**).

3.1 Small RNA Isolation: For Plants Rich in Polyphenols and Polysaccharides

This procedure is adapted from Peng et al. [7]

1. Add frozen powder to CTAB-PVPP lysis buffer (for 2–3 g tissue 20 mL buffer), homogenize by vortexing to remove the clumps for at least 30 s (*see* **Note 8**). Keep the homogenate at room temperature for 3–5 min, and followed by centrifugation at $10,000 \times g$ for 5 min at 4 °C.

2. After centrifugation, transfer the upper aqueous phase carefully to an RNase-free tube.

3. Add equal volume of Trizol reagent and thoroughly mix by vortexing, and place the mixture at room temperature for 5–10 min.

4. And then, add 4 mL chloroform–isoamyl alcohol (24:1, v/v), vortex vigorously and centrifuge at $10,000 \times g$ for 10 min at 4 °C.

5. Transfer resulting upper aqueous phase into an RNase-free centrifuge tube.

6. Then, add an equal volume of pre-heated PEG8000 precipitation buffer and incubate at 65 °C for 15 min, keep at room temperature for 5–10 min, and chill on ice immediately for 30–45 min to precipitate the high molecular weight (HMW) RNAs, using 4 M of LiCl overnight and centrifuge at $10,000 \times g$

for 15 min at 4 °C, collect the supernatant for the enrichment of small RNAs.

7. Recover the aqueous phase after centrifugation and transfer into a new centrifuge tube.

8. Precipitate the low molecular weight (LMW) RNAs with 1/10 volume of 3 M sodium acetate (pH 5.2) and 2.5 volume of precooled absolute ethanol at −20 °C overnight.

9. Collect pellet by centrifugation at $8000 \times g$ for 20 min at 4 °C, then rinse with 80 % ice-cold ethanol and collect by centrifugation at $8000 \times g$ for 5 min at 4 °C (*see* **Note 9**).

10. Resuspend air-dried pellet in an appropriate volume of sterile DEPC-treated double-distilled water and store at −80 °C (*see* **Note 10**).

11. Measure the OD of the RNA. Good-quality RNA should have A260/A280 and A260/A230 ratios > 1.8.

12. Separate all RNA samples by electrophoresis using 17 % polyacrylamide (19:1) gel cast in 7 M urea using 0.5× TBE buffer.

13. Run gels at 300 V for 3–4 h to separate small RNAs till the bromophenol blue dye extend the end of the gel, employing a miRNA marker as control.

3.2 High-Quality Small RNA Isolation Using Combined CTAB and Qiagen miRNeasy Mini Kit [9]

1. Pre-warm extraction buffer (CTAB; *see* **Note 11**) (5 mL+ 100 μL β-mercaptoethanol) in 65 °C water bath; 1 mL extraction buffer for 100 mg young leaves (*see* **Note 12**).

2. Transfer the ground materials into a frozen 2 mL RNase-free microfuge tube and add 1 mL pre-warmed CTAB extraction buffer (freshly added β mercaptoethanol). Vortex for about 1 min to mix thoroughly. Incubate the tubes in 65 °C water bath for 30 min. Vortex six to eight times during incubation. Cool down the tubes at room temperature (RT) for 2 min.

3. Add 840 μL chloroform:isoamyl alcohol (24:1). Vortex the samples vigorously (1–2 min). Centrifuge the homogenate at $10,000 \times g$ for 15 min at 4 °C. The aqueous layer is transferred to a fresh tube (*see* **Note 13**).

4. To the supernatant add 820 μL 8 M lithium chloride. Mix thoroughly by inverting the tube. Store at −80 °C for 30 min. Centrifuge at $12,000 \times g$ for 15 min at 4 °C.

5. Recover the pellet and proceed to miRNeasy Mini Kit.

6. Add 700 μL QIAzol Lysis Reagent to the tube containing the pellet. Vortex to dissolve the pellet. Incubate the tube containing the homogenate at room temperature (15–25 °C) for 5 min.

7. Add 140 μL chloroform to the tube containing the homogenate and shake the tube vigorously for 20 s. Incubate the tube

containing the homogenate at RT for 2–3 min. Centrifuge for 15 min at $10,000 \times g$ at 4 °C.

8. Transfer the aqueous layer (~650 μL) to a new collection tube (supplied with kit). Add 1.5 volumes of 100% ethanol and mix thoroughly by pipetting up and down several times. Proceed to next step without delay.

9. Pipette up to 700 μL of the sample, including any precipitate that may have formed into an RNeasy Mini spin column in a 2 mL collection tube (supplied). Close the lid gently and centrifuge at $\geq 8000 \times g$ for 15 s at RT (15–25 °C). Discard the flow-through.

10. Proceed to on-column DNase digestion according to the manufacturer's instruction.

11. Proceed to wash steps instructed in miRNeasy Mini Kit with RWT and RPE wash buffers. Elute the total RNA enriched with small RNAs using 30 μL nuclease-free water (reuse the elute for second elution to retain high-quality RNA in good concentration). The above method can use in all tissues of a plant for example, leaf 100 mg, stem 250 mg, flower and flower buds 250 mg, fruits 250 mg and root 250 mg.

3.3 Isolation of LMW RNA Using Low Salt Concentration Buffer (LSC) [10]

3.3.1 Small-Scale Extraction Protocol

1. Grind 50 mg tissue into fine powder.

2. Transfer the sample into 0.5 mL LSC extraction buffer and vortex vigorously for 1 min.

3. Incubate at 65 °C for 10 min with occasionally swirling, centrifuge at $20,000 \times g$ for 10 min at 4 °C.

4. Transfer the upper liquid phase (about 400 μL to new tube).

5. Add 200 μL of isopropanol and mix well.

6. Transfer the mixture into an RNase-free silica spin column, and centrifuge for 30 s at $6500 \times g$.

7. Add 700 μL washing buffer and centrifuge for 30 s at $6500 \times g$; discard the flow through and repeat step 7; centrifuge for 1 min at $12,000 \times g$.

8. Add 50 μL TE buffer onto the silica membrane and elute the low molecular weight RNA into a new RNase-free tube.

3.3.2 Large-Scale Extraction Protocol

1. Grind 1 g tissue into fine powder.

2. Transfer the sample into 10 mL LSC extraction buffer and incubate at 65 °C for 10 min, then place the tube on ice.

3. Add 10 mL PCI, vortex vigorously for 1 min; centrifuge at $30,000 \times g$ for 10 min at 4 °C.

4. Transfer the supernatant into new tube; add 10 mL CI, vortex and centrifuge at $30,000 \times g$ for 10 min at 4 °C.

5. Recover the supernatant, add 10 mL ice-cooled isopropanol and incubate at −20 °C for more than 1 h.

6. Centrifuge at 30,000×g for 20 min at 4 °C, and discard the supernatant.

7. Resuspend the precipitate with 0.5 mL LSC buffer and transfer to a 1.5 mL tube.

8. Extract the sample sequentially with 0.5 mL PCI and CI, and collect the supernatant.

9. Add 0.5 mL isopropanol and incubate at −20 °C for more than 30 min.

10. Centrifuge at 20,000×g for 10 min at 4 °C, and discard the supernatant.

11. Wash the precipitant twice with 80% ethanol, and dissolve in 50 μL TE buffer.

12. For electrophoresis, denature 3 mg LMW RNA of each sample and load onto urea (8%) 15% polyacrylamide gels. After electrophoresis, stain the gels with 1 mg/L ethidium bromide for 30 min and visualized under ultraviolet light.

3.4 An Economical Method for Low Molecular Weight RNA Isolation

1. Pre-warm the extraction buffer to 65 °C and add 200 μL of β mercaptoethanol to the tube.

2. Mix by vigorously inverting the tube and let it stand for 5 min at RT.

3. Transfer the powder to a clear 15 mL polypropylene centrifuge tube and add 5 mL extraction buffer.

4. Add an equal volume of acid-saturated phenol and vortex vigorously for 1 min. Centrifuge at 10,000×g for 15 min at 4 °C.

5. Transfer the supernatant to a fresh 15 mL centrifuge tube.

6. Add an equal volume of chloroform:isoamyl alcohol (24:1) and vortex vigorously for 1 min. Centrifuge at 10,000×g for 10 min at 4 °C and transfer the supernatant to a fresh 15 mL centrifuge tube. Repeat **step 6**.

7. Add ¼ volumes of 30% PEG 8000 and chill on ice for 10 min at 4 °C. Centrifuge at 10,000×g for 10 min at 4 °C.

8. Transfer the supernatant to a clear 15 mL centrifuge tube, and add ¾ volume of absolute ethanol. Mix by inverting the tube and incubate at −20 °C for 30 min at 4 °C.

9. Wash the pellets with 70% ethanol twice. Briefly, dry and resuspend the pellets in 80 μL of DEPC treated water. Store at −80 °C.

10. The quality of low molecular weight RNA was determined by running the samples on 1.2% formaldehyde agarose gel and 15% urea PAGE.

3.5   RNA Quality Analyses

3.5.1   Concentration and Purity

The concentration and purity of isolated RNA can be analyzed either by NanoDrop or by BioPhotometer which measures the amount of RNA and estimate protein–phenol contamination. The RNA has to be diluted in RNase-free water to make dilution factor 50 (1 μL RNA sample + 49 μL RNase-free water). For the assessment of purity, record the absorbance level at 280, 260, and 230 nm. The A260/230 denotes extend of polysaccharide and polyphenol interference, whereas the A260/280 ratio indicates the considerable protein precipitation [12]. It was reported that A260/280 value below 2 indicates protein contamination and A260/230 value below 2 indicates the presence of polysaccharides and polyphenols in the extracted RNA sample [13].

3.5.2   Agarose Gel Electrophoresis

The integrity of total RNA isolated and the extent of genomic DNA contamination can be analyzed through agarose gel electrophoresis (1.2% agarose gel containing 0.5 μg/mL ethidium bromide). The running buffer (1× TBE) containing Tris base, boric acid, and EDTA has to be prepared in RNase-free water using RNase-free glassware (overnight incubation of glass wares using 0.1% DEPC followed by autoclaving at 121 °C for 20 min). Use a gel loading buffer such as 40% sucrose prepared using RNase-free water. 2 μg RNA with 3 μL gel loading buffer can be loaded to the agarose gel, and run the gel at 65 V for 20 min (for 1.4% 100 mL gels). The gel can be visualized using a gel documentation system. On non-denaturing agarose gels, partly deteriorated RNA samples will be visible as outspreaded smear, with dull bands representing the 28S and 18S rRNA molecules as expected in eukaryotic samples whereas the fully degraded RNA will be observed as a very low molecular weight smear.

3.5.3   Polyacrylamide Gel Electrophoresis

Small RNA analysis can be done on polyacrylamide gel. For this, prepare a denaturing 12.5% polyacrylamide gel and polyacrylamide should be allowed to polymerize for not less than 30 min and later the combs can be removed; gels may be kept at 4 °C (Note: The polymerization time influences the running excellence, and it has been shown that gels prepared 2 days before use are of refined band clarification). Pre-run the gel(s) in 0.5× TBE buffer (to discard ammonium persulfate residues) for 2 h at 90 V.

Sample preparation: For 2 μg LMW RNA, add 0.3 (v/v) loading buffer (calibrate to equal volume in all samples with RNase-free water). Incubate samples at 65 °C for 5 min to denature RNA and right away place on ice for 1 min. Prior to loading samples in the gel, wash each gel slot with 0.5× TBE using a syringe. Load the samples in the gel (cover empty slots with loading buffer) and run for about 2 h at 90 V in 0.5× TBE buffer (running should be continued till the bromophenol blue of the loading buffer reaches the end of the gel). When the electrophoresis run has completed, take the gel out and stain in 15 mL 0.5× TBE buffer with 0.001%

SYBR Gold for 30 min. Eventually, rinse for 5 min with RNase-free water. Visualize the gel under UV light [14].

3.5.4 Detect RNA Integrity Number (RIN)

The distribution and size of the purified RNA molecules can be assessed using instrument such as Agilent 2100 BioAnalyzer. The BioAnalyzer performs capillary electrophoresis through a chip and determines both RNA concentration and integrity by using a fluorescent dye, which gets bound to RNA. The basic principle of capillary electrophoretic analysis through a chip is similar to gel electrophoresis principles, besides the chip format conveniently minimizes the sample requirement and running time. The BioAnalyzer generates an electropherogram of the filled total RNA by representing two well-defined ribosomal peaks correlated to 18S and 28S rRNA and a flat baseline holding between the 5S and 18S ribosomal peaks. For accepting RNA as good quality, the peak height of the 28S rRNA should be twice of the 18S rRNA peak. Apart from the 18S to 28S ribosomal RNAs ratio, the BioAnalyzer is provided with a software algorithm, which captures the complete electrophoretic trace into report for rating the integrity of total RNA samples. The electrophoretic trace by the software algorithm creates the RNA Integrity Number (RIN) and systematize the RNA sample on the basis of RIN value from 1 to 10 [15]. The RNA samples with RIN value of 1 are considered as being the most degraded and the RIN value of 10 being the most intact (*see* **Note 14**).

4   Notes

1. Baking of glassware and other utensils owned for RNA works must be baked at 160–200 °C for at least 5 h to get rid of functional nucleases. Utensils that would not resist these temperatures must be treated with 1% hydrogen. Gel tanks and combs used for RNA analysis should be treated similarly. Plastic wares used should be RNase-free. RNase-free solutions can be prepared by treating with 0.1% DEPC overnight at RT in a fume hood and then autoclaving at 121 °C for 15 min; still, solutions containing Tris [Tris(hydroxymethyl)aminomethane] are not compatible with DEPC. Preferably, commercially available products, such as RNase Zap, RNase AWAY may be used for cleaning RNA workbench and other instruments. Autoclaving is recommended for detergents.

2. To reduce the presence of RNase, it is essential to keep equipment for RNA extraction use only. Electrophoresis equipment can be set for use only for RNA. Keep everything RNase-free by not using them in other procedures.

3. Wear gloves all the time and proper sterile approaches should be pursued while managing samples and reagents. Certainly,

RNase may contaminate the surface of gloves following contacts with RNase-contaminated objects like test tube racks, pipettes, freezer door handles, human skin, etc.

4. Since plant tissues are more prone to degradation, it is highly recommended to immediately freeze them in liquid nitrogen once separated from whole live plant; reduce environmental exposure once the process starts.

5. As soon as the cells or tissues are disrupted, endogenous RNase will get discharged from the complexes and organelles that usually separate them from RNA in the cell. For preserving integrity of the RNA, these discharged RNases must be deactivated rapidly and entirely, as cells are broken.

6. Sample disruption and homogenization are commonly executed in the presence of high guanidine concentration, which denatures proteins and thus transiently inactivates RNase. The presence of SDS in extraction buffer can reduce RNase contamination within the cells. PVP solves the problem with high levels of polyphenols.

7. Complete the RNA isolation work quickly and try to keep every step under cold condition as far as possible to reduce RNA degradation.

8. Strictly do not let the plant tissue to thaw until the addition of extraction buffer. Also it is quite important to safeguard the tissues not to form lumps during the addition of buffer. Add tissue slowly to the hot extraction buffer using a pre-cooled spatula. Make sure to incubate for 5 min at room temperature after homogenization.

9. Do not allow RNA pellet to dry completely. Do not lyophilize or vacuum dry samples. Clear pellet indicates over-drying.

10. To improve solubilization, RNA pellet should be pipetted up and down in DEPC-treated water.

11. miRNeasy Mini Kit alone will not remove the polysaccharides and polyphenols, and can be removed only with a detergent-based extraction buffer.

12. Incubation at high temperature in the presence of detergents is a good way of removing polysaccharides in most of the plants, by making them more soluble.

13. As soon as cells are lysed, acidified phenol:chloroform:isoamyl alcohol organic extraction is a better option for refining total RNA.

14. RIN values are considered to be the best quality check for RNA samples. For downstream applications such as those involving NGS, RIN value of 7 can be considered good for plant RNA samples.

References

1. MacRae E (2007) Extraction of plant RNA. In: Hilario E, Mackay J (eds) Protocols for nucleic acid analysis by nonradioactive probes, vol 353, 2nd edn, Methods in molecular biology. Humana Press, Totowa, pp 15–24

2. Wang SX, Hunter W, Plant A (2000) Isolation and purification of functional total RNA from woody branches and needles of Sitka and white spruce. Biotechnique 28:292–296

3. Geuna F, Hartings H, Scienza A (1998) A new method for rapid extraction of high quality RNA from recalcitrant tissues of grapevine. Plant Mol Biol Rep 16:61–67

4. Salzman RA, Fugita T, Zhu-Salzman K et al (1999) An improved RNA isolation method for plant tissues containing high levels of phenolic compound or carbohydrates. Plant Mol Biol Rep 17:11–17

5. Tai HH, Pelletier C, Beardmore T (2004) Total RNA isolation from Pica mariana dry seed. Plant Mol Biol Rep 22:93a–93e

6. Yeh K, Juang R, Su J (1991) A rapid and efficient method for RNA isolation from plant with high carbohydrate content. Focus 13:102–103

7. Peng J, Xia Z, Chen L et al (2014) Rapid and efficient isolation of high-quality small RNAs from recalcitrant plant species rich in polyphenols and polysaccharides. PLoS One 9(5), e95687. doi:10.1371/journal.pone.0095687

8. Yockteng R, Almeida AMR, Yee S, et al (2013) A method for extracting high-quality rna from diverse plants for next generation sequencing and gene expression analysis. Appl Plant Sci 1: Article ID: 13000700

9. Nadiya F, Anjali N, Gangaprasad A, Sabu KK (2015) High-quality RNA extraction from small cardamom tissues rich in polysaccharides and polyphenols. Anal Biochem 485:25–27

10. Cheng H, Gao J, An ZW, Huang HS (2010) A rapid method for isolation of low molecular-weight RNA from Arabidopsis using low salt concentration buffer. Int J Plant Biol 1, e14

11. Zewei AN, Li Y, XiE L et al (2013) A rapid and economical method for low molecular weight RNA isolation from a wide variety of plant species. Biosci Biotechnol Biochem 77(7):1599–1601

12. Logemann J, Schell J, Willmitzer L (1987) Improved method for the isolation of RNA from plant tissues. Anal Biochem 163:16–20

13. Asif MH, Dhawan P, Nath P (2000) Plant Mol Biol Rep 18:109–115

14. Rosas-Cárdenas Fde F, Durán-Figueroa N, Vielle-Calzada JP, Cruz-Hernández A, Marsch-Martínez N, de Folter S (2011) A simple and efficient method for isolating small RNAs from different plant species. Plant Methods 7:4

15. SchroederA MO, StockerS SR, Leiber M, Gassmann M, Lighfoot S, Menzel W, Granzow M, Ragg T (2006) BMC Mol Biol 7:3

Chapter 5

MicroRNA Profiling of Exosomes

Melissa Daly and Lorraine O'Driscoll

Abstract

Exosomes are nano-sized membrane-bound vesicles released by a range of different cell types. Exosomes have been shown to specifically package certain membrane and cytosolic proteins and nucleic acids. Furthermore, it has been shown that their contents can be transferred to secondary cells, affecting the recipient cells' cellular processes. Exosomes are present in a multitude of body fluids and so represent a novel source of circulating biomarkers. Here, we describe ultracentrifugation methods suitable for the isolation of exosomes from serum and plasma. We also detail transmission electron microscopy, nanoparticle tracking analysis, and immunoblotting methods suitable for the characterization of exosomes.

Key words Exosomes, Serum, Plasma, Ultracentrifugation, Characterization

1 Introduction

Exosomes are nano-sized (30–120 nm), membrane-bound vesicles released by a range of different cell types. Exosomes are released when multi-vesicular bodies fuse with the cell membrane and expel their contents into the extracellular space [1]. Exosomes represent an exciting area of biomarker research, as their contents are a wealth of information on the state of their cell of origin and they are present in a multitude of body fluids, including blood, semen, and saliva; to name but a few [2]. Exosomes are also thought to be important mediators in intercellular communication. Indeed, many studies have found evidence that their contents, including membrane and cytosolic proteins, DNA and various types of RNA, can be transferred to cells either through membrane–membrane interaction or direct uptake of the exosome and that they can directly influence the cellular processes of the recipient cell [3–5]. Exosomes appear particularly relevant to the area of microRNA (miRNA) research as, not only have they been shown to be enriched in miRNA, their lipid membrane structure acts as a protective barrier from RNase degradation. Studies have identified exosomal miR-NAs as potential diagnostic and prognostic biomarkers in many

Sweta Rani (ed.), *MicroRNA Profiling: Methods and Protocols*, Methods in Molecular Biology, vol. 1509,
DOI 10.1007/978-1-4939-6524-3_5, © Springer Science+Business Media New York 2017

cancers including lung [6], brain [7], breast [8], ovarian [9, 10], and prostate cancer [11].

The success of such studies is dependent on good exosome isolation and characterization techniques. Herein we outline the use of ultracentrifugation, and a variation using a density gradient, for the isolation of exosomes from serum and plasma and the use of transmission electron microscopy (size and morphology), nanoparticle tracking analysis (size and concentration), and immunoblots (presence of exosome markers) as standard methods for exosome characterization [12].

2   Materials

2.1 Serum Collection

1. Non-heparinized tube(s) for blood collection (by trained Phlebotomist).
2. Bench-top centrifuge.
3. Cryovial tubes.
4. –80 °C freezer.

2.2 Ultra-centrifugation

1. Ultracentrifuge and appropriate fixed-angle or swinging bucket rotor (for details on Beckman Coulter ultracentrifuge rotors and accessories see: http://www.labplan.ie/admin/documents/Ultracentrifuge_Rotors_Tubes_Accs_06.pdf).
2. Polyallomer or polycarbonate centrifuge tubes appropriate for rotors mentioned in **Item 1**.
3. Phosphate-buffered saline (PBS): sodium chloride 8 g/L, potassium chloride 0.2 g/L, di-sodium hydrogen phosphate 1.15 g/L, and potassium dihydrogen phosphate 0.2 g/L pH 7.3 at 25 °C.
4. 0.22 μm low protein binding syringe filters.
5. 10 mL Syringes.
6. 18-G syringe needles.
7. 30 mL universal tubes.
   For the Optiprep density gradient variation
8. Optiprep density gradient medium (60% w/v) (Sigma-Aldrich).
9. Dilution buffer: 0.25 M sucrose, 1 mM EDTA and 10 mM Tris–HCl, pH 7.4. (There are a number of similar dilution buffers for this type of gradient. For details please see: http://www.axis-shield-density-gradient-media.com/Preparation%20of%20gradient%20solutions.pdf).

2.3 Transmission Electron Microscopy

1. Transmission electron microscope (TEM).
2. Formvar/carbon-coated nickel or copper grids.

3. PBS: sodium chloride 8 g/L, potassium chloride 0.2 g/L, disodium hydrogen phosphate 1.15 g/L, and potassium dihydrogen phosphate 0.2 g/L pH 7.3 at 25 °C.

4. 4% glutaraldehyde: Dilute glutaraldehyde in 0.1 M sodium phosphate buffer, pH 7.4, to a final concentration of 4%.

5. 2% uranyl acetate, pH 4.0: Dissolve 1 g in 50 mL distilled H_2O. This may be stored at 4 °C in the dark for up to 6 months. Prior to use, filter required volume through a 0.22 μm filter.

6. Parafilm.

7. Whatman no. 1 filter paper.

8. Forceps.

2.4 Nanoparticle Tracking Analysis

1. NanoSight NS300 (or NS500).

2. 100 nm polystyrene latex calibration nanoparticles.

3. PBS.

4. 1 mL syringes.

2.5 SDS-Polyacrylamide Electrophoresis

1. Resolving buffer (4×): 1.5 M Tris–HCl, pH 8.8, 0.4% SDS. Stored at room temperature.

2. Stacking buffer (4×): 0.5 M Tris–HCl, pH 6.8, 0.4% SDS. Stored at room temperature.

3. Sample buffer (4×): 4 mL stacking buffer, 2 mL β-mercaptoethanol, 6 mL glycerol, 1 g SDS and 50 mg bromophenol blue. Aliquot and store at –20 °C.

4. Acrylamide/bis-acrylamide, 30% solution (Sigma-Aldrich). Stored at 4 °C.

5. *N, N, N, N'*-Tetramethyl-ethylenediamine (TEMED).

6. Ammonium persulfate: 10% solution in distilled water, freshly prepared.

7. Running buffer (10×): 25 mM Tris pH 8.3, 192 mM glycine, and 0.1% SDS. Stored at room temperature.

8. Prestained molecular weight markers: SeeBlue®Plus2 Prestained protein standard (Bio-Sciences, Ireland).

9. 1-D Electrophoresis system (ATTO Corporation, Tokyo, Japan).

2.6 Immunoblotting

1. Blotting buffer: buffer (10×): 25 mM Tris pH 8.3, 192 mM glycine, and 20% (v/v) methanol. Stored at 4 °C.

2. Immun-Blot PVDF membrane and extra thick blot paper.

3. Ponceau S solution.

4. Phosphate buffered saline (PBS, 1×): 0.01 M phosphate buffer, 0.0027 M potassium chloride and 0.137 M sodium chloride, pH 7.4.

5. Washing buffer (PBS-T): 1× PBS supplemented with 0.1 % Tween-20.

6. Blocking buffer: 5 % (w/v) bovine serum albumin (BSA) solution in PBST.

7. Antibody dilution buffer: 1× PBS supplemented with 3 % (w/v) BSA and 0.1 % Tween-20. Aliquots frozen at −20 °C.

8. Primary antibodies: rabbit anti-Grp94 antibody (Cell Signalling Technology Europe, The Netherlands) diluted 1:1000 in antibody dilution buffer, mouse anti-TSG101 antibody (Abcam, Cambridge, UK) diluted 1:1000 in antibody dilution buffer and rabbit anti-CD81 (Santa Cruz Biotechnology Inc., CA) diluted 1:200 in antibody dilution buffer.

9. Secondary antibodies: Anti-rabbit and anti-mouse IgG HRP-conjugated (Cell Signalling) diluted 1:1000 in antibody dilution buffer.

10. Enhanced chemiluminescent reagent: SuperSignal West Pico Chemiluminescent Substrate (ThermoFischer Scientific).

11. Stripping buffer: 62.5 mM Tris–HCl, pH 6.8, 2 % (w/v) SDS. Before use warm to 70 °C and add 100 mM β-mercaptoethanol.

12. Semi-dry transfer system (BioRad Laboratories Inc.).

13. Imaging system: ChemiDoc XRS system (BioRad Laboratories Inc.).

3   Methods

3.1   Serum Collection

1. Allow blood in non-heparinized tube(s) to clot for 30 min minimum to 1 h maximum.

2. Centrifuge at $1000 \times g$ for 10 min at room temperature.

3. Gently remove the serum and aliquot into labeled cryovial tubes.

4. Store at −80 °C within <3 h of procurement.

3.2   Ultra-centrifugation

The most commonly used and preferred method by which exosomes are isolated from serum or plasma is ultracentrifugation. The procedure outlined here is an adaptation of a technique previously described for conditioned media and bodily fluids [13].

1. Dilute a known volume (*see* **Note 1**) of serum or plasma to 5 mL in PBS.

2. Filter this suspension through a 0.22 μm syringe filter.

3. Using a fresh syringe place the filtrate in an ultracentrifuge tube. Using a waterproof marker place a mark on the bottom/side of the tube where the pellet will be found following cen-

trifugation. For swinging bucket rotors the pellet will be found at the bottom and for fixed angle rotors the pellet will be found on the side facing out.

4. Fill the ultracentrifuge tube with PBS and centrifuge at 110,000 × g for 75 min at 4 °C.

5. Remove the supernatant and carefully resuspend the exosome pellet in 1 mL PBS (*see* **Note 2**).

6. Place the resuspended exosome pellet into a fresh centrifuge tube and fill with PBS.

7. Centrifuge at 110,000 × g for 75 min at 4 °C.

8. Carefully remove the supernatant. Resuspend exosome pellet in 200 μL PBS and store at –80 °C.

3.2.1 Ultracentrifugation with Optiprep Density Gradient

The procedure outlined above is considered adequate for exosomes isolation. If, after characterization, the exosomes are not of acceptable purity or yield is deemed insufficient for preferred profiling methods, the addition of a density gradient using a medium such as iodixanol is recommended.

1. Prepare 40, 20, 10, and 5 % solutions of Optiprep density gradient medium using dilution buffer (0.25 M sucrose, 1 mM EDTA, and 10 mM Tris–HCl, pH 7.4).

2. Using a syringe, carefully layer the gradient in an ultracentrifuge tube with equal volumes of 40, 20, and 10 % solutions and 0.5 mL less of the 5 % solution.

3. Filter a known volume of serum (or plasma) through a 0.22-μM filter and place on top of the gradient.

4. Centrifuge at 100,000 × g for 18 h at 4 °C.

5. Collect 1 mL fractions starting from the top of the gradient.

6. Centrifuge individual fractions at 100,000 × g for 3 h at 4 °C.

7. Resuspend exosome pellets in 100 μL PBS.

8. Assess fractions for the presence of exosomes and if necessary pool exosome positive fractions before proceeding to miRNA profiling.

3.3 Transmission Electron Microscopy

The procedure outlined here is an adaptation of a previously described technique sufficient for transmission electron microscopy (TEM) analysis of exosome preparations [14]

1. Place a drop (~30 μL) of intact EVs on parafilm.

2. Using a forceps gently place a formvar/carbon-coated grid, coated side down, on top of the drop. Leave for 30–60 min (*see* **Note 3**).

3. Place three drops, >30 μL each, of PBS on parafilm and wash the grid by placing the grid on top of each droplet for 5 min

each using absorbent paper in between (*see* **Note 3**). Fix the sample by placing the grid on a drop of 4% glutaraldehyde for 10 min.

4. Repeat wash as **step 3**.

5. Contrast the sample by placing a drop of 2% uranyl acetate onto parafilm and placing the grid on top of the drop for 15 min.

6. Remove excess liquid using absorbent paper and allow the grids to air dry.

7. Once dry, grids can be examined by TEM immediately or can be stored in a suitable grid box for up to 2 weeks.

3.4 Nanoparticle Tracking Analysis

Nanoparticle tracking analysis uses light scattering and Brownian motion to measure the size and concentration of particles in solution. A laser light is used to illuminate particles and a series of videos are taken. The software analyses the videos tracking individual particles to assess their size and give the overall concentration of particles in the solution (Fig. 1).

1. Calibrate the system with 100 nm polystyrene latex calibration nanoparticles.

2. Dilute EV sample 1/10 to 1/100 in filtered PBS. It is advisable to analyze the PBS used to verify that it is particle free.

3. Place the sample in instrument. If using the NanoSight NS300 system the sample is manually placed inside the sample chamber using a 1 mL syringe. If using the NanoSight NS500 system place the sample tube on the platform and insert the inlet tube. The sample will be automatically pumped into the sample chamber during analysis.

4. Set temperature to 23 °C.

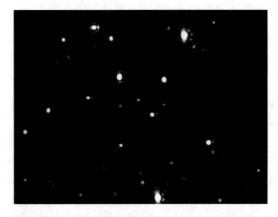

Fig. 1 Screenshot of video from Nanosight analysis of exosomes, isolated using ultracentrifugation, showing a suitable number (between 20 and 100) of particles per frame

5. Start camera and adjust camera level to 15. Samples should be clearly visible

6. Capture 5 60 s videos using a 30 s delay to make sure movement of particles can only be attributed to Brownian motion. If using the NanoSight NS300 system you will be prompted to manually pass the solution through the chamber between each video.

3.5   SDS-PAGE

1. The protocol here refers to the use of a mini gel 1-D gel electrophoresis system (ATTO Corporation) but can be adapted to other formats.

2. Clean the glass plates thoroughly with 70% (v/v) ethanol and assemble the front and back plates in the clamps. Ensure there is no leakage by pouring water inside the plates and leaving for at least 5 min. Remove the water.

3. Prepare a 10% gel solution using 2 mL of resolving buffer (4×), 2.5 mL of 30% acrylamide/bis-acrylamide solution, 75 μL of 10% SDS and 3 mL water. Add 40 μL of ammonium persulfate and 3 μL of TEMED. Mix and immediately pour the gel, taking care to leave enough room for the stacking gel. Slowly pour a small amount of distilled water (or ethanol) on top of the gel.

4. Pour off the water (or ethanol). Prepare the stacking gel using 250 μL of stacking buffer, 340 μL 30% acrylamide/bis-acrylamide solution, 20 μL of 10% SDS, and 1.4 mL water. Add 20 μL of ammonium persulfate and 2 μL of TEMED. Pour the stacking gel solution and immediately insert the combs.

5. Remove the plates from the holder and assemble the gasket. Fill the gasket and the outer chamber with running buffer and remove the comb.

6. Load the samples and the molecular weight marker in the wells.

7. Assemble the unit and connect to the power source. Use constant voltage up to 80 mV through the stacking gel and up to 100 mV through the resolving gel. Once the bromophenol blue dye has run off the gel, turn off and disconnect the power supply.

3.6   Immunoblotting

It is recommended to assess isolated exosomes for the presence of at least two extracellular vesicle positive markers (*e.g.* TSG101, 42 kDa; CD81, 26 kDa) and one negative marker (*e.g.* Grp94, 96 kDa) (Fig. 2). At present there are no protein markers verified as specific to exosomes, only those associated with extracellular vesicles (exosomes and microvesicles).

1. The protocol here refers to a semi-dry transfer method using a Bio-Rad Trans-blot system.

2. Cut a sheet of PVDF paper to slightly larger than the gel size and soak in methanol for 1 min to activate the membrane.

Once activated leave to soak in transfer buffer until needed. Soak two sheets of extra thick paper in transfer buffer.

3. Carefully remove the gel from the gel unit. Remove the stacking gel and soak the resolving gel in transfer buffer. Note the orientation of the gel.

4. Prepare the transfer cell placing a sheet of extra thick paper and placing the membrane on top. Place the gel on top of the membrane and cover with the second sheet of extra thick paper. Ensure there are no air bubbles between the gel and the membrane.

5. Place the lid on top and connect the unit to the power supply. Transfer at 20 mV for 1 h.

6. Disconnect the power supply and carefully remove the lid of the transfer unit. Remove the paper and gel and check that the corresponding markers from the prestained marker are visible on the membrane.

7. Incubate the membrane in Ponceau S staining solution for 1 min.

8. Wash the membrane in three washes of PBST, 5 min each, with vigorous shaking to remove the stain.

9. Incubate the membrane in blocking buffer for 1 h at room temperature on a gently shaking (~30 rpm) rocker.

10. Wash the membrane in three washes of PBST, 5 min each, with vigorous shaking.

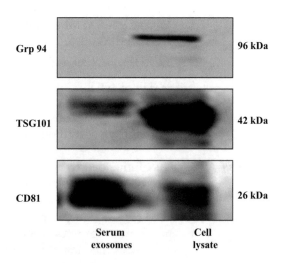

Fig. 2 Immunoblot analysis of samples of exosomes isolated from serum using ultracentrifugation for extracellular vesicle positive markers TSG101 and CD81 and negative marker GRP94. Cell lysate, here BT474, is typically used as a positive control for extracellular vesicle negative marker

11. Incubate the membrane in primary antibody overnight at 4 °C with gentle shaking or at room temperature for 3 h.

12. Remove the primary antibody (*see* **Note 4**) and wash the membrane three times, 5 min each, in PBST with vigorous shaking.

13. Incubate the membrane in secondary antibody for 1 h at room temperature with gentle shaking.

14. Remove the secondary antibody (*see* **Note 4**) and wash the membrane three times, 5 min each, in PBST with vigorous shaking.

15. Place the blot in the tray of the imaging system. Mix the ECL reagents at a ratio of 1:1 and apply evenly to the blot for 3 min. Proceed with imaging.

16. After a suitable signal has been obtained, wash the blot once more with PBST to remove any excess ECL solution. If necessary carry out the stripping procedure before probing for another extracellular vesicle marker.

17. For the stripping procedure, warm 30 mL of stripping buffer to 70 °C and then add 100 mM of β-mercaptoethanol. Incubate the membrane in just enough buffer to cover it for 10 min. Replace the buffer with fresh buffer for a further 10 min. Wash the membrane twice, 10 min each, with PBS and once, 10 min, with PBST. Repeat the blocking step before re-probing with primary antibody.

4   Notes

1. Use a minimum of 250 μL of serum or plasma for exosomes isolation.

2. Exosomes are nano-sized and so the pellet produced may not be visible to the naked eye. For this reason, it is important to mark the tube prior to ultracentrifugation so as to be aware of where the pellet is placed.

3. During the washing and fixing steps ensure that the grid is not allowed to dry out while keeping the back of the grid dry. Remove excess solution by gently touching the circumference of the grid against a Whatman no.1 filter paper.

4. Antibody dilutions can be used several times. Store antibody dilutions at –20 °C.

Acknowledgements

Irish Cancer Society's support of Breast-Predict [CCRC13GAL] and HEA PRTLI Cycle 5 funding of TBSI.

References

1. Kowal J, Tkach M, Théry C (2014) Biogenesis and secretion of exosomes. Curr Opin Cell Biol 29:116–125. doi:10.1016/j.ceb.2014.05.004, http://dx.doi.org

2. Raposo G, Stoorvogel W (2013) Extracellular vesicles: exosomes, microvesicles, and friends. J Cell Biol 200(4):373–383. doi:10.1083/jcb.201211138

3. Montecalvo A, Larregina AT, Shufesky WJ et al (2012) Mechanism of transfer of functional microRNAs between mouse dendritic cells via exosomes. Blood 119(3):756–766. doi:10.1182/blood-2011-02-338004

4. Lai CP, Kim EY, Badr CE et al. (2015) Visualization and tracking of tumour extracellular vesicle delivery and RNA translation using multiplexed reporters. Nat Commun 6. doi:10.1038/ncomms8029

5. Valadi H, Ekstrom K, Bossios A et al (2007) Exosome-mediated transfer of mRNAs and microRNAs is a novel mechanism of genetic exchange between cells. Nat Cell Biol 9(6):654–659. doi:10.1038/ncb1596

6. Silva J, Garcia V, Zaballos A et al (2011) Vesicle-related microRNAs in plasma of nonsmall cell lung cancer patients and correlation with survival. Eur Respir J 37(3):617–623. doi:10.1183/09031936.00029610

7. Zhang L, Zhang S, Yao J et al (2015) Microenvironment-induced PTEN loss by exosomal microRNA primes brain metastasis outgrowth. Nature 527(7576):100–104. doi:10.1038/nature15376, http://www.nature.com/nature/journal/v527/n7576/abs/nature15376.html#supplementary-information

8. O'Brien K, Lowry MC, Corcoran C et al (2015) miR-134 in extracellular vesicles reduces triple-negative breast cancer aggression and increases drug sensitivity., Oncotarget

9. Vaksman O, Trope C, Davidson B et al (2014) Exosome-derived miRNAs and ovarian carcinoma progression. Carcinogenesis 35(9):2113–2120. doi:10.1093/carcin/bgu130

10. Taylor DD, Gercel-Taylor C (2008) MicroRNA signatures of tumor-derived exosomes as diagnostic biomarkers of ovarian cancer. Gynecol Oncol 110(1):13–21. doi:10.1016/j.ygyno.2008.04.033

11. Corcoran C, Rani S, O'Driscoll L (2014) miR-34a is an intracellular and exosomal predictive biomarker for response to docetaxel with clinical relevance to prostate cancer progression. Prostate 74(13):1320–1334. doi:10.1002/pros.22848

12. Lötvall J, Hill AF, Hochberg F et al (2014) Minimal experimental requirements for definition of extracellular vesicles and their functions: a position statement from the international society for extracellular vesicles. J Extracell Vesicles 3:26913

13. Rani S, O'Brien K, Kelleher FC et al (2011) Isolation of exosomes for subsequent mRNA, MicroRNA, and protein profiling. Methods Mol Biol 784:181–195. doi:10.1007/978-1-61779-289-2_13

14. Lässer C, Eldh M, Lötvall J (2012) Isolation and characterization of RNA-containing exosomes. J Vis Exp 59:3037. doi:10.3791/3037

Chapter 6

MiRNA Profiling in Human Induced Pluripotent Stem Cells

Erica Hennessy

Abstract

Human iPS cells are capable of differentiation towards all three germ layer lineages. As well as being of use for the study of developmental biology, these cells also provide an excellent resource for disease modeling and cell replacement therapies. iPS cells derived from an individual with a disease type of interest can be differentiated towards the cell type afflicted in that particular disease. Such differentiated cell types can be used to test patient-specific drug responses *in vitro*, for generation of replacement cells for transplantation, or as a starting material for gene editing to correct disease-causing mutations/deletions. With such a vast array of potential applications, there is a great need to understand the exact mechanisms controlling the maintenance of pluripotency, and the distinct cues signaling these cells to differentiate towards lineages of interest. This chapter focuses on microRNA profiling using TaqMan Human MicroRNA Arrays to examine expression of 754 miRNAs in human iPS cells in the pluripotent state, and iPS derived definitive endoderm.

Key words iPS cells, miRNA profiling, Pluripotency, Definitive endoderm, TaqMan MicroRNA Arrays

1 Introduction

Generation of induced pluripotent stem (iPS) cells from somatic cells by forced overexpression of reprogramming factors—oct4, sox2, c-myc, and klf4 [1, 2]—represented a significant advancement in stem cell research. iPS cells possess key characteristics of their embryonic stem cell counterparts, with the additional benefit of allowing derivation of patient-specific pluripotent stem cells for studying a disease type of interest [3].

Definitive endoderm is formed *in vivo* during the gastrulation stage of embryonic development; it undergoes a series of morphogenetic movements generating the primitive gut tube, which is then patterned along the dorsal/ventral and anterior/posterior axis. From the primitive gut tube organs such as the lungs, liver, pancreas, stomach, and intestine are derived [4]. Many developmental disorders can arise during the formation of these endodermal derivatives leading to congenital gastrointestinal malformations. Using the iPS platform, patient-specific pluripotent cells can be

Sweta Rani (ed.), *MicroRNA Profiling: Methods and Protocols*, Methods in Molecular Biology, vol. 1509,
DOI 10.1007/978-1-4939-6524-3_6, © Springer Science+Business Media New York 2017

differentiated towards disease affected lineages allowing *in vitro* modeling of disease development [5].

miRNAs are involved in a diverse range of biological processes such as cell differentiation, proliferation, and metabolism [6] and have been shown to be intimately involved in the iPS reprogramming process [7–10]. Studying the molecular mechanisms controlling differentiation to definitive endoderm and subsequent endodermal lineages, in healthy and disease affected iPS lines will allow a greater understanding of the impact of disease processes on normal cell development and function, and how miRNAs may play a role in these processes.

This chapter describes feeder-free culture of human iPS cells, and a directed differentiation to definitive endoderm. This directed differentiation protocol, developed by ViaCyte/Novocell involves treatment of iPS cells with Activin A and Wnt3a in the presence of low serum, mimicking signaling pathways driving *in vivo* definitive endoderm formation [11, 12]. RNA samples can be taken from iPS cells (Subheading 3.1), and iPS-derived definitive endoderm (Subheading 3.2), allowing comparison of miRNA expression changes related to pluripotency and definitive endoderm differentiation.

A range of technologies are available for examination of miRNA expression, including small RNA sequencing, microarrays and RT-PCR based methods. This chapter focuses on miRNA profiling using the TaqMan MicroRNA Array Card Set V3.0 (Subheading 3.4), this RT-PCR based technology allows simultaneous measurement of 754 miRNAs using a streamlined workflow, with high miRNA specificity capable of deciphering closely related miRNA family members differing by as little as a single base and achieving a dynamic range of 6–7 logs.

TaqMan MicroRNA Array Card Set V3.0 is composed of two 384-well microfludic cards (A and B), with each well representing a unique miRNA assay or endogenous control. MegaPlex RT primers consisting of two pools (A and B) of 380 stem-looped RT primers, allow simultaneous reverse transcription of 380 miRNA species to cDNA. The MegaPlex PreAmp Primers (Pool A and B) then allow unbiased pre-amplification of the miRNA cDNA prior to loading the array. MegaPlex RT and PreAmp Primer pools A and B correspond to the TaqMan MicroRNA Array cards A and B. Each sample to be analyzed will be run on card A and B to profile the maximum 754 miRNA targets, it is also recommended to run biological triplicates of all samples to allow normalization of biological noise.

2   Materials

2.1   Human iPS Cell Culture

1. Human iPS cells: available from stem cell banks such as WiCell.

2. iPS media: StemPro hESC SFM (Thermo Fisher). To prepare 100 mL of 1× iPS media—90.8 mL DMEM/F12 + GlutaMAX,

2 mL StemPro hESC Supplement, 7.2 mL BSA 25%, 8 ng/μL bFGF, 0.1 mM 2-mercaptoethanol.

3. Basic fibroblast growth factor: reconstitute in PBS 0.1% BSA to 10 μg/mL.

4. 2-mercaptoethanol.

5. Matrigel hES-qualified matrix (Corning): diluted in DMEM/F12 (*see* **Note 1**).

6. Phosphate-buffered saline (PBS).

7. Dispase.

8. Cell scraper.

2.2 Human iPS Cell Differentiation to Definitive Endoderm

1. Matrigel GFR (Growth Factor Reduced; Corning).

2. RPMI.

3. HyClone FBS.

4. Activin A—reconstitute in PBS 0.1% BSA to a concentration of 50 μg/mL (500X).

5. Wnt3A—reconstitute in PBS 0.1% BSA to a concentration of 25 μg/mL (1000X).

2.3 RNA Isolation

1. TriReagent.

2. Chloroform.

3. Isopropanol.

4. 75% ethanol.

5. RNase-free water.

6. NanoDrop 2000.

2.4 TaqMan Human MicroRNA Arrays

1. TaqMan MicroRNA Reverse Transcription Kit (Thermo Fisher).

2. Megaplex RT Primers (Thermo Fisher).

3. Megaplex PreAmp Primers (Thermo Fisher).

4. TaqMan PreAmp Master Mix (Thermo Fisher).

5. TaqMan Universal PCR Master Mix, No Amperase UNG (2X) (Thermo Fisher).

6. TE buffer—dilute to 0.1X with RNase-free water.

7. TaqMan Array Human MicroRNA A+B Cards Set v3.0 (Thermo Fisher).

8. Low density array sealer (Thermo Fisher).

9. Low density array centrifuge adapters and buckets (Thermo Fisher).

10. Applied Biosystem 7900HT Fast Real-Time Instrument.

3   Methods

3.1   Human iPS Culture (See Note 2)

1. Prepare a 10 cm tissue culture dish coated with 6 mL diluted Matrigel hES-qualified (*see* **Note 2**), incubate for 1 h at 37 °C.

2. Thaw a vial of iPS cells in a 37 °C water bath until only a small ice crystal remains; slowly add 9 mL of iPS media with 10 μM RhoKi. Centrifuge at $200 \times g$ for 5 min.

3. Remove supernatant from iPS cell pellet, gently resuspend pellet in 10 mL iPS media with 10 μM RhoKi by pipetting up and down once so as not to break up the cell clusters. Transfer to prepared 10 cm dish. Incubate at 37 °C. Feed daily with iPS media (no RhoKi).

4. When cells reach approximately 80 % confluency (*see* **Note 3**), prepare 3 wells of a 6-well plate to passage cells. Add 1 mL of diluted Matrigel hES-qualified matrix per well (*see* **Note 1**), incubate at 37 °C for 1 h, remove excess Matrigel and add 1.5 mL iPS media.

5. Remove media from confluent iPS cells, rinse with PBS, add 3 mL dispase and incubate for 5 min at 37 °C.

6. Remove dispase, rinse with 5 mL iPS media and discard, add 6 mL iPS media and remove cells using a cell scraper. Pipette up and down three to four times to achieve uniform colony size.

7. Add 400 μL of cell suspension to each Matrigel ES-qualified coated well. Ensure cell suspension is dispersed evenly over well surface. Incubate at 37 °C. Proceed to Subheading 3.2 with remaining cell suspension to seed wells for definitive endoderm differentiation. Biological triplicate cultures should be set up for pluripotent iPS cultures and definitive endoderm differentiation and maintained separately to allow for normalization of biological variation.

8. Feed daily with fresh iPS media until colonies reach 60–70 % confluence (*see* **Note 3**).

9. Harvest 2 wells for RNA (A), and 1 well for immunofluorescence (B). One well is analyzed by immunofluorescence for pluripotency marker expression as a quality control measure. A variety of pluripotency markers may be used for this application such as Oct4, Nanog, Tra-1-81, and Tra-1-60 (*see* **Note 4**).

   (a) To harvest RNA, remove media and rinse wells with 1 mL PBS. Add 500 μL TriReagent per well, allow to sit at room temperature for 5 min. Combine TriReagent lysed cells from these two wells into a single Eppendorf and store at −80 °C until required (Subheading 3.3).

   (b) To fix for immunofluorescence, remove media and rinse well with 1 mL PBS. Add 1 mL 10 % formalin, incubate at room temperature for 30 min, remove and discard formalin, add 2 mL PBS and store at 4 °C until ready to proceed with immunofluorescence staining. Perform immunofluorescence staining as per antibody specifications.

3.2 Human iPS Differentiation to Definitive Endoderm

1. Thaw aliquot of Matrigel GFR, dilute 100 μL in 3 mL DMEM/F12. Add 1 mL per well to 3 wells of a 6-well plate. Incubate at 37 °C for 1 h.

2. Remove Matrigel GFR and add 1.5 mL iPS media per well. Using iPS cell suspension from **step 7**, Subheading 3.1, add 400 μL to each of 3 wells. Ensure colonies are well dispersed over well surface.

3. Feed with 2 mL iPS media daily until cells reach 60–70% confluence.

4. Remove media and rinse with 1X PBS, initiate differentiation by adding 2 mL RPMI with 1X GlutaMAX, 100 ng/mL Activin A, and 25 ng/mL Wnt3A to each well.

5. After 24 h differentiation, remove media, to each well add 2 mL RPMI with 1X GlutaMAX, 0.2% HyClone FBS, and 100 ng/mL Activin A.

6. After 24 h, feed wells with same media from **step 5** above.

7. After 24 h, remove media and rinse wells with 1X PBS. Harvest 2 wells for RNA (A), and 1 well for immunofluorescence (B). One well is analyzed by immunofluorescence for definitive endoderm marker expression (such as Sox17 and Foxa2) as a quality control measure (*see* **Note 4**).

   (a) To harvest RNA add 500 μL TriReagent per well, allow to sit at room temperature for 5 min. Combine TriReagent lysed cells from these two wells into a single Eppendorf and store at −80 °C until required.

   (b) To fix for immunofluorescence, add 1 mL 10% formalin, incubate at room temperature for 30 min, remove and discard formalin, add 2 mL PBS and store at 4 °C until ready to proceed with immunofluorescence staining. Ensure to use primary antibodies raised in different species when analyzing expression of more than one marker in a single well. Proceed with immunofluorescence staining as per antibody specifications.

3.3 RNA Isolation

1. Remove samples in TriReagent from −80 °C storage and allow to thaw on ice.

2. Add 0.2 mL chloroform to each sample, shake vigorously for 15 s, and allow to stand for 15 min at room temperature.

3. Centrifuge for 15 min at $8000 \times g$ at 4 °C. Remove the color-less upper aqueous phase (containing RNA) to a fresh tube (*see* **Note 5**).

4. Add 0.5 mL ice-cold isopropanol and mix; incubate at room temperature for 10 min.

5. Centrifuge for 30 min at $8000 \times g$ at 4 °C to pellet the precipi-tated RNA.

6. Taking care not to disturb the RNA pellet, remove and discard the supernatant.

7. Wash pellet by adding 750 μL of 75 % ethanol and vortex. Centrifuge for 5 min at $8000 \times g$ at 4 °C. Remove and discard the supernatant.

8. Repeat wash **step 8**.

9. Allow RNA pellet to air-dry for 10 min and then resuspend in 50 μL of RNase-free water. Pipette up and down to ensure complete resolubilization of RNA pellet (*see* **Note 6**).

10. Check RNA concentration using a NanoDrop 2000, store RNA at –80 °C until required.

3.4 TaqMan Low Density MiRNA Arrays

1. Remove RNA samples from –80 °C, Megaplex RT primers and TaqMan MicroRNA Reverse Transcription Kit from –20 °C storage and thaw on ice.

2. Prepare MicroRNA Reverse Transcription reaction according to the Table 1 (*see* **Note 7**). Prepare separate reaction mixes with MegaPlex RT Primer Pool A and B, i.e., 2 reverse tran-scription reactions per sample being analyzed.

3. Pipette up and down to mix components and centrifuge for 10 s.

4. Transfer 4.5 μL of reverse transcription mix to fresh 0.2 mL Eppendorfs. Add 3 μL of RNA (1–350 ng) to each tube, pipette up and down to mix RNA and reverse transcription reaction mix.

5. Centrifuge briefly to bring all reagents to the bottom of the tube. Incubate on ice for 5 min.

6. Load plate onto thermocycler using cycling parameters from Table 2.

7. Prepare the Pre-amplification reaction according to the Table 3. Prepare separate reaction mixes with MegaPlex PreAmp Primer Pool A and B.

8. Pipette up and down to mix components, and centrifuge for 10 s.

9. To 2.5 μL of RT product from **step 6**, add 22.5 μL of Pre-Amplification reaction mixture. Adding PreAmp mastermix A and B to the corresponding cDNA samples reverse transcribed with Pool A and B.

Table 1
MicroRNA reverse transcription reaction mixture

Components	Volume for 1 reaction (µL)	Volume for 6 reactions (+10 % excess)[a] (µL)
Megaplex RT Primers (10×) Pool A or B	0.8	5.28
dNTPs (100 mM)	0.2	1.32
MultiScribe Reverse Transcriptase (50 U/µL)	1.5	9.9
10X RT Buffer	0.8	5.28
$MgCl_2$ (25 mM)	0.9	5.94
RNase Inhibitor (20 U/µL)	0.1	0.66
RNase-free water	0.2	1.32
Total	4.5	29.7

[a]Six reactions—biological triplicates of pluripotent iPS cells and definitive endoderm differentiated iPS cells. Allow extra 10 % for pipetting losses. Prepare reverse transcription reaction mix for 6 reactions with MegaPlex RT Primer Pool A, and 6 reactions with Primer Pool B

Table 2
MicroRNA reverse transcription thermocycler settings

Stage	Temperature (°C)	Time
Cycle (40 cycles)	16	2 min
	42	1 min
	50	1 s
Hold	85	5 min
Hold	4	Hold

10. Pipette up and down to mix, and centrifuge for 10 s. Incubate on ice for 5 min.

11. Load plate onto thermocycler using cycling parameters from Table 4.

12. Add 75 µL of 0.1X TE buffer to each tube, pipette up and down to mix, centrifuge for 10 s.

13. Remove TaqMan Low Density Arrays from 4 °C storage and allow to reach room temperature before use. To run the experiment described above, 6 TaqMan MicroRNA Array-A cards, and 6 Array-B cards will be required.

14. Prepare TaqMan Array reaction mixture according to Table 5.

15. To 9 µL of diluted pre-amp product from **step 12**, add 891 µL of TaqMan Array reaction mix. Pipette up and down to mix. Centrifuge for 10 s.

Table 3
MicroRNA Pre-amplification reaction mixture

Components	Volume per reaction (μL)	Volume for 6 reactions (+10% excess)[a] (μL)
TaqMan Pre-Amp Master Mix (2×)	12.5	82.5
Megaplex PreAmp Primers (10×) Pool A or B	2.5	16.5
RNase-free water	7.5	49.5
Total	22.5	148.5

[a]Six reactions—biological triplicates of pluripotent iPS cells and definitive endoderm differentiated iPS cells. Allow extra 10% for pipetting losses. Prepare pre-amplification reaction mix for 6 reactions with MegaPlex PreAmp Primer Pool A, and 6 reactions with Primer Pool B

Table 4
MicroRNA Pre-amplification thermocycler settings

Stage	Temperature (°C)	Time
Hold	95	10 min
Hold	55	2 min
Hold	72	2 min
Cycle (12 cycles)	95	15 s
	60	4 min
Hold	99.9	10 min
Hold	4	Hold

16. Add 100 μL of reaction mix from **step 15** to each port of the TaqMan Array, RT and PreAmp pool A samples to card A, and RT and PreAmp pool B samples to card B. Place loaded array cards in centrifuge bucket adapters, centrifuge at $200 \times g$ for 1 min, allow centrifuge to come to a stop, and repeat 1 min spin at $200 \times g$. Remove cards from centrifuge and ensure reaction mix has been dispersed into the card. A minimal amount of reaction mix should be visible in the sample port, and this volume should be uniform between all sample ports.

17. Place TaqMan Array card in plate sealer with the foil side facing up. Pull sealer along the entire length of the TaqMan Array card, remove plate and cut off sample ports.

18. Load card onto the 7900HT Real-Time PCR instrument, fitted with the 384-well card block.

19. Import the SDS file from the CD supplied with the TaqMan Array cards, this file contains all the cycling parameters and

Table 5
TaqMan array reaction mixture

Component	Volume for 1 array (μL)	Volume for 12 arrays (+10 % excess)[a] (mL)
TaqMan Universal PCR Master Mix, No Amperase UNG (2×)	450	5.94
RNase-free water	441	5.82
Total	891	11.76

[a]12 arrays—6 Card-A arrays and 6 Card-B arrays. Allow extra 10 % for pipetting losses

plate mapping required to run the TaqMan MicroRNA Array real-time PCR reaction.

20. The remaining TaqMan Array cards can be stored at 4 °C until ready to run on the instrument.

21. Analyze resulting data using the relative quantification (ΔΔCt) method. Compare average miRNA ΔCt for the pluripotent biological triplicate samples to the average miRNA ΔCt for the definitive endoderm biological triplicate samples to identify miRNAs differentially expressed between these two populations. Calculating $2^{ΔΔCt}$ allows assessment of the fold change difference in miRNA expression.

4   Notes

1. Human iPS cells may also be cultured under feeder-dependent conditions using irradiated mouse embryonic fibroblast (iMEF) feeder cells. An iMEF depletion should be carried out before plating iPS cells for differentiation (Subheading 3.2). An iMEF RNA sample should be processed as per the human iPS and definitive endoderm samples and run on a separate TaqMan Array card to rule out any miRNA expression changes derived from contaminating iMEFs.

2. Protein concentration of Matrigel hES-Qualified matrix differs between batches, and should be diluted according to each batch specification; in general 270–350 μL is diluted in 25 mL DMEM/F12, this volume is sufficient to coat 4 × 10 cm dishes, or 4 × 6-well plates.

3. If pluripotent iPS cultures display any areas of differentiation they should be removed from the plate by visualizing under a dissection microscope in a laminar flow hood, and removed by gently scraping away using a 200 μL pipette tip.

4. One well of pluripotent iPS cells and definitive endoderm differentiated iPS cells should be stained for pluripotent or definitive endoderm markers to determine the purity of the cultures. iPS cell lines may vary in their propensity to form certain cell lineages. If low yield of definitive endoderm (Sox17 and Foxa2) is achieved, alternative iPS lines should be tested. FACS may be used to sort pure populations of a desired cell type (definitive endoderm) for microRNA profiling.

5. When removing the upper aqueous phase containing RNA, ensure not to disturb the interphase to avoid phenol contamination, which may inhibit downstream PCR reactions.

6. Once pellet begins to change from white to transparent add RNase-free water, if RNA pellet is allowed to air-dry completely it may be difficult to get back into solution.

7. Excess RNA not used for TaqMan Array processing can be stored at −80 °C. This RNA can be used in single-plex TaqMan MicroRNA assays to validate targets identified in the TaqMan Array profiling.

References

1. Takahashi K, Yamanaka S (2006) Induction of pluripotent stem cells from mouse embryonic and adult fibroblast cultures by defined factors. Cell 126(4):663–676

2. Takahashi K, Tanabe K, Ohnuki M, Narita M, Ichisaka T, Tomada K, Yamanaka S (2007) Induction of pluripotent stem cells from adult human fibroblasts by defined factors. Cell 131(5):861–872

3. Robinton DA, Daley GQ (2012) The promise of pluripotent stem cells in research and therapy. Nature 481:295–305

4. Wells JM, Melton DA (1999) Vertebrate endoderm development. Annu Rev Cell Dev Biol 15:393–410

5. Unternaehrer JJ, Daley GQ (2011) Induced pluripotent stem cells for modelling human diseases. Philos Trans R Soc Lond B Biol Sci 366(1575):2274–2285

6. Bartel DP (2004) MicroRNAs: genomics, biogenesis, mechanism, and function. Cell 116:281–297

7. Choi YJ, Lin CP, Ho JJ, He X, Okada N, Bu P, Zhong Y, Kim SY, Bennett MJ, Chen C, Ozturk A, Hicks GG, Hannon GJ, He L (2011) Mir-34 miRNAs provide a barrier for somatic cell reprogramming. Nat Cell Biol 13:1253–1260

8. Melton C, Judson RL, Blelloch R (2010) Opposing microRNA families regulate self-renewal in mouse embryonic stem cells. Nature 463:621–626

9. Subramanyam D, Lamouille S, Judson RL, Liu JY, Bucay N, Derynck R, Blelloch R (2011) Multiple targets of mir-302 and mir-372 promote reprogramming of human fibroblasts to induced pluripotent stem cells. Nat Biotechnol 29:443–448

10. Judson RL, Babiarz JE, Venere M, Blelloch R (2009) Embryonic stem cell-specific microRNAs promote induced pluripotency. Nat Biotechnol 27:459–461

11. D'Amour KA, Agulnick AD, Eliazer S, Kelly OG, Kroon E, Baetge EE (2005) Efficient differentiation of human embryonic stem cells to definitive endoderm. Nat Biotechnol 23(12):1534–1541

12. D'Amour KA, Bang AG, Eliazer S, Kelly OG, Agulnick AD, Smart NG, Moorman MA, Kroon E, Carpenter MK, Baetge EE (2006) Production of pancreatic hormone-expressing endocrine cells from human embryonic stem cells. Nat Biotechnol 24(11):1392–1401

Chapter 7

MiRNA Expression in Cystic Fibrosis Bronchial Epithelial Cells

Irene K. Oglesby and Paul J. McKiernan

Abstract

Bronchial epithelial cells represent an invaluable tool to elucidate molecular signaling regulation in cystic fibrosis (CF). CF is a lethal genetic condition characterized by chronic inflammation in which bronchial epithelial cells play a pivotal role. Here we describe their use in analysis of microRNA (miRNA) and their target genes following a two-step RT-PCR miRNA profiling method in bronchial cell specimens from CF and control individuals where 667 human miRNA were examined. We also describe an approach to experimental modulation of these miRNA in vitro.

Key words Cystic fibrosis, miRNA, Array, Bronchial cells, qRT-PCR, Transfection

1 Introduction

CF is a multifaceted disorder making the design of therapeutic strategies extremely challenging. With the advent of the discovery of miRNA and the exponential level of research in this area it is likely that these small noncoding RNAs also play a role in the pathology of CF [1]. We performed miRNA expression profiling in CF and non-CF bronchial brushing RNA by a stem-loop real-time PCR-based method using TaqMan MicroRNA Arrays from Applied Biosystems (see user bulletin [2] for detailed protocol). The content is derived from the miRBase microRNA registry, providing comprehensive coverage of miRNA and allows relative quantitation (RQ) of targets using the comparative CT (ddCT) method [3]. Of 667 miRNA examined 93 were differentially expressed with 56 being downregulated (Relative Quantification (RQ) ≤ 0.7) and 36 upregulated (RQ ≥ 1.5) in CF versus non-CF controls [4]. Essential array validation and analysis was performed via qRT-PCR in bronchial epithelial cells ex vivo and using an in vitro cell model for specific miRNA and their respective target gene expression. Transfection of cell lines was optimized and performed for miRNA upregulation and inhibition studies.

Sweta Rani (ed.), *MicroRNA Profiling: Methods and Protocols*, Methods in Molecular Biology, vol. 1509,
DOI 10.1007/978-1-4939-6524-3_7, © Springer Science+Business Media New York 2017

2   Materials

2.1 *Bronchial Brush Sampling Components*

1. 10 mm × 1.2 mm bronchial brush (Olympus Medical Systems Corp, Japan).

2. Sterile 0.9% NaCl.

3. Complete media: To a 500 mL bottle of Minimal Essential Media + GlutaMAX (MEM) add 50 mL (10%) heat-inactivated fetal calf serum (FCS) and 5 mL (25,000 U—1%) penicillin/streptomycin. Heat to 37 °C prior to use (*see* **Note 1**).

4. TRI Reagent—keep at 4 °C prior to use.

5. Ice for transport of samples.

2.2 *Cell Culture*

Cell lines used are CF (CFBE41o-) and non-CF (16HBE14o-) airway epithelial cells (Fig. 1) obtained from the Gruenert lab [5] cultured on fibronectin/BSA-coated flasks.

2.2.1 *Coating Tissue Culture Flasks*

1. Coating solution; in a sterile container mix 100 mL LHC-8 basal medium, 10 mL bovine serum albumin (BSA, 1 mg/mL), 1 mL collagen I, bovine (2.9 mg/mL), 1 mL human fibronectin (1 mg/mL) in a sterile container. Aliquot and freeze at –20 °C (*see* **Note 2**).

2.2.2 *Cell Growth and Subculture*

1. Culture media as per complete media, No. 3 in Subheading 2.1.

2. T75 vented tissue culture flasks.

3. PET modified trypsin solution for cell detachment; 50 mL of PET contains 10% polyvinylpyrrolidone (5 mL) and 0.2%

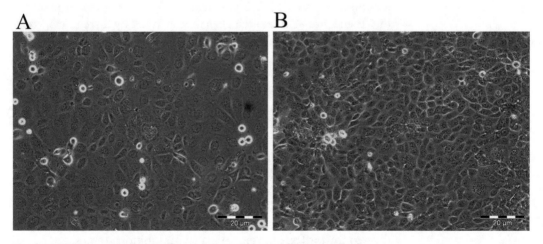

Fig. 1 (**a**) CFBE41o- and (**b**) 16HBE14o- cell monolayer at 20× magnification

EGTA (5 mL) (made in distilled H_2O and Hepes Buffered Saline (HBSS), respectively and filter-sterilized), 4 mL trypsin–EDTA, and 36 mL of HBSS (*see* **Note 3**).

4. Dulbecco's phosphate buffered saline (DPBS).

2.3 RNA Isolation and Quantification

1. Chloroform.

2. Prepare a 75 % ethanol solution using molecular grade water. For 100 mL add 25 mL of water to 75 mL of ethanol. Scale this down to just above the amount required depending on number of samples and make fresh each time.

3. Isopropanol.

4. Molecular grade nuclease-free water.

5. 1.5 mL Eppendorf tubes.

6. Prepare a 0.1 % solution of diethylpyrocarbonate (DEPC) H_2O by adding 0.1 mL of DEPC to 100 mL of deionized water. Autoclave and keep sterile.

7. NanoDrop or equivalent spectrophotometer.

2.4 Validation of microRNA Expression

1. TaqMan® MicroRNA assays.

2. TaqMan® MicroRNA Reverse Transcription Kit.

3. TaqMan® Universal PCR Master Mix II (2×), no UNG (uracil-N-glycosylase).

4. Molecular grade nuclease-free water.

5. 96-well PCR plates and seals.

6. Centrifuge with 96-well plate holders.

2.5 Identification of Predicted mRNA Targets of microRNA and Expression Analysis

1. Quantitect® Reverse Transcription Kit (Qiagen).

2. SYBR Green master mix (Roche).

3. Specific oligonucleotide primers (*see* Subheading 3.5.2).

2.6 miRNA and siRNA Transfection

1. RiboJuice™ transfection reagent.

2. Specific synthetic miRNA mimics or inhibitors and non-targeting controls.

3. siRNA and non-targeting controls.

4. OptiMEM® reduced serum media.

5. Fluorescently labeled miRIDIAN mimic negative control.

6. Minimum Essential Media +GlutaMax supplemented with FCS.

7. 6/24-well tissue culture plates.

8. 10 mL sterile pipettes.

9. 1.5 mL sterile Pasteur pipettes.

10. Hemocytometer for cell counts.

3 Methods

3.1 Obtaining Bronchial Brushings from CF Patients/ Controls Undergoing Routine Bronchoscopy

Bronchial brush samples can be taken from participants who have given informed consent (CF and controls) undergoing diagnostic and/or therapeutic fiber-optic flexible bronchoscopy as part of routine care. A trained physician samples brushings.

1. Following completion of the bronchoscopy and prior to the withdrawal of the bronchoscope, select an area 2 cm distal to the carina (medially located) in either the right or left main bronchus and wash twice with 10 mL sterile 0.9 % NaCl.

2. Following this, insert a sterile 10 mm × 1.2 mm bronchial brush through the appropriate port on the bronchoscope and obtain sample from the chosen area with two consecutive brushes by scraping the area gently.

3. Withdraw the brush immediately and place in 5 mL complete media.

4. Gently agitate brushes to dislodge cells into the media and centrifuge at $150 \times g$ for 5 min.

5. Resuspend cell pellets in 0.5 mL of TRI Reagent and transfer to 1.5 mL Eppendorf tubes prior to RNA extraction.

3.2 Cell Culture

Cell lines should be maintained in 75 cm² flasks with vented lids at 37 °C in a humidified 5 % CO_2 incubator and fed every 2–3 days. Cells should also be routinely cultured in the presence of 1 % penicillin/streptomycin to prevent bacterial contamination.

3.2.1 Coating of Flasks

For optimal growth of cells obtained from the Grunert laboratory culture flasks were coated with a fibronectin/collagen/BSA coating solution.

1. Add 3–4 mL of coating solution aseptically into 75 cm² flask. Swirl back and forth to ensure complete coverage of the flask base.

2. Place flasks into incubator for a minimum of 2 h and then remove any excess solution into a sterile tube (*see* **Note 4**).

3. Wrap and store at room temperature for up to 1 month.

3.2.2 Thawing/Reviving Cells from Liquid Nitrogen

Thawing of cells from liquid nitrogen must be performed rapidly to reduce exposure time to the dimethyl sulfoxide (DMSO) freezing solution, which is toxic at room temperature.

1. Remove cryovial from liquid nitrogen storage and thaw rapidly in a 37 °C water bath. Ensure lid stays above water to prevent contamination (*see* **Note 5**).

2. When almost fully thawed, transfer the DMSO-cell suspension into a sterile 15 mL tube containing 5 mL of pre-warmed culture media.

3. Centrifuge at $150 \times g$ for 5 min, remove the DMSO-containing supernatant, and resuspend the pellet in 1 mL of pre-warmed fresh complete media.

4. Transfer to a pre-coated 75 cm² tissue culture flask with 9 mL of media and allowed to attach overnight.

5. After 24 h, re-feed cells with fresh media to remove any residual traces of DMSO.

3.2.3 Subculture of Adherent Cells

During routine subculturing or harvesting of adherent lines, cells were removed from their flasks by enzymatic detachment using PET.

1. Aseptically remove waste media, cells and rinse cell monolayer with pre-warmed DPBS to remove any naturally occurring trypsin inhibitor present in residual serum in culture media.

2. Add 3–5 mL of PET to one 75 cm² flask, swirl to cover monolayer and incubate at 37 °C, 5% CO_2 for 5 min. Remove to waste and add a fresh 3–5 mL of PET incubate for a further 5 min until the cells have detached (*see* **Note 6**).

3. The PET is inactivated by addition of an equal volume of complete growth media (i.e., containing 10% FCS) (*see* **Note 7**).

4. Transfer cell suspension to a 15 mL tube and centrifuge at $250 \times g$ for 5 min.

5. Remove supernatant to waste and resuspend cell pellet in pre-warmed (37 °C) fresh growth media, count and use to re-seed a flask at the required cell density or to set up a given assay (*see* **Note 8**).

3.3 RNA Isolation

This procedure is based on a single step liquid phase separation resulting in the simultaneous isolation of RNA, DNA and protein. Volumes listed are based on 0.5 mL of TRI Reagent per sample. This procedure is carried out according to the protocol outlined in the Sigma datasheet for TRI Reagent.

1. For phase separation leave samples to stand at room temperature for ~5 min after which add 100 µL chloroform.

2. Cover samples and shake vigorously for 15 s after which stand tubes at room temp for 2–15 min.

3. Centrifuge tubes at $12,000 \times g$ for 15 min at 4 °C to separate the mixture into three phases (a red organic phase, an interphase, and a colorless upper aqueous phase containing protein, DNA, and RNA respectively).

4. Transfer the aqueous phase to a new tube, taking care not to disturb either layer below and add 0.25 mL isopropanol.

5. Shake to mix samples then stand at room temperature for 5–10 min. Centrifuge again at $12,000 \times g$ for 10 min at 4 °C

for RNA to precipitate and form a pellet at the side/bottom of the tube.

6. Remove supernatant carefully taking care not to disturb the pellet.

7. Add 0.5 mL 75 % EtOH to wash the RNA pellet then vortex and centrifuge at $12,000 \times g$ for 5 min at 4 °C.

8. Remove supernatant carefully and allow samples to air-dry for ~5–10 min (*see* **Note 9**). Then resuspend in a 0.1 % autoclaved solution of diethyl pyrocarbonate (DEPC) H_2O.

3.3.1 RNA Quantification

Quantification of RNA is performed spectrophotometrically, this method describes the use of an 8 channel NanoDrop 8000 for this purpose. The amount of RNA present is calculated using the following formula:

$$OD_{260\,nm} \times \text{Dilution factor} \times 40 = \mu g\,/\,mL\ RNA$$

1. Sample pedestals (upper and lower) must be cleaned before and after use with nuclease-free H_2O. To read the samples select "Nucleic acid" on the NanoDrop software and perform initialisation of the instrument using 1–2 μL of nuclease-free H_2O followed by 1–2 μL of DEPC H_2O to blank instrument.

2. Clean both the upper and lower pedestals between samples. Samples are loaded (1–2 μL) onto the lower pedestal where up to eight samples can be measured at any one time.

3. The upper pedestal is then closed on top and when reading samples the droplet is stretched between pedestals. Using DEPC H_2O as a diluent an A_{260}/A_{280} ratio of 1.6 is indicative of pure RNA, although RNA with ratios from 1.6 to 1.8 were routinely observed and used in subsequent experiments (*see* **Note 10**). RNA yield (ng/μL) from a 24-well culture plate was typically between 100 and 300 μg for cell lines used. RNA samples were stored at −80 °C.

3.4 MiRNA Expression Profiling Validation in CF Bronchial Brushings and Cell Lines

Following in situ PCR in CF and non-CF bronchial brushing RNA using 384-well TaqMan Arrays (*see* **Note 11**) validation of results was performed in additional clinical samples and cell lines. Particular attention must be placed on normalization of the large amounts of data that profiling generates. To this end we found that the expression of miR-16 and miR-218 remained unchanged between CF and non-CF samples and these were subsequently were used as controls. Array data is deposited in the National Center for Biotechnology Information Gene Expression Omnibus (21) and are accessible through Gene Expression Omnibus Series accession number GSE19431 [6].

3.4.1 miRNA Reverse Transcription

Generation of cDNA from extracted RNA for microRNAs of interest is performed using miRNA specific stem loop reverse transcription (RT) primers from TaqMan® MicroRNA assays and reagents from the TaqMan® MicroRNA Reverse Transcription kit (*see* **Note 12**). Dilute RNA samples to 40 ng/μL and aliquot 2.5 μL into a PCR microfuge tube giving a final amount of 100 ng total RNA per tube.

1. Prepare a mastermix of reagents (1–5) in Table 1 in a separate tube including a 10 % excess to allow for loss due to pipetting. Total volume per sample is 3.5 μL.

2. Prepare a mastermix of the RT specific primer (1.5 μL per sample) and add to RT mastermix. Centrifuge briefly at <400×g.

3. Aliquot 5 μL of mastermix (RT plus probe) to tube containing RNA, mix gently and centrifuge briefly at <400×g and then incubate on ice for 5 min.

4. Perform the RT reaction on a thermal cycler using a program consisting of incubation at 16 °C for 30 min, followed by 42 °C for 30 min. The RT enzyme should then be inactivated by heating to 85 °C for 5 min, followed by a cooling step to 4 °C. If not doing PCR immediately store the cDNA at –20 °C until required.

3.4.2 Quantitative Real-Time PCR (qRT-PCR): miRNA Expression

A robust means of measuring mature microRNA expression by qRT-PCR is by use of the well-characterized TaqMan® miRNA assays according to the manufacturer's instructions. This section describes the TaqMan® miRNA assay qRT-PCR protocol on a LightCycler® instrument using a 480 mono color hydrolysis probe program.

1. Thaw and prepare reagents as per Table 2. Scale up accordingly, allowing an extra 10 % volume due to pipetting loss.

Table 1
miRNA RT reaction components

Reagent	Volume (μL)
1. dNTP mix 100 mM	0.075
2. Multiscribe Transcriptase	0.05
3. 10× RT Buffer	0.75
4. RNase Inhibitor	0.19
5. Nuclease-free water	2.08
Total RNA	2.5 (40 ng/μL)
RT specific primer	1.5
Total volume	**7.5**

Table 2
Components of the TaqMan® microRNA qRT-PCR reaction

Component	Volume per 20 µL reaction
TaqMan® Universal PCR Master Mix II (2×), no UNG	10
miRNA specific probe Master Mix (20×)	1
Nuclease-free Water	7.67
Mix well and dispense 18.67 µL per well	
Product from RT reaction	1.33

2. Briefly centrifuge at low speed and add 18.67 of master mix to wells of a suitable PCR plate.

3. Add 1.33 µL of the appropriate RT product for miRNA of interest.

4. Perform PCR reaction. This program consists of pre-incubation at 95 °C × 10 min for enzyme activation. The PCR cycles are (1) denaturation at 95 °C × 15 s and (2) annealing/extension at 60 °C × 60 s. This two step cycle is repeated 40–45 times in which measurement of fluorescence that was achieved by cleavage of probes hybridized to the target resulting in separation of the MGB reporter dye (FAM) from the quencher is determined at the end of each cycle.

5. Relative quantification of gene expression is determined using the comparative cycle threshold method ($2^{-\Delta\Delta Ct}$) as previously described [3].

3.5 Identification of Predicted mRNA Targets of microRNA and Expression Analysis

In silico analysis of miRNA target prediction databases can be performed for identification of predicted microRNA targets of interest. Various online tools aid in these predictions and some well-known examples include TargetScan v7.0, MicroCosm Targets v5.0 (formally miRBase Targets), microRNA.org (formally miRANDA), picTar, DIANA-microT, PITA, RNA Hybrid, and RNA22, all of which utilize different algorithms, and different sources of mRNA sequences.

3.5.1 Synthesis of cDNA for Gene Expression Analysis Using SYBR Green Chemistry

Equal quantities of total RNA extracted using TRI Reagent or other RNA isolation approaches should be reverse transcribed into complementary DNA (cDNA) to use as a template for RT-PCR reactions, using the Quantitect® Reverse Transcription Kit following the manufacturer's protocol. This is a two-step protocol where removal of genomic DNA contamination is performed in part 1 and reverse transcription in part 2 using the components and volumes outlined in Table 3. The cDNA should be stored at –20 °C until required.

Table 3
Components of cDNA reverse transcription for gene expression analysis

Part 1—Components	Volume/reaction
gDNA wipeout buffer	2 μL
Template RNA	5 μL (variable) (1–1000 ng)
Nuclease-free water	7 μL (variable)
Total volume	14 μL
Part 2—Components	Volume/reaction
Quantiscript Reverse Transcriptase	1 μL
Quantiscript RT Buffer	4 μL
RT Primer mix	1 μL
Part 1 reaction contents	14 μL
Total volume	20 μL

3.5.2 Primer Design

PCR primers can be designed using various online tools such as Primer 3 [7, 8] and NCBI Primer-BLAST [9]. Synthesized primers should be desalted; however, there is no need for higher purification such as by HPLC. Primer selection should be based on fulfilling the following criteria as much as possible:

1. Primer length of 18–22 bp.

2. Melting temperature in the range of 52–58 °C.

3. GC content of 40–60 %.

4. More than 3 G's or C's avoided in the last 5 bases at the 3′ end of the primer.

5. Primer secondary structures such as hairpins, self-dimer and cross-dimer avoided.

6. Product size of 100–200 bp spanning 2 exons.

7. Not targeting other transcripts in the human genome as determined by Homo sapiens nucleotide BLAST Sequence Analysis Tool (nBLAST) [10].

3.5.3 Quantitative Real-Time PCR (qRT-PCR): Gene Expression

qRT-PCR can be performed on any suitable instrument, this protocol details the experimental setup for the LightCycler® 480 (Roche) using a SYBR Green master mix. This master mix contains FastStart Taq DNA Polymerase, reaction buffer, dNTPs, SYBR Green I dye and magnesium chloride ($MgCl_2$). Optimal primer concentrations should be empirically determined, but 10 pmol per 20 μL reactions can be used as a starting point. Template cDNA should be used at a concentration of no more than 10 % of the total reaction volume.

Table 4
Reaction mixture for gene expression qRT-PCR

Components	Volume/20 µL reaction
SYBR Green 2×	10
Primer (F) (10 pmol- variable)	1
Primer (R) (10 pmol- variable)	1
Nuclease-free water	6
Mix and plate 18 µL/well	
Add template cDNA	2

1. Components in Table 4 should be thawed, mixed, and 18 µl dispensed into a white LightCycler® 480 multiwell plate.

2. Template cDNA should then be added and the plate sealed with LightCycler® 480 sealing foil.

3. Loaded plates should be centrifuged at $250 \times g$ for 2 min to concentrate the mixture at the bottom of the wells.

4. A typical SYBR Green qRT-PCR program consists of pre-incubation at 95 °C × 5 min to activate the FastStart Taq DNA Polymerase enzyme. Amplification, annealing of primers, and elongation are at 95 °C × 10 s, 57 °C × 10 s (temperature here is primer dependent), and 72 °C × 10 s (25 bases/s), respectively. This three-step cycle is repeated 40–45 times and at the end of each cycle measurement of fluorescence is performed to monitor increasing amounts of amplified DNA. Fluorescence is achieved by incorporation of the SYBR Green dye into the DNA helix and is directly proportional to the amount of double stranded DNA generated. Melting curve analysis for PCR product identification is performed at the end of the program by heating the reaction mixture slowly to 97 °C to melt the double stranded DNA resulting in a corresponding decrease in fluorescence which is continuously monitored and displayed as a peak (www.roche applied-science.com).

3.6 miRNA Transfection

Transfection conditions need to be optimized for each cell type to determine optimal seeding density, and miRNA concentrations. Optimal transfection conditions used for both siRNA and miRNA transfection were determined in CFBE41o- and 16HBE14o- cell lines using a GAPDH siRNA which routinely exhibits ~80% knock down compared to a negative control siRNA (both at a concentration of 30 nM). Varying cells densities and volumes of transfection reagent were assessed. Conditions selected were based on the greatest knockdown achieved with minimal toxicity for each cell

Table 5
Optimal transfection conditions

Cell line	Cell density/mL		Volume of Ribojuice		OptiMEM®	
	24-well	6-well	24-well	6-well	24-well	6-well
CFBE41o-	8×10^4	3×10^5	2 μL	6 μL	48 μL	244 μL
16HBE14o-	1×10^5	3×10^5	2 μL	6 μL	48 μL	244 μL

line and are shown in Table 5. RiboJuice™ was used as the transfection reagent of choice for delivery of miRNA mimics to airway epithelial cell lines.

3.6.1 Transfection Procedure

1. Seed cells 24 h prior to transfection and feed with fresh media on the day of transfection—(250 μL/24-well plate; 1,250 μL/6-well plate).

2. Transfection should be performed under optimal conditions with Ribojuice according to the manufacturer's instructions using Table 5 as a guide if transfecting airway epithelial cells.

3. Dilute Ribojuice™ in OptiMEM® reduced serum media, vortex gently, and incubate at room temperature for 5 min.

4. Add siRNA/miRNA (pre-miR mimics or anti-miR antagmoirs) and relevant negative controls at a final concentration of 30 nM to the Ribojuice/OptiMEM® solution, mix gently and incubate for a further 10 min at room temperature (*see* **Note 13**).

5. Add 50 μL or 100 μL of the transfection mix to 24-well or 6-well plates, respectively.

6. Plates should be mixed gently by rocking and incubated at 37 °C for 24 h or 48 h. After 24 h, remove the transfection mixture from the cells and the feed cells with fresh complete media (48 h transfections only).

7. Sample collection is dependent on subsequent analysis. For example, TRIzol can be utilized for RNA extraction for gene expression/miRNA studies; supernatant can be removed for ELISA analysis of secreted protein or the cells may be lysed for cellular protein analysis.

4 Notes

1. For heat inactivation of FCS place bottle in water bath at 56 °C for 30 min. Ensure water does not come in contact with top of bottle, wrap lid in Parafilm to prevent as a precaution. Always use fresh media for collection of brushing specimens and avoid repeated reheating of media.

2. Human fibronectin comes as a frozen solution and needs to be handled carefully and not disturbed during thawing process. Aliquot coating solution into 15 mL sterile tubes and freeze until required.

3. PET can either be prepared fresh or can be aliquoted and stored at −20 °C. 10 mL of PET is required for detachment of one T75 flask of cells. PET solution volumes can be scaled up to allow aliquots of 25–50 mL be frozen.

4. Excess solution can be refrozen and reused for the same cell line once it is kept sterile.

5. Hold cryovial in warm water using a tweezers or tin foil wrapped around lid.

6. Always look at flask under microscope between addition of first and second round of PET as occasionally a lot of cells can become detached upon first addition of PET. Gently tap flask to detach cells after second round of PET. Always used freshly thawed PET and pre-warm just prior to use to ensure best enzymatic activity.

7. Add pre-warmed media immediately after cell detachment to prevent degradation of cells if overexposed to PET.

8. If subculturing only, cells can be split 1:3 or 1:5 without counting, i.e., resuspend pellet in 1.5 mL media and transfer 0.5 mL to a new flask containing 9 mL media.

9. Remove majority of supernatant with a P1000 pipette leaving a small amount in tube (approx. 20 μL) to ensure pellet not sucked up. Check if pellet visible on side of tube, then gently decant remaining supernatant onto a tissue and leave tube open to air-dry for 10 min.

10. Using DEPC-treated H_2O as the reference diluent, an A260/A280 ratio of >1.6 is indicative of pure RNA. This depends on the diluent, as for example RNA resuspended in TE buffer (pH 8.0) should have a ratio of >2.0. The A260/A230 ratio should be close to 2.0, as absorbance at 230 nm is indicative of contamination by protein, and chaotropic agents such as phenol and guanidinium thiocyanate.

11. We used 30 ng RNA from clinical samples thereby needing to perform a pre-amplification step. If the total RNA amount available is 350–1000 ng a pre-amplification step is not required.

12. TaqMan® assays contain miRNA specific RT primers in one tube (used for the RT reaction) and forward and reverse miRNA specific PCR primers and miRNA specific TaqMan minor groove binder (MGB) probe combined in a second tube (used in the PCR reaction mix).

13. We recommend using a non-targeting fluorescently labeled miRNA mimic or inhibitor to monitor transfection efficiency in

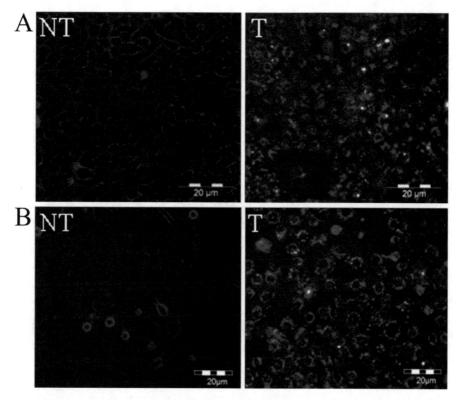

Fig. 2 (**a**) 16HBE14o-cells non-transfected (NT) and transfected (T) and (**b**) CFBE41o-cells non-transfected (NT) and transfected (T) with pierce dye547-labeled negative control

pre-miR and anti-miR experiments (Fig. 2). We used miRID-IAN mimic negative control fluorescently labeled with Thermo Scientific Pierce Dy547 (Dharmacon, CP-004500-01-0).

References

1. Oglesby IK, McElvaney NG, Greene CM (2010) MicroRNAs in inflammatory lung disease--master regulators or target practice? Respir Res 11:148

2. Applied Biosystems (2010). Applied Biosystems TaqMan® Low Density Array. Available via Applied Biosystems https://www3.appliedbiosystems.com/cms/groups/mcb_support/documents/generaldocuments/cms_042326.pdf. Accessed 14 Nov 2015

3. Livak KJ, Schmittgen TD (2001) Analysis of relative gene expression data using real-time quantitative PCR and the $2^{-\Delta\Delta CT}$ method. Methods 25:402–408

4. Oglesby IK, Bray IM, Chotirmall SH et al (2010) miR-126 is downregulated in cystic fibrosis airway epithelial cells and regulates TOM1 expression. J Immunol 184:1702–1709

5. Gruenert DC, Willems M, Cassiman JJ, Frizzell RA (2004) Established cell lines used in cystic fibrosis research. J Cyst Fibros 3(Suppl 2):191–196

6. Gene Expression Omnibus. NCBI. www.ncbi.nlm.nih.gov/geo/query/acc.cgi?acc=GSE19431

7. Primer3 Database (v4.0.0). http://frodo.wi.mit.edu. Accessed 15 Nov 2015

8. Untergrasser A, Cutcutache I, Koressaar T et al (2012) Primer3—new capabilities and interfaces. Nucleic Acids Res 40(15), e115

9. NCBI. Primer-BLAST. Available via http://www.ncbi.nlm.nih.gov/tools/primer-blast. Accessed 15 Nov 2015

10. NCBI. Basic Local Alignment Search Tool. Available via http://www.ncbi.nlm.nih.gov/blast. Accessed 15 Nov 2015

Chapter 8

TaqMan Low Density Array: MicroRNA Profiling for Biomarker and Oncosuppressor Discovery

Keith O'Brien

Abstract

MicroRNAs (miRNAs) have gained a lot of interest as biomarkers and biotherapeutics in recent years. The discovery of miRNAs in circulation as recently as 2008, aided by rapid advances in high-throughput profiling techniques initiated an explosion of investigations dedicated to discovering circulating miRNAs as minimally invasive biomarkers. As miRNAs regulate many cellular processes, investigators are actively exploring their relevance in disease treatment by miRNA restoration. This chapter demonstrates an approach to discover miRNAs of biomarker and therapeutic potential by isolating miRNAs from cell lines, performing global miRNA profiling, investigating miRNA expression in clinical specimens and examining their therapeutic relevance by restoring miRNA expression using Lipofectamine in vitro.

Key words microRNA, Biomarker, TaqMan low density array, miRNA mimic, Transfection, RNAi, Clinical, In vitro

1 Introduction

miRNAs are small (18–25 nucleotides) noncoding RNAs that function intracellularly to halt messenger RNA (mRNA) translation [1, 2] subsequently regulating a plethora of cellular processes and phenotypes associated with development and disease progression [3–5]. The discovery of circulating miRNAs in 2008 stimulated a new field of biomarker research [6]. miRNAs have since been observed to be circulating in blood encapsulated within exosomes [7], microvesicles [8], part of lipoprotein–miRNA complexes [9] or as free unbound miRNA [10]. They are attractive entities for the use as biomarkers as they can be obtained minimally invasively, are stable in circulation and storage, resistant to RNAses, can be detected sensitively and specifically (by qPCR), show disease-specific expression, are evolutionarily conserved, and represent epigenetic alterations reflecting microenvironmental and cellular changes prior to and throughout disease progression [6–8].

Sweta Rani (ed.), *MicroRNA Profiling: Methods and Protocols*, Methods in Molecular Biology, vol. 1509,
DOI 10.1007/978-1-4939-6524-3_8, © Springer Science+Business Media New York 2017

There remain challenges in discovering effective circulating miRNAs as biomarkers. Of paramount importance to developing a reproducible, specific and sensitive biomarker is the absolute observance of the established standard operating procedure (SOP) developed by the Early Detection Research Network, as will be presented in this chapter [11]. Variables such as processing time, temperature, sample hemolysis, additives in blood collection tubes, sample storage, and excessive freeze–thaw cycles can interfere with the discovery of effective biomarkers [12]. Extra care must be taken to standardize preanalytical variables as miRNA expressions are highly sensitive to environmental alterations, including, but not limited to, exercise [13], eating patterns [14], smoking [15], and sleeping patterns [16]. Lack of following standardized protocols has, at least partly, led to difficulties in producing rugged data in miRNA biomarker research [17].

An on-going challenge in the field of miRNA biomarker research is the lack of consensus on the most appropriate endogenous control to normalize relative miRNA expressions [12]. Four options are available to researchers for miRNA expression normalization: (a): normalization to housekeeping miRNAs, however there is a lack of consensus of their accuracy due to apparent disease specific expression patters [18] (b): Global mean normalization: however, this is only statistically accurate for large datasets [19] (c): Direct C_T versus C_T normalization: this requires extremely precise measurements and can be used to determine relative miRNA expression per mL of serum and (d): Spike-in reference miRNA: 1.6×10^8 copies of Cel—miR-39 are spiked-in to the serum specimen during RNA isolation [12]. Here, we recommend using the spiked-in approach as it allows the researcher to normalize the data in three ways: (a): relative miRNA level per volume of starting serum, (b): quantification of miRNA copy number and (c): relative miRNA expression compared to the spiked-in control [12].

miRNA expression is typically and vastly downregulated in cancerous tumors, suggesting that loss of miRNA expression is partly responsible for tumor progression by allowing increased oncoprotein translation [20]. As miRNAs can act as potent oncosuppressors, this leaves the possibility for the use of miRNAs therapeutically as a miRNA restoration approach to cancer treatment [21]. This field of research is showing much promise, with the first miRNA restoration therapy entering a phase 1 clinical trial in 2013 for treatment of solid tumors and hematological malignancies and is well tolerated [22].

In this chapter, we present global miRNA profiling as a method to identify downregulated miRNAs, which may have therapeutic potential in control versus experimental samples. We recommend restoring miRNA expression using miRNA mimics with Lipofectamine®, a liposome forming reagent, to investigate their therapeutic potential in vitro.

To discover miRNAs of biomarker and therapeutic potential one can employ the use of global miRNA profiling by TaqMan Low Density Array (TLDA). TLDA is a quantitative reverse transcription PCR (RT-qPCR) based profiling method using 384-well micro-fluidic cards, where each well represents a miRNA of interest. The system offers a user friendly, straightforward workflow for the profiling of hundreds of miRNAs, which come either as standard or customizable cards. The TLDA procedure begins with reverse transcription (RT) of total RNA (350–1000 ng) using MegaPlex miRNA RT primers. The system also allows for the use of as little as 1 ng of RNA if performed with a pre-amplification PCR step. The RT product is then combined with TaqMan universal master mix, loaded onto the micro-fluidic cards and global miRNA profiling is performed. To identify miRNAs of biomarker/therapeutic potential the C_T values are normalized to the endogenous controls (included on the cards) and relative miRNA expressions are calculated using the $\Delta\Delta C_T$ method as will be described.

Here we outline a complete protocol detailing a translational approach to miRNA biomarker discovery, developing on in vitro profiling to clinical samples. We also present standardized protocols for serum collection to aid in the discovery of rugged miRNA based biomarkers. This method is intended to collate SOPs and best methods determined from extensive investigations to discover robust and rugged miRNA biomarkers. In addition, we also present an approach to discover oncosuppressive miRNAs by global miRNA profiling and how these miRNAs may be exploited in preclinical investigations in vitro as miRNA restoration therapies.

2   Materials

2.1   Collection of Cell Pellets

1. ~70% confluent cells (control and experimental cell lines, e.g., Hs578T and Hs578Ts(i)$_8$ triple-negative breast cancer isogenic variants).

2. Phosphate buffered saline (PBS).

3. Trypsin.

4. 15 mL polypropylene centrifuge tubes.

5. 1.5 mL Eppendorfs-RNase free.

6. Microcentrifuge.

2.2   Isolation of Total RNA (Including miRNA) from Cells

1. RNAseZap.

2. miRNeasy mini kit (Qiagen). Contents: RNeasy® Mini Spin columns, 1.5 mL collection tubes, 2.0 collection tubes, QIAzol® lysis regent, Bufer RWT, Buffer RPE, RNase-free water.

3. Chloroform—Harmful and should only be used in a fume hood.

4. Vortex.

5. 100% molecular grade ethanol.

6. Sterile, RNase-free pipette tips.

7. Microcentrifuge.

8. 1.5 mL or 2 mL microcentrifuge tubes.

2.3   TaqMan Low Density Array

1. microRNA reverse transcription kit (for this study we used from Applied Biosystems). Contents: 100 mM dNTPs, MultiScribe reverse transcriptase 50 U/μL, 10× RT buffer and RNase inhibitor 20 U/μL.

2. MegaPlex™ RT primers (10×).

3. 1.5 mL eppendorfs—RNase free.

4. 96-well MicroAmp® optical reaction plate.

5. MicroAmp® clear adhesive film.

6. Thermocycler.

7. TaqMan miRNA array cards (Applied Biosystems).

8. TaqMan Universal PCR master mix, no AmpErase UNG (Applied Biosystems).

9. Nuclease-free water.

10. Sorvall or Heraeus centrifuge.

11. TaqMan® Array Micro Fluidic Card Sealer.

12. ViiA™ 7 Real Time PCR System.

2.4   Obtaining and Biobanking Serum Specimens

1. Red top Vacutainer.

2. Swinging bucket centrifuge.

3. Sterile cryovials.

4. RNase-free, filter tips.

2.5   Isolation of Total RNA (Including miRNA) from Serum

1. Serum/plasma miRNA isolation kit (we used miRNeasy Kit, Qiagen). Contents: RNeasy® MinElute® Spin columns, 1.5 mL collection tubes, 2 mL collection tubes, QIAzol® lysis regent, Buffer RWT, Buffer RPE, Ce-miR-39_1 miScript® primer assay, RNase-free water.

2. miRNeasy Serum/Plasma Spike-in Control (Qiagen).

3. Chloroform-Harmful and should only be used in a fume hood.

4. 100% molecular grade ethanol.

5. Nuclease-free water.

6. Sterile, RNase-free pipette tips.

7. Microcentrifuge.

8. RNAseZap.

9. 1.5 mL or 2 mL microcentrifuge tubes.

2.6 Preparation of miRNA cDNA from Serum RNA

1. TaqMan microRNA Reverse transcription kit (Applied Biosystems). Contents: 100 mM dNTPs, MultiScribe reverse transcriptase 50 U/μL, 10× reverse transcription buffer, RNase inhibitor 20 U/μL.

2. RNase-free water.

3. 1.5 mL eppendorfs-RNase free.

4. TaqMan microRNA assay (Applied Biosystems).

5. TaqMan microRNA assay kit for Cel-miR-39.

6. MicroAmp® optical reaction plate 96-well (Applied Biosystems).

7. MicroAmp® clear adhesive film (Applied Biosystems).

8. TaqMan Universal PCR master mix, no AmpErase UNG (Applied Biosystems).

9. MicroAmp® fast optical 96-well reaction plate with barcode 0.1 mL (Applied Biosystems).

10. MicroAmp® optical adhesive film (Applied Biosystems).

11. Real time PCR system (e.g., ViiA™7 Real Time PCR System).

2.7 Transfection of Cell Lines with miRNA Mimics

1. Lipofectamine® 2000 reagent (ThermoFischer).

2. mirVana™ miRNA mimic and negative control mimics (Applied Biosystems).

3. 6-well tissue culture plates.

4. Opti-MEM medium.

3 Methods

3.1 Collection of Cell Pellets

1. 24 h before collection, feed cells with their recommended volume of complete media.

2. Collect cell pellets from 70% confluent, healthy cells. Do not use more than 1×10^7 cells.

3. Aspirate the medium from the cells and wash cell layer with 5 mL of PBS twice.

4. Aspirate PBS and add 5 mL of trypsin for 5 min.

5. Neutralize trypsin with 5 mL of media containing FBS.

6. Centrifuge the cell suspension at $300 \times g$ for 5 min.

7. Discard supernatant and resuspend the cell pellet in 1 mL of PBS.

8. Centrifuge at $300 \times g$ for 5 min. Aspirate PBS and resuspend in 1 mL of PBS.

9. Transfer to a 1.5 mL RNase-free eppendorf and centrifuge for 5 min at $13,000 \times g$ and 4 °C using a microcentrifuge. Remove all traces of PBS and use immediately or store at –80 °C until required.

3.2   Isolation of Total RNA (Including miRNA) from Cells

1. Clean all surfaces and equipment with RNAseZap®.

2. Dilute buffer RWT and RPE with 100% ethanol, as indicated on their bottles, to obtain a working solution.

3. Cool microcentrifuge to 4 °C.

4. Add 700 μL of QIAzol® Lysis Reagent to the cell pellet and vortex for 1 min. Allow to stand at 15–25 °C for 5 min.

5. Add 140 μL of chloroform and vortex for 15 s. Allow to stand at 15–25 °C for 3 min.

6. Centrifuge 12,000×g for 15 min at 4 °C.

7. Warm the microcentrifuge to 22 °C.

8. Post centrifugation, three phases have developed (*see* **Note 1**). Carefully transfer the upper aqueous phase to a new collection tube and record the transferred volume. Ensure not to disrupt the interphase as this will result in reduced RNA purity. Discard interphase and lower organic phase.

9. Add 1.5 volumes of 100% molecular grade ethanol to the aqueous phase and mix by pipetting up and down.

10. Immediately add 700 μL of the sample to a spin column and centrifuge at 8000×g for 15 s at 22 °C. Discard the flow through.

11. Add the remaining solution to the spin column. Repeat centrifugation at 8000×g for 15 s at 22 °C.

12. Add 700 μL of buffer RWT to the spin column, close the lid and centrifuge at 8000×g for 15 s at 22 °C. Discard flow through.

13. Add 500 μL of buffer RPE to the spin column, close the lid and centrifuge at 8000×g for 15 s at 22 °C. Discard flow through.

14. Add another 500 μL of buffer RPE to the spin column, close the lid and centrifuge at 8000×g for 2 min at 22 °C. Discard flow through.

15. To dry the spin column membrane, place the spin column in a new 2 mL collection tube, open the lid of the spin column and centrifuge at 13,000×g for 1 min at 22 °C.

16. Finally, to elute the captured RNA, place the spin column in a new 1.5 mL collection tube and add 50 μL of RNase-free water carefully to the center of the membrane. Centrifuge for 1 min at 13,000×g to collect the RNA.

17. The eluted RNA can be assessed spectrophotometrically using NanoDrop to determine RNA yield and purity. A pure RNA sample is indicated by a 260/280 ratio of 2.0 (*see* **Note 2**).

3.3   TaqMan Low Density Array

1. Prepare RNA dilutions in 3 μL of RNase-free water per reaction so that it contains 350–1000 ng of RNA (116.67 ng/μL–333.33 ng/μL).

2. Prepare the RT master mix according to Table 1.

3. Gently mix the samples and briefly centrifuge.

4. Pipette 4.5 μL of RT master mix as appropriate to each well of a 96-well MicroAmp® Optical Reaction Plate.

5. Add 3 μL of diluted RNA sample to each well as appropriate.

6. Seal the plate using MicroAmp® clear adhesive film.

7. Briefly centrifuge the plate and place on ice for 5 min.

8. Run the RT-PCR under the conditions in Table 2.

9. Store cDNA at –20 °C until needed.

10. Allow the TaqMan microRNA array card to reach room temperature.

11. Thaw the RT product on ice, invert gently and briefly centrifuge.

12. Prepare the PCR reaction according to Table 3.

Table 1
Reverse transcription master mix

Component	Volume per reaction (μL)	Volume per ten reactions (Includes 12.5 % excess) (μL)
MegaPlex RT primers (10×)	0.80	9.00
dNTPs with dTTP (100 mM)	0.20	2.25
MultiScribe reverse transcriptase (50 U/μL)	1.50	16.88
Reverse transcriptase buffer (10×)	0.80	9.00
MgCl$_2$ (25 mM)	0.90	10.13
RNase inhibitor (20 U/μL)	0.10	1.13
Nuclease-free water	0.20	2.25

Table 2
RT-qPCR program

40 cycles	2 min	16 °C
40 cycles Hold	1 min	42 °C
	1 s	50 °C
	5 min	85 °C
Hold	∞	4 °C

13. Gently mix the samples and briefly centrifuge using a Sorvall or Hereaus centrifuge.

14. Add 100 μL of the PCR reaction mix into each port of the TaqMan array card.

15. Centrifuge the array card at $331 \times g$ for 1 min twice using a Sorvall or Hereaus centrifuge.

16. Seal the micro fluidic cards using the TaqMan® micro fluidic card sealer

17. Load onto the ViiA™ 7 Real-Time PCR System and run using the predefined TLDA thermal cycling conditions for your TaqMan MicroRNA Array of use.

18. Analyze the C_T values to determine relative miRNA expressions (*see* **Notes 3** and **4**).

3.4 Obtaining and Biobanking Serum Specimens

1. Blood specimens should sit at room temperature for a minimum of 30 min and a maximum of 60 min to allow the clot to form.

2. Centrifuge the blood specimens at $1200 \times g$ for 20 min at room temperature.

3. Aliquot the serum in 250 μL volumes using RNase-free pipette. Pipette to labeled cryovials and secure cap tightly (*see* **Note 5**).

4. Ensure no hemolysis has occurred as would be indicated by a pink/red hue in the serum. Hemolysed specimens cannot be used for RNA analysis.

5. Promptly transfer all specimens to a labeled −80 °C box and place at −80 °C.

3.5 Total RNA Isolation Using Qiagen miRNeasy Serum/Plasma Kit

1. Clean all surfaces and equipment with RNAseZap®.

2. Dilute buffer RWT and RPE with 100% ethanol, as indicated on their bottles, to obtain a working solution.

3. Prepare a solution of 80% ethanol using molecular grade ethanol and RNase-free water.

Table 3
Master mix for TaqMan low density array

Component	Volume for one array card (μL)
TaqMan® Universal PCR Master Mix, No AmpErase® UNG, 2×	450
RT product (cDNA)	6
Nuclease-free water	444
Total	900

4. Cool microcentrifuge to 4 °C.

5. Prepare the miRNeasy Serum/Plasma spike-in control according to Table 4.

6. Thaw all serum specimens on ice.

7. Using 200 µL (*see* **Note 6**) of serum, add 1000 µL of QIAzol® lysis reagent and mix by pipetting up and down. Allow to stand at 15–25 °C for 5 min.

8. Add 3.5 µL of the spike-in control working solution and mix thoroughly.

9. Add 200 µL of chloroform and vortex for 15 s. Allow to stand at 15–25 °C for 3 min.

10. Centrifuge at $12,000 \times g$ for 15 min at 4 °C.

11. Warm the centrifuge to 22 °C post centrifugation to prepare for subsequent steps.

12. Carefully transfer the upper aqueous phase to a new collection tube and record the transferred volume. Ensure not to disrupt the interphase as this will result in reduced RNA purity. Discard interphase and lower organic phase (*see* **Note 1**).

13. Add 1.5 volumes of 100% molecular grade ethanol to the aqueous phase and mix by pipetting up and down.

14. Immediately add 700 µL of the sample to an RNeasy MinElute spin column and centrifuge at $8000 \times g$ for 15 s at 22 °C. Discard the flow through and add the remaining solution to the spin column. Repeat centrifugation at $8000 \times g$ for 15 s at 22 °C.

15. Add 700 µL of buffer RWT to the spin column, close the lid, and centrifuge at $8000 \times g$ for 15 s at 22 °C. Discard flow through.

16. Add 500 µL of buffer RPE to the spin column, close the lid, and centrifuge at $8000 \times g$ for 15 s at 22 °C. Discard flow through.

Table 4
Preparation of the working solution of the Cel-miR-39 spike-in control miRNA

Solution	Volumes	Copies/µL	Storage
Stock solution	Add 300 µL of RNase-free water to lyophilized Ce-miR-39	2×10^{10}	Aliquot avoid freeze–thaw cycles. Store at –80 °C.
Dilution 1	Add 4 µL of stock to 16 µL RNase-free water	4×10^{9}	Use immediately.
Working solution	Add 2 µL of Dilution 1 to 48 µL RNase-free water	1.6×10^{8}	Use immediately.

17. Add 500 µL of 80 % ethanol to the spin column, close the lid, and centrifuge at $8000 \times g$ for 2 min at 22 °C. Discard flow through and the collection tube.

18. Place the spin column in a new 2 mL collection tube, open the lid of the spin column, and centrifuge at $13,000 \times g$ for 5 min at 22 °C.

19. Place the spin column in a new 1.5 mL collection tube and add 14 µL of RNase-free water carefully to the center of the membrane. Centrifuge for 1 min at $13,000 \times g$.

20. The yield, size distribution and quality of the RNA can be assessed using the Agilent Small RNA Analysis Kit. Using spectrophotometric systems are not recommended due to their inability to accurately quantify low concentrations of RNA obtained from serum.

3.6   RT-qPCR of Serum Derived miRNA

1. Prepare 5 µL of a 2 ng/µL dilution of RNA with RNase-free water.

2. Add the 5 µL RNA sample to the 96-well MicroAmp® Optical Reaction Plate.

3. Prepare the RT master mix according to Table 5.

4. Flick and briefly centrifuge the RT master mix and place on ice.

5. Add 7 µL of RT master mix to the 5 µL RNA sample. Briefly centrifuge.

6. Briefly centrifuge the TaqMan RT primer and add 3 µL of it to the RNA/RT master mixture. Briefly centrifuge.

7. Seal the plate using MicroAmp® clear adhesive film and briefly centrifuge.

8. Run the PCR under the conditions in Table 6.

9. Store the samples at –20 °C until required or keep on ice if immediately performing the qPCR step.

10. Perform all qPCR assays in triplicate per miRNA and include the endogenous control/spike-in control (Cel-miR-39) on the same plate for each sample. A "no template" control should also be included on each well for each miRNA on the plate.

11. Prepare the qPCR master mix for each miRNA primer according to Table 7.

12. Flick and briefly centrifuge the RT product and place on ice.

13. Add 1.33 µL of the RT product (cDNA) to each well as appropriate.

14. Add 18.67 µL of the qPCR master mix to each well MicroAmp® fast optical 96-well reaction plate as appropriate.

15. Seal the plate with the MicroAmp® optical adhesive film and run the qPCR according to Table 8.

16. Analyze the data using the $\Delta\Delta C_T$ method (*see* **Note 3**) normalizing C_T values to the Cel-miR-39 spike-in control.

Table 5
Reverse transcription master mix for serum miRNA expression analysis

Component	Volume per reaction (µL)	Volume per ten reactions (Includes 12.5 % excess) (µL)
100 mM dNTPs (with dTTP)	0.15	1.69
Multiscribe™ reverse transcriptase, 50 U/µL	1.00	11.25
10× reverse transcription buffer	1.50	16.88
RNase inhibitor, 20 U/µL	0.19	2.14
Nuclease-free water	4.16	46.80
Total volume	7.00	78.75

Table 6
Reverse transcription PCR program

Hold	30 min	16 °C
Hold	30 min	42 °C
Hold	5 min	85 °C
Hold	∞	4 °C

Table 7
Master mix for RT-qPCR of serum miRNAs

Component	Volume per reaction (µL)	Volume per ten reactions (Includes 12.5 % excess) (µL)
TaqMan universal PCR master mix II (2×), no UNG	10.00	112.50
Nuclease-free water	7.67	86.29
TaqMan miRNA assay primer (20×)	1.00	11.25
Total volume	18.67	210.04

Table 8
qPCR program

Hold	10 min	95 °C
40 cycles	15 s	95 °C
	60 s	60 °C

3.7 Transfection of Cell Lines with miRNA Mimics

1. Briefly centrifuge the mirVana mimics.

2. Reconstitute the 5 nmol lyophilized miRNA mimic in 50 μL of nuclease-free water to prepare a 100 μM stock solution. Store at –20 °C.

3. Seed cells in 2 mL of antibiotic-free (*see* **Note 7**) media in a 6-well plate to be ~60% confluent.

4. Allow to grow for 24 h at 37 °C.

5. 24 h later, prepare a 10 μM working stock of the miRNA mimic and negative control (NC) mimics with nuclease-free water for immediate use.

6. Dilute 5 μL of Lipofectamine® in 250 μL Opti-MEM per well and mix by inverting once.

7. Incubate at room temperature for 5 min.

8. Dilute 10 nM (*see* **Note 8**) of miRNA mimic in 250 μL Opti-MEM and mix by inverting.

9. Incubate at room temperature for 5 min. Proceed immediately to **step 10**.

10. Combine the Lipofectamine/Opti-MEM mix and the miRNA mimic/Opti-MEM mix.

11. Incubate at room temperature for 20 min.

12. Add the 500 μL mixture drop by drop to the cells (*see* **Note 9**).

13. Culture for 48–72 h at 37 °C depending on downstream applications (*see* **Note 10**).

14. Transfected cells can be analyzed for phenotypic alterations and protein expression analyses (*see* **Note 11**) for investigation of their therapeutic effects.

4 Notes

1. Three phases develop after centrifugation: (1) an upper, colorless, aqueous phase containing the RNA; (2) a mid, white interphase containing DNA, and (3) a lower, red, organic phase containing proteins. When removing the RNA aqueous phase, care must be taken to not remove any of the other phases, as this will contaminate your sample.

2. To determine RNA purity and quantity the NanoDrop system measures sample absorbance at 260 nm and 280 nm. A ratio of 2.0 indicates a pure, high-quality RNA sample. A lower 260/280 ratio indicates protein/phenol contamination.

3. Using the C_T values are automatically determined by the SDS software on your ViiA™ 7 Real Time PCR System, relative quantities of miRNAs are calculated using the $\Delta\Delta C_T$ method by

Table 9
How to calculate fold changes using the $\Delta\Delta C_T$ method

C_T	Cycle threshold where miRNA is detected
ΔC_T	C_T of control sample miRNA *(minus)* C_T of control sample endogenous control
$\Delta\Delta C_T$	C_T of experimental sample miRNA *(minus)* ΔC_T of control sample
$2^{(-\Delta\Delta C_T)}$	Relative fold change of expression

normalization to one of the predefined endogenous controls on your array card (MammU6, RNU44, or RNU48) or your spiked- in control Cel-miR-39. An outline of how to calculate fold changes using the $\Delta\Delta C_T$ method is shown in Table 9.

4. To identify miRNAs of clinical relevance and to strengthen the study after miRNA expression profiling, one can use Gene Expression Omnibus (GEO2R) to analyze publically available miRNA profiles of previously performed studies on tumor/serum/plasma specimens relevant to one's work.

5. Aliquots of 250 µL per cryovial are recommended to prevent freeze–thaw cycles.

6. It is of paramount importance to ensure that the volumes of all specimens used are kept absolutely consistent when using the spike-on approach for accurate normalization.

7. Do not use antibiotics in medium during transfection as they can interfere with Lipofectamine.

8. A considerable amount of protocol optimization may be required depending on the nature of the cell line used. Some cell lines are easily transfected, while others require more optimization. We present here the recommended starting point concentrations and time-points outlined by the manufacturer. If difficulty is observed with transfection, one can alter the mimic concentration, Lipofectamine concentration and incubation time.

9. Ensure to add the Lipofectamine mixture drop-by-drop to minimize the chance of cells undergoing osmotic shock.

10. Lipofectamine may also cause some adverse toxic effects on some cell lines. If considerable toxicity observed due to the presence of Lipofectamine in culture, one can replace the media on the transfected cells after 6 h to remove the Lipofectamine without substantially affecting transfection efficiency.

11. To investigate the predicted mRNA targets of your miRNA of interest, there are free online bioinformatics tools to predict miRNA-mRNA interactions including miRWalk, miRTarBase, TargetScan, and DianaLab.

References

1. Esquela-Kerscher A, Slack FJ (2006) Oncomirs—microRNAs with a role in cancer. Nat Rev Cancer 6(4):259–269. doi:10.1038/nrc1840

2. Bartel DP (2004) MicroRNAs: genomics, biogenesis, mechanism, and function. Cell 116(2):281–297. doi:S0092867404000455

3. Calin GA, Dumitru CD, Shimizu M et al (2002) Frequent deletions and downregulation of micro- RNA genes miR15 and miR16 at 13q14 in chronic lymphocytic leukemia. Proc Natl Acad Sci U S A 99(24):15524–15529. doi:10.1073/pnas.242606799

4. Miska EA (2005) How microRNAs control cell division, differentiation and death. Curr Opin Genet Dev 15(5):563–568. doi:10.1016/j.gde.2005.08.005

5. O'Brien K, Lowry MC, Corcoran C et al (2015) miR-134 in extracellular vesicles reduces triple-negative breast cancer aggression and increases drug sensitivity. Oncotarget 20;6(32):32774–89. doi: 10.18632/oncotarget.5192.t

6. Chen X, Ba Y, Ma L et al (2008) Characterization of microRNAs in serum: a novel class of biomarkers for diagnosis of cancer and other diseases. Cell Res 18(10):997–1006. doi:10.1038/cr.2008.282

7. Valadi H, Ekström K, Bossios A et al (2007) Exosome-mediated transfer of mRNAs and microRNAs is a novel mechanism of genetic exchange between cells. Nat Cell Biol 9(6):654–659. doi:10.1038/ncb1596

8. Skog J, Würdinger T, van Rijn S et al (2008) Glioblastoma microvesicles transport RNA and proteins that promote tumour growth and provide diagnostic biomarkers. Nat Cell Biol 10(12):1470–1476. doi:10.1038/ncb1800

9. Vickers KC, Palmisano BT, Shoucri BM et al (2011) MicroRNAs are transported in plasma and delivered to recipient cells by high-density lipoproteins. Nat Cell Biol 13(4):423–433. doi:10.1038/ncb2210

10. Wang K, Zhang S, Weber J et al (2010) Export of microRNAs and microRNA-protective protein by mammalian cells. Nucleic Acids Res 38(20):7248–7259. doi:10.1093/nar/gkq601

11. Tuck MK, Chan DW, Chia D et al (2009) Standard operating procedures for serum and plasma collection: early detection research network consensus statement standard operating procedure integration working group. J Proteome Res 8(1):113–117. doi:10.1021/pr800545q

12. Farina NH, Wood ME, Perrapato SD et al (2014) Standardizing analysis of circulating microRNA: clinical and biological relevance. J Cell Biochem 115(5):805–811. doi:10.1002/jcb.24745

13. McLean CS, Mielke C, Cordova JM et al (2015) Gene and MicroRNA expression responses to exercise; relationship with insulin sensitivity. PLoS One 10(5), e0127089. doi:10.1371/journal.pone.0127089

14. Zhang L, Hou D, Chen X et al (2012) Exogenous plant MIR168a specifically targets mammalian LDLRAP1: evidence of cross-kingdom regulation by microRNA. Cell Res 22(1):107–126. doi:10.1038/cr.2011.158

15. Vucic EA, Thu KL, Pikor LA et al (2014) Smoking status impacts microRNA mediated prognosis and lung adenocarcinoma biology. BMC Cancer 14:778. doi:10.1186/1471-2407-14-778

16. Davis CJ, Bohnet SG, Meyerson JM et al (2007) Sleep loss changes microRNA levels in the brain: a possible mechanism for state-dependent translational regulation. Neurosci Lett 422(1):68–73. doi:10.1016/j.neulet.2007.06.005

17. Leidner RS, Li L, Thompson CL (2013) Dampening enthusiasm for circulating microRNA in breast cancer. PLoS One 8(3), e57841. doi:10.1371/journal.pone.0057841

18. Paola Tiberio MC, Valentina Angeloni, Maria Grazia Daidone, and Valentina Appierto (2015) Challenges in Using Circulating miRNAs as Cancer Biomarkers. BioMed research international 2015 (Article ID 731479):10 pages. doi:http://dx.doi.org/10.1155/2015/731479

19. Kang K, Peng X, Luo J et al (2012) Identification of circulating miRNA biomarkers based on global quantitative real-time PCR profiling. J Anim Sci Biotechnol 3(1):4. doi:10.1186/2049-1891-3-4

20. Jansson MD, Lund AH (2012) MicroRNA and cancer. Mol Oncol 6(6):590–610. doi:10.1016/j.molonc.2012.09.006

21. Eva van Rooij SK (2014) Development of microRNA therapeutics is coming of age. EMBO Mol Med 6(7):851–864. doi:10.15252/emmm.201100899

22. Mirna Therapeutics I A Multicenter Phase I Study of MRX34, MicroRNA miR-RX34 Liposomal Injection. https://www.clinicaltrials.gov/ct2/show/NCT01829971?term=mrx34&rank=1.

Chapter 9

Detection of MicroRNAs in Brain Slices Using In Situ Hybridization

Sean Quinlan, Christine Henke, Gary P. Brennan, David C. Henshall, and Eva M. Jimenez-Mateos

Abstract

MicroRNAs are key posttranscriptional regulators of protein levels in cells. The brain is particularly enriched in microRNAs, and important roles have been demonstrated for these noncoding RNAs in various neurological disorders. To this end, visualization of microRNAs in specific cell types and subcellular compartments within tissue sections provides researchers with essential insights that support understanding of the cell and molecular mechanisms of microRNAs in brain diseases. In this chapter we describe an in situ *hybridization* protocol for the detection of microRNAs in mouse brain sections, which provides cellular resolution of the expression of microRNAs in the brain.

Key words microRNA, Brain, Neurodegenerative disorders, In situ hybridization, Staining, CNS

---

1 Introduction

MicroRNAs (miRNA) are small noncoding RNAs (~23 nt) that regulate gene expression at the posttranscriptional level resulting in repression of protein production [1]. MiRNAs create an additional layer of complexity in cell signaling with roles in the fine-tuning of almost all cellular functions from development to programmed cell death [2, 3]. These noncoding RNAs are transcribed from DNA to generate a primary microRNA (pri-miRNA) sequence; this then undergoes micro-processing by Drosha to produce the precursor miRNA (pre-miR). In the cytoplasm, Dicer cleaves the precursor isoform to generate the mature miRNA [3]. This mature miRNA will be recruited to the RNA-induced silencing complex (RISC), binding to a member of the Argonaute family and pairing with the 3′ UTR on the target mRNA [3]. Typically miRNAs in the CNS binds incompletely to mRNA along a 7–8 "seed" sequence [3]. As a result, mRNA destabilization and degradation occurs or translation is inhibited.

Sweta Rani (ed.), *MicroRNA Profiling: Methods and Protocols*, Methods in Molecular Biology, vol. 1509,
DOI 10.1007/978-1-4939-6524-3_9, © Springer Science+Business Media New York 2017

Experimental animal models have been essential in our understanding of the role of miRNAs in the complex functioning of the CNS. The use of genetic tools has shown the critical role of miRNAs in the brain whereby disruption of key enzymes in the miRNA biogenesis pathway is embryonically lethal or induces severe developmental defects [4–6]. For example, conditional loss of *Dicer* at different stages of development impacts on cortical development, progenitor proliferation, migration, and differentiation indicating the profound temporal and spatial importance of miRNA regulation in brain maturation [7]. Notably, aberrant miRNA expression has been seen in neurodevelopmental and neuropsychiatric diseases such as autism and schizophrenia [8, 9].

Approximately 70 % of all known miRNAs are expressed in the human nervous system [10]. Neural tissue is very heterogeneous, with different cell types including neurons, astrocytes, microglia, and oligodendrocytes. MiRNAs show specific enrichment in these cell types, such as the brain specific miRNA, miR-134 is expressed exclusively in neurons [11]. Through accurate visualization of miRNA in the brain, we will improve our understanding of miRNA function. Techniques such as in situ *hybridization* will facilitate our understanding of miRNA cellular localization (neuronal, astrocytes or microglia) or changes in the cellular expression after a brain insult. Furthermore, miRNA can translocate between the different intracellular compartments [12]. Thus in situ *hybridization* can determine any translocation in neurodegenerative disorders or after a brain insult. In this chapter we describe an easy in situ *hybridization* protocol for brain tissue sections or slices, which can be applied to human and experimental animal models of neurological conditions.

2 Materials

Prepare all solutions using ultrapure RNAse-free water. You may use DEPC-treated water for making the solutions. Use double-autoclaved glassware and magnetic stirrer or disposable plasticware. All chemicals should be reserved exclusively for RNA work, and avoid placing spatulas into RNA-reserved chemicals. Autoclave solutions when possible (solutions containing detergent or toxic chemical should not be autoclaved). All solutions should be stored at 4 °C.

2.1 Equipment

1. Ventilation hood.

2. Incubator or bath.

3. Rocking platform.

4. Slide containers.

5. Air-tight incubation chambers.

6. Super-frost microscope slides.

7. RNAse-free and filtered tips.

2.2 General Solutions

1. *PBS 1×*: It is recommended to use already prepared mixes to reduce the risk of contamination of reagents.

2. *PBS–Tween 20*: 0.05 % Tween 20 in PBS 1×.

3. *RIPA buffer*: 150 mM NaCl, 1 % IGEPAL (NP-40), 0.5 % Na deoxycholate, 0.1 % SDS, 1 mM EDTA pH 8, and 50 mM Tris–HCl pH 8.

4. *Paraformaldehyde*: For a final volume of 100 mL, heat up 70 mL of RNAse-free autoclaved H_2O to 60 °C; add 4 g of paraformaldehyde and mix gently. Adjust pH to 7.5 using NaOH. Add 10 mL of RNAse-free autoclaved 10× PBS and fill up to 100 mL with RNAse-free autoclaved H_2O.

5. *Triethanolmine solution*: 100 mM of triethanolmine in RNAse-free autoclaved H_2O. Adjust pH to 8 with Acetic Acid.

6. *10× Saline Solution*: 1.95 M NaCl, 89 mM Tris–HCl, 11 mM Tris base, 65 mM NaH_2PO_4, 50 mM Na_2HPO_4, and 0.05 mM EDTA pH 8.

2.3 Solutions for Probes Hybridization

1. *Pre-hybridization solution*: 1× saline solution, 50 % formamide, and 1× Denhardt's solution. Keep the pre-hybridization solution at –20 °C.

2. *Hybridization solutions*: 1× saline solution, 50 % formamide, 1× Denhardt's solution, and 10 % dextran sulfate. Keep the hybridization solution at –20 °C.

3. *FAM buffer*; 2× SSC, 50 % formamide, and 0.1 % Tween 20.

2.4 Solutions for Antibody Incubation

1. *B1 buffer*: 150 mM NaCl, 100 mM maleic acid, and 0.04 % Tween 20. Adjust pH to 7.5 with NaOH. Make it fresh every time.

2. *B2 Buffer*: 2 % Blocking Reagent (Sigma-Aldrich) and 10 % fetal calf serum or goat serum in B1 solution. Make it fresh every time.

3. Anti-DIG-PA (Roche).

2.5 Development Signal Solution

1. *B3 buffer*: 100 mM NaCl, 100 mM Tris Base pH 9.5, 50 mM $MgCl_2$, and 0.05 % Tween 20.

2. *NBT/BCIP solution*: 45 μL of NBT and 35 μL of BCIP in 10 mL of B3 solution.

3   Methods

3.1 Preparation of Brain Tissue for In Situ

Please be informed that ethical approval from the appropriate authority is required for animal experimentation, which can only be undertaken under license from the competent authority. In our case, animal experiments have been performed in accordance with the European Communities Council Directive (86/609/EEC) and approval from the Research Ethics Committee of the Royal College of Surgeons in Ireland, under license from the HPRA office.

1. Deeply anesthetise mice (e.g., pentobarbital) and perfuse the mice intra-cardially with autoclaved ice-cold 1× PBS to remove blood component followed by 4% paraformaldehyde (PFA).

2. Remove brains and leave them in 4% PFA at 4 °C overnight (16–20 h) in a 15 mL Falcon tube.

3. Remove 4% PFA and submerge brains in a 30% sucrose solution until they sink to in the bottom of the 15 mL falcon tubes. This will take around 48 h.

4. Remove brains from the sucrose solution, freeze them in OCT glue at −20 °C and leave them in −80 °C until they will be micro-sliced.

5. Cut the brain at 12 μm on a cryostat and mounted on super-frost microscope slides (*see* **Note 1**). Return the slices to −80 °C.

3.2 Preparation of Slices for Hybridization

From **step 2**, each step is performed at room temperature and rocking in a shaker.

1. Let the slides dry for 20 min in the bench or 10 min under a fume hood.

2. Rinse the slides in 1× PBS for 10 min.

3. Treat the slides with RIPA buffer two times, 10 min each time.

4. Post-fix the slides with 4% PFA for 10 min.

5. Wash the slides with 1× PBS for 5 min, repeat three times.

6. Treat the slides with triethanolamine for 15 min. While rocking, add acetic anhydride dropwise to a final concentration of 0.43% (*see* **Note 2**).

7. Wash slides with PBS–Tween 20 for 5 min, and repeat it three times.

8. Treat the slides with 5 μg/mL of Proteinase K for 4 min (*see* **Note 3**).

9. Wash with PBS for 5 min.

3.3 Hybridization of the Probes

The incubation temperature (T.inc) for the next steps is calculated on the basis of the melting temperature (Tm) of the probes. Generally, the incubation temperature (T.inc) is between 15 °C and 25 °C degrees less than the RNA-Tm of the probes. We used the following formula:

$$T.inc = Tm + 16.6 * \log 10 \big([Na+] / (1.0 + 0.7[Na+]) \big) + 0.7 * (\%GC) -$$
$$0.35 * (\%\text{formamide}) - 500 / (\text{duplex length}) - 1°C / (\%\text{mismatch})$$

In our buffers, $16.6*\log 10([Na^+]/(1.0+0.7[Na^+])) = -15.87$; and $0.35*(\%\text{formamide}) = 17.5$

1. Pretreat the slides for 1 h in pre-hybridization buffer at the calculated T.inc.

2. Prepare the probes for the hybridization step. We recommend the LNA-5′-3′ DIG labeled probes. Dilute the probes in hybridization buffer at the correct concentration (between 10 nM and 20 nM) (*see* **Notes 4** and **5**). Heat up the probes solution at 80 °C for 5 min, and quickly place them on ice (*see* **Note 6**).

3. Incubate the slides with the probes overnight at the correct T.inc in an air-tight incubation chamber (*see* **Notes 7** and **8**).

4. Wash the slides with FAM solution at the T.inc for 1 h. Repeat this step twice (*see* **Notes 9** and **10**).

3.4 Incubation with Primary Antibody

1. Rinse the slides in B1 buffer at room temperature for 1 h.

2. Block the slides with the B2 buffer for 30 min at room temperature.

3. Incubate the anti-DIG-PA antibody at 1/1000 in B2 buffer overnight at 4 °C.

3.5 Incubation with NBT/BCIP Solution

1. Wash the slides with B1 for 5 min. Repeat this step three times.

2. Rinse the slides in B3 for 30 min at room temperature.

3. Transfer the slides into an incubation chamber and incubate with the NBT/BCIP substrate until signal appears. This step could be from 4 h to 4 days (*see* **Note 11**).

4. Once the signal appears; stop the reaction by washing three times in B3 buffer (Figs. 1 and 2).

5. Rinse the slides in 1× PBS. Mounted with Fluor-Save Reagent.

6. Visualize under a light microscope.

4 Notes

1. To ensure quality of the tissue, it is recommended to perform a Nissl or hematoxylin staining of the tissue before the in situ *hybridization*.

2. The recommendation is 0.43% of acetic anhydride. For an incubation volume between 25 mL and 30 mL, 60 µL of acetic anhydride are necessary.

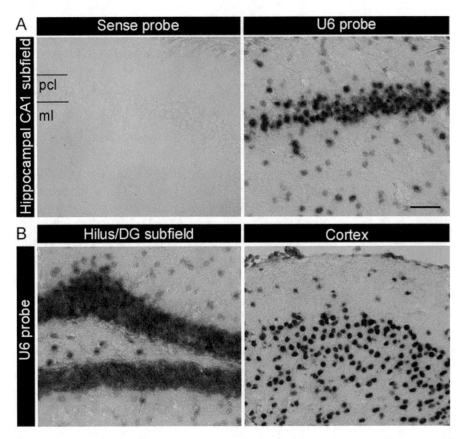

Fig. 1 RNU6 in situ *hybridization*. (**a**) Representative in situ *hybridization* images of the hippocampal CA1 sub-field for the sense probe (*left*) or U6 probes (*right*). (**b**) Representative images for the U6 probes in hilus/DG subfield (*left*) and cortex (*right*). Scale bar: 50 μm. Note: pcl, pyramidal cell layer; ml, molecular layer

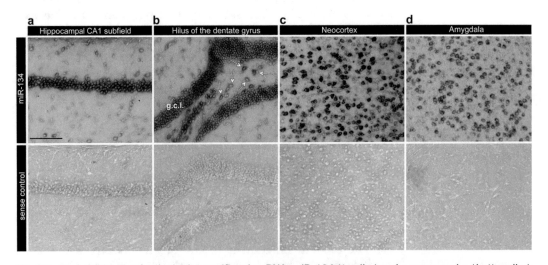

Fig. 2 In situ hybridization for the brain specific microRNA, miR-134 (*top line*) and a sense probe (*bottom line*). (**a**) Hippocampal CA1 subfield. (**b**) Hilus of the dentate gyrus. (**c**) Neocortex. (**d**) Amygdala. Image has been adapted from Jimenez-Mateos et al., Nature Medicine. 2012. Jul; 18(7):1087–94. (Supplementary Fig. 1)

3. If after Proteinase K incubation, the tissue looks damaged, reduce incubation time to 2–3 min.

4. Concentration of the probes needed for high quality staining will vary between different microRNAs. It is recommended to use two different concentrations to set up the proper conditions.

5. It is recommended to use a probe against a highly expressed small noncoding RNA in the brain, such as RNU6 or RNU19. Signal from the positive control will appear (Subheading 3.5) from 4 h to 24 h after NBT/BCIP incubation.

6. If probes do not cool really quickly, no signal will appear. A bucket of ice should be left next to the heater-block.

7. If no signal appears or the signal is too faint, reduce slightly (~2 °C) the incubation temperature.

8. If the background signal is too high, increase slightly (~2 °C) the incubation temperature.

9. If the signal is too faint, reduce slightly (~2 °C) the FAM temperature.

10. If the background signal is too high, increase slightly (~2 °C) the FAM temperature.

11. The NBT/BCIP solution should be changed at least twice daily to avoid the formation of precipitates over the slices.

References

1. Guo H, Ingolia NT, Weissman JS et al (2010) Mammalian microRNAs predominantly act to decrease target mRNA levels. Nature 466: 835–840

2. Schratt G (2009) microRNAs at the synapse. Nat Rev Neurosci 10:842–849

3. McNeill E, Van Vactor D (2012) MicroRNAs shape the neuronal landscape. Neuron 75:363–379

4. Bartel DP (2004) MicroRNAs: genomics, biogenesis, mechanism, and function. Cell 116:281–297

5. Wang Y, Medvid R, Melton C et al (2007) DGCR8 is essential for microRNA biogenesis and silencing of embryonic stem cell self-renewal. Nat Genet 39:380–385

6. Tang F, Kaneda M, O'Carroll D et al (2007) Maternal microRNAs are essential for mouse zygotic development. Genes Dev 21:644–648

7. Giraldez AJ, Cinalli RM, Glasner ME et al (2005) MicroRNAs regulate brain morphogenesis in zebrafish. Science 308:833–838

8. Kawase-Koga Y, Otaegi G, Sun T (2009) Different timings of Dicer deletion affect neurogenesis and gliogenesis in the developing mouse central nervous system. Dev Dyn 238:2800–2812

9. Sun E, Shi Y (2015) MicroRNAs: Small molecules with big roles in neurodevelopment and diseases. Exp Neurol 268:46–53

10. Nowak JS, Michlewski G (2013) miRNAs in development and pathogenesis of the nervous system. Biochem Soc Trans 41:815–820

11. Jimenez-Mateos EM, Engel T, Merino-Serrais P et al (2012) Silencing microRNA-134 produces neuroprotective and prolonged seizure-suppressive effects. Nat Med 18: 1087–1094

12. Bicker S, Khudayberdiev S, Weiss K et al (2013) The DEAH-box helicase DHX36 mediates dentritic localization of the neuronal precursor-microRNA-134. Genes Dev 27: 991–996

Chapter 10

Exosomal MicroRNA Discovery in Age-Related Macular Degeneration

Hanan Elshelmani and Sweta Rani

Abstract

Age-related macular degeneration (AMD) is a common condition causing progressive visual impairment, leading to irreversible blindness. Existing diagnostic tools for AMD are limited to clinical signs in the macula and the visual assessment of the patient. The presence of circulating microRNAs (miRNAs) in the peripheral circulatory system with potential as diagnostic, prognostic and/or predictive biomarkers has been reported in a number of conditions/diseases. miRNAs are key regulators of several biological processes, and miRNA dysregulation has been linked with numerous diseases, most remarkably cancer. miRNAs have been shown to be involved in AMD pathology and several miRNAs target genes and signaling pathways were identified in relation to AMD pathogenesis. Exosomes are 50–90 nm membrane microvesicles (MVs), released by several cell types. Although exosomal functions are not completely understood, there is much evidence to suggest that exosomes play an essential role in cell–cell communication. They may stimulate target cells by transferring different bioactive molecules such as miRNA. Here we discuss methods to isolate exosome using serum specimens from AMD patients and miRNA profiling for the better understanding of the disease.

Key words Age-related macular degeneration, MicroRNA, Exosomes, Serum, Atrophic AMD, Neovascular AMD, Retinal pigment epithelium

1 Introduction

AMD is a multifactorial disease, associated with a complex interaction of genetic and environmental factors. The early stage of AMD is characterized by dysfunction of retinal pigment epithelium (RPE) cells, which are essential for the function of the photoreceptors, whereas neovascularization and geographical atrophy are the manifestations of the late stages of AMD [1]. MiRNAs are small noncoding RNA molecules that have shown an inhibitory effect on the expression of several genes. Therefore, it is suggested that miRNAs are controlling a variety of normal physiological and pathological processes [2, 3]. Understanding the mechanisms by which miRNAs affect RPE cells is fundamental for understanding RPE dysfunction, and to discovering novel treatment targets for AMD.

Sweta Rani (ed.), *MicroRNA Profiling: Methods and Protocols*, Methods in Molecular Biology, vol. 1509, DOI 10.1007/978-1-4939-6524-3_10, © Springer Science+Business Media New York 2017

It is challenging to link certain groups of miRNAs to particular cellular activities and to identify a single key miRNA as a biomarker. Should this be achieved, it will undoubtedly lead to development of new screening tools, which may aid in diagnosis and possibly treatment for AMD. In addition, using samples that are easily obtained, such as serum, to acquire AMD biomarkers by the least invasive methods will have a large impact on clinical research and trials.

Profiling of miRNA has become a vital technology, which could provide potential biomarkers. It might also contribute to elucidating pathogenesis of many diseases, which, in turn, will give valuable diagnostic and prognostic information and reveal promising treatment targets. Furthermore, it has been reported that miRNAs have a great potential to work as biomarkers for numerous human diseases, most notably cancer [4]. With regard to AMD, recent miRNA studies focused on therapeutic research but have not shown any specific miRNAs directly linked with pathology of AMD. For example, miR-126 can control vascular integrity and angiogenesis, which may provide a novel target for neovascular AMD [3]. However, according to some in vivo and in vitro studies, it is suggested that numerous miRNAs are associated with the pathological process involved in AMD such as pathological angiogenesis, oxidative stress, and inflammation, which suggests that miRNAs might be potential therapeutic targets for neovascular and atrophic AMD [3]. miRNAs provide promising biomarkers because of their significant stability in blood and their distinctive expression in different diseases [5].

Computational approaches have been used recently to predict miRNA targets and their signaling pathways; this effective tool was adopted to analyze the function of miRNAs [6]. miRNA–target interactions were validated experimentally by reporter assays, western blot, or microarray experiments with over-expression or knock-down of miRNAs. Computational approaches have been classified into two types: one type such as miRanda and DIANA-microT, use a selective rule-based approach to predict miRNA targets from features of experimentally validated targets. The approach with miTarget and miRTar is more data-driven, as it is generated from sequence features of miRNAs, and so it is more accurate in separating the true miRNAs targets from false ones [7, 8]. These miRNA-related database systems give further insight into miRNAs and their target genes [9]. According to experimental and computational evidence, miRNAs have several target genes and regulatory functions, and so the biological role of miRNAs and their therapeutic potential need to be further explored by the integration of computational and experimental approaches [6].

Target genes and signaling pathways correlation with the expression of miRNAs may increase our understanding of the pathological role of the detected miRNAs that are differentially expressed in AMD; this approach is more powerful than miRNA expression testing alone. However, the computational prediction tools of miRNA targets and signaling pathways become challenging, as the current computational tools for target prediction are based on the gene level. Gene expression controlled by miRNAs is an essential mechanism for the regulation of several biological processes [8, 9]. According to experimental and computational evidence, miRNAs have several target genes and regulatory functions, and so the biological role of miRNAs and their therapeutic potential need to be further explored by the integration of computational and experimental approaches [6].

Exosomes are 50–90 nm membrane micro-vesicles (MVs) [10], released by several cell types, including tumor cells. These small vesicles are created by inward budding of endosomal membranes (endocytosis), which results in vesicle-containing endosomes that are termed multivesicular bodies (MVBs). When the MVBs fuse with the cell membrane and release their intraluminal vesicles (ILVs) into the extracellular environment (exocytosis), the vesicles are then termed "exosomes" [11]. Exosomes contain genetic materials, such as mRNAs and miRNAs, which play an important role in cell–cell communication. Exosomes are endocytic vesicles containing miRNAs and are secreted into the extracellular space by cells in both physiological and pathological situations, including pathological angiogenesis, the oxidative stress response, immune response, inflammation, and tumors [12]. In vitro and in vivo studies revealed that exosome transfer from cell to cell mediating disease progression [12]. It has been reported that miRNAs play critical roles in AMD pathology processes. Furthermore, several miRNA candidates that are involved in choroidal neovascularization or retinal pigment epithelium atrophy are considered as AMD therapeutic targets. It is noteworthy that choroidal neovascularization can be induced by angiogenic factors, which are produced from apoptotic RPE and inflammatory cells. Anti-angiogenic therapy has been considered as mandatory treatment for wet AMD; a group of specific miRNAs (angiomiRs) have been demonstrated to play a major role in angiogenesis. These include the miR-15/107 group, the miR-17~92 cluster, miR-21, miR-132, miR-296, miR-378, and miR-519c. It has also been shown that there is an increased expression of apoptosis-inducing ligand in the photoreceptors of exudative AMD and the patient with geographic atrophy. Apoptosis is believed to be increased by miR-23a, and inhibited or decreased by miR-23a mimic [3, 13]. Also, it is known that drusen is a hallmark of AMD; it is a common early sign and is a risk factor for developing atrophic (dry) AMD. An aged RPE of an AMD patient is believed to be more susceptible to genetic mutations due to the alteration of biological processes [14]. Drusen formation is hypothesized to result from the release of intracellular proteins via exosomes by the old RPE. In addition, drusen in AMD donor eyes contain markers for exosomes. Exosome markers were also found in the region of Bruch's membrane in the retinas of old mice; they were also upregulated in RPE cells exposed to rotenone (inducing mtDNA damage) [14, 15].

2 Materials

2.1 Total RNA Extraction from Serum

1. TriReagent™ store at 4 °C.
2. Chloroform, store at room temperature.
3. Isopropanol, store at room temperature.
4. 120 µg/mL glycogen, store at –20 °C.
5. 75% ethanol, store at room temperature.
6. DEPC-treated H_2O (Ambion).
7. NanoDrop ND-1000.

2.2 The miRCURY LNA™ Universal RT microRNA PCR for Serum (Exiqon)

1. miRCURY LNA™ Universal RT microRNA PCR cDNA synthesis kit (Exiqon)

   (a) 5× Reaction buffer, store at –20 °C.

   (b) Enzyme mix, store at–20 °C.

   (c) Synthetic RNA spike-in, store at –20 °C.

   (d) Nuclease-free water, store at either room temperature or –20 °C.

   (e) Thermocycler (Biometra).

2. microRNA real-time qPCR amplification

   - PCR master mix, store at –20 °C.

   - PCR primer mix5, store at –20 °C.

   - The Applied Biosystems 7500 Real-Time PCR System platform.

   - The amplification curves were analyzed using the AB 7500 software

2.3 Cell Culture of Retinal Pigment Epithelium Cells

1. The human retinal pigment epithelial cell line (ARPE-19).
2. Dulbecco's modified Eagle's medium (DMEM).
3. 4 mMl-glutamine.
4. 10% fetal bovine serum (FBS).
5. 100 U/mL penicillin.
6. 100 µg/mL streptomycin.
7. Trypsin.
8. Cell culture flasks.
9. Sterile pipettes.

10. Hemocytometer.

11. Incubator (37 °C in 5% CO_2 in air).

12. Biosafety Cabinet for cell culture.

2.4 Exosomes Isolation from Serum

1. ExoQuick Exosome Precipitation (SBI) store at 4 °C.

2. Centrifuge.

3. Nuclease-free water.

2.5 Validated Antibody Systems for Confirmation of Exosomes (Western Blot Analysis)

1. Exosome specific primary antibody (CD63, CD9, CD81 or Hsp70) store at 4 °C.

2. Exosome validated secondary antibody (goat anti-rabbit HRP) store at 4 °C.

3. RIPA (radioimmunoprecipitation assay) buffer: 25 mM Tris–HCl pH 7.6, 150 mM NaCl, 1% NP-40, 1% sodium deoxycholate, 0.1% SDS along with 1× protease inhibitor cocktail.

4. TBS-T: 50 mM Tris. 150 mM NaCl. 0.05% Tween 20.

5. Laemmli buffer (with beta-mercaptoethanol).

6. Standard SDS-PAGE electrophoresis.

7. PVDF (polyvinylidene difluoride) membrane.

8. Blocking buffer: 5% dry milk in Tris Buffered Saline + 0.05% Tween in TBS-T.

9. The blot was then incubated overnight at 4 °C with specific primary antibody (CD63, CD9, CD81, and Hsp70; SBI) at 1:1000 dilution (5% dry milk in TBS-T).

10. The secondary antibody (Goat-Rabbit-HRP; SBI) at 1:20,000 dilution (5% dry milk in TBS-T).

11. Chemiluminescent substrate.

12. LAS-3000 imaging equipment system.

2.6 RNA Extraction from Cells

1. 6-well plates.

2. Trypsin.

3. Centrifuge.

4. 1× Phosphate Buffered Saline (PBS): 10 mM PO_4^{3-}, 137 mM NaCl, and 2.7 mM KCl.

5. GenElute™ Mammalian Total RNA Miniprep kit.

2.7 Cytotoxicity Assays

Cytotoxicity assays for exosomes were performed on RPE-19 cells using the acid phosphatase assay to determine the apoptotic activity for these exosomes.

1. 96-well plates.

2. Phosphatase substrate (10 mM p-nitrophenol phosphate).

3. 0.1 M sodium acetate.

4. 0.1% Triton X-100 (pH 5.5).

5. 1 M NaOH.

6. Dual beam plate reader at 405 nm with a reference wavelength of 620 nm.

2.8 The Human Apoptosis miScript miRNA PCR Array (Qiagen)

1. RNase-free water store at room temperature.

2. 10× miScript Nucleics Mix, store at −20 °C.

3. 5× miScript HiSpec Buffer, store at −20 °C.

4. Reverse-transcription mix, store at −20 °C.

5. Thermocycler (Biometra).

2.8.1 Reverse Transcription for Quantitative Real-Time PCR (qRT-PCR)

2.8.2 Real-Time PCR for Mature miRNA Expression Profiling

1. 2× QuantiTect SYBR Green PCR Master Mix.

2. 10× miScript Universal Primer.

3. RNase-free water.

2.9 Angiogenesis Assays

1. V2a Kit™ (Vasculogenesis to Angiogenesis).

2. Angiogenesis Basal Medium (provided with the kit), store at 2–8 °C.

3. Angiogenesis Seeding Supplement (provided with the kit), store at −20 °C.

---

3 Methods

3.1 Human Serum Preparation

1. Serum is the liquid fraction of whole blood that is collected after the blood is allowed to clot (*see* **Note 1**). Non-fasting blood specimens must be collected following consent given by the patients.

2. From the collected blood samples, allow the red blood cells to clot naturally, then process within 3–4 h of blood draw (*see* **Note 2**).

3. Centrifuge the tubes at 4 °C for 15 min at $400 \times g$ (relative centrifugal force).

4. After centrifugation carefully remove the blood serum and aliquot to a 1.8 mL CryoPure-Tube (*see* **Note 3**).

5. Store the serum immediately at −80 °C until analysis.

3.2 RNA Extraction

3.2.1 RNA Isolation and Quantification

1. Isolate total RNA from serum samples using TRI Reagent.

2. Defrost the serum and transfer 0.25 mL to clean Eppendorf tubes. Add 0.75 mL of TRI Reagent to the serum and incubate at RT for 10 min.

3. Add 0.2 mL of chloroform to each sample and shake vigorously for 15 s, followed by incubation at room temperature for 15 min.

4. Centrifuge the mix at $13,400 \times g$ for 15 min at 4 °C. Remove the aqueous phase containing RNA (upper layer) and transfer into a fresh RNAse-free 1.5 mL Eppendorf tube.

5. Add isopropanol (0.5 mL) and glycogen (final concentration 120 µg/mL), then incubate at room temperature for 5–10 min before storing at –20 °C overnight, to ensure maximum RNA precipitation.

6. Centrifuge the Eppendorf tubes at $13,400 \times g$ for 30 min at 4 °C to pellet the precipitated RNA.

7. Taking care not to disturb the RNA pellet. Remove the supernatant and wash the pellet subsequently by the addition of 750 µL of 75 % ethanol and vortex. Following centrifugation at $5400 \times g$ for 5 min at 4 °C, remove the supernatant and repeat this washing step.

8. Allow the RNA pellet to air-dry for 5–10 min, and resuspend subsequently in 10 µL of DEPC-treated H_2O (Ambion). To assess the quantity and quality of extracted RNA, an aliquot of each should be read at 260 nm, 280 nm and 230 nm using a NanoDrop ND-1000.

3.2.2 Interpretation of Results

1. *A260/280*: The ratio of absorbance at 260 and 280 nm provides an estimate of the purity of RNA with respect to contaminants that absorb in the UV spectrum. A ratio of ~2.0 is generally accepted as "pure" for RNA. If the ratio is appreciably lower in either case, it may indicate the presence of protein, phenol or other contaminants that absorb strongly at or near 280 nm. The A260/280 ratio is considerably influenced by pH; lower pH results in a lower ratio and reduced sensitivity to protein contamination.

2. *A260/230*: Ratio of sample absorbance at 260 and 230 nm. This is a secondary measure of nucleic acid purity, being usually higher than the respective 260/280 values for "pure" nucleic acids. It is usually in a range of 1.8–2.2; if lower, it may indicate co-purified contamination.

3. *Concentration (ng/µL)*: Sample concentration in ng/µL based on absorbance at 260 nm minus the absorbance at 340 nm (i.e., normalized at 340 nm) and the selected analysis constant.

3.3 The miRCURY LNA™ Universal RT microRNA PCR

The Exiqon platform is selected as the platform for microRNA discovery using serum specimen for this study. It is based on proprietary LNA™ detection technology and is a complete system for microRNA qPCR analysis from sample to results (*see* **Note 4**). The miRCURY LNA™ Universal RT microRNA PCR protocol was used for conducting first-strand cDNA synthesis and real time PCR, using the Pick-&-Mix microRNA PCR Panel, 96-well plates. The miRCURY LNA™ Universal RT microRNA PCR was performed in two-steps, consisting of (1) first-strand cDNA synthesis and (2) microRNA real-time qPCR amplification.

3.3.1 First-Strand cDNA Synthesis

1. Reverse-transcribe 2 μL RNA in 10 μL reactions using the miRCURY LNA™ Universal RT microRNA PCR cDNA synthesis kit, as shown in Table 1. Perform the reverse transcription reaction in thermocycler (Biometra®).

2. Mix the reagents by very gentle vortexing or pipetting. After mixing, spin down at $15{,}000 \times g$ for 1 min and then incubate for 60 min at 42 °C.

3. Heat-inactivate the reverse transcriptase for 5 min at 95 °C, and then immediately cool to 4 °C and store at 4 °C or freeze.

3.3.2 microRNA Real-Time qPCR Amplification

1. Dilute the cDNA 50× and assay in 10 μL PCR reactions according to the protocol for miRCURY LNA™ Universal RT microRNA PCR (Exiqon).

2. Assay each miRNA in triplicate by qPCR on the Ready-to-Use PCR custom Pick-&-Mix panel (*see* **Note 5**).

3. Perform the amplification in the Applied Biosystems 7500 Real-Time PCR System platform.

4. Analyze the amplification curves using the AB 7500 software, to determine the Ct value. Prepare the reaction mix as shown in Table 2.

5. Mix the reagents thoroughly by gentle pipetting. After mixing, seal the plate with optical sealing, as recommended by the manufacturer. Spin down in a centrifuge ($1500 \times g$ for 1 min) to bring the content to the bottom of the plate. The Real-time PCR cycle conditions are shown in Table 3.

Table 1
RT reaction mix components

Reagent	Volume (μL)
5× reaction buffer	2
Nuclease-free water	4.5
Enzyme mix	1
Synthetic RNA spike ins, optional	0.5
Template total RNA	2
Total volume	10

6. Export the raw CT data (SDS file format) from the Plate Centric View and calculate the fold change values according to the following formula using Excel:

$$\Delta CT = CT \text{ target} - CT \text{ control}$$
$$\text{Fold change} = 2 - \Delta CT$$

3.3.3   Data Quality Control

1. Use the RNA spike-in for quality control of the cDNA synthesis and qPCR experiment to ensure that the quality of the input RNA is high enough for effective amplification (*see* **Note 6**).

2. Use RNA spike-in control UniSp6 (CP) to evaluate the RT reaction. The expression level of this assay indicates that the reverse transcription is successful; UniSp3 (IPC) evaluates the qPCR reaction, which indicated good technical performance of the experiment.

3.3.4   Identification of Consistent Normalizer (Endogenous Control)

1. In order to select and validate the appropriate reference genes to normalize the data (*see* **Note 7**), use both geNorm and Normfinder programs available through GenEx software. We chose two endogenous controls (without considering groups) based on their relative stability on the microarrays (*see* **Note 8**).

2. miR-323-3p and miR-324-3p as controls were recommended by Applied Biosystems, TLDA manufacturer, as normalizers for Real-Time quantification of miRNA Using TaqMan MiRNA Assays and also they have been identified as potential normalizers in previous serum/blood studies. These include miR-323-3p and miR-324-3p [16–19].

Table 2
qPCR amplification components

Reagent	Volume (µL)
PCR Master mix	5
PCR primer mix5	1
Diluted cDNA template	4
Total volume	10

Table 3
Thermal cycling conditions

• Polymerase activation/denaturation	95 °C, 10 min
• Amplification	40 amplification cycles
	95 °C, 10 s
	60 °C, 1 min

3. The two best endogenous controls miR-323-3p and miR-324-3p were the most consistent miRNAs among the whole samples to be used for normalization. Perform the normalization based on the average of the normalizer assays CT, which included miR-323-3p and miR-324-3p.

4. Use the following formula to calculate the normalized Ct values is:

$$\text{Normalized Ct}\,(\text{dCt}) = \text{assay Ct}\,(\text{sample}) - \text{average Ct}\,(\text{Normalizer assays}).$$

3.3.5 Normalization

Normalization is performed based on the average of the normalizer assays. For the present study, has-miR-323-3p and miR-324-3p is used.

The formula used to calculate the normalized Ct values is:

$$\text{Normalized Ct}\,(\text{dCt}) = \text{assay Ct}\,(\text{sample}) - \text{average Ct}\,(\text{Normalizer assays}).$$

3.3.6 Data Analysis

Raw CT data (SDS file format) were exported and fold change values were calculated according to the following formula using Excel:

1. Normalized ct (ct sample—ct endo).

2. Calibrator ct (ct of control after normalizing).

3. ΔΔct (normalized ct—calibrator ct).

4. RQ on normalized ct (=POWER (2,—ΔΔCt)).

3.4 Bioinformatics

1. Use a web-based computational tool (DIANA-mirPath micro-T 4.0) to identify potential protein coding mRNA targets and potential molecular pathways that are altered by the expression of some of the validated miRNAs.

2. Identify the predicted targets from DIANA-miRpath software. Use the miR-TarBase database to see the target genes of the three validated miRNAs. Integrate the detected miRNAs gene targets with their signaling pathways using KEGG (Kyoto Encyclopedia of Genes and Genomes) Pathways enrichment (*see* **Note 9**).

3.5 Functional Analysis

3.5.1 Experimental Design

The study follows a linear process of exosomes isolation, cell culture and treatment, and applying the proper assay followed by analysis.

3.5.2 Cell Culture of Retinal Pigment Epithelium Cells

1. Maintain the human retinal pigment epithelial cell line ARPE-19 in Dulbecco's modified Eagle's medium (DMEM) supplemented with 4 mM l-glutamine, 10 % fetal bovine serum (FBS),

100 U/mL penicillin, and 100 μg/mL streptomycin at 37 °C in 5 % CO_2 in air.

2. Replace the culture medium at least twice weekly. In all experiments, maintain cells at 70–80 % confluency (Fig. 1) and seed the day before treatment.

3.5.3 Exosome Isolation from Serum Using ExoQuick

1. Transfer 250 μL of serum into a sterile vessel and 63 μL of ExoQuick Exosome Precipitation (SBI), and then mix well by inverting or flicking the tube.

2. Incubate the mix at room temperature for 30 min and then centrifuge (ExoQuick–serum mixture) at $1500 \times g$ for 30 min.

3. Centrifugation can be performed at either room temperature or 4 °C with similar results. After centrifugation, the exosomes may appear as a white pellet at the bottom of the vessel.

4. Aspirate the supernatant and spin down the residual ExoQuick solution by centrifugation at $1500 \times g$ for 5 min. Remove all traces of fluid by aspiration, taking great care not to disturb the precipitated exosomes.

5. Resuspend the exosome pellet in 1/10 (25 μL) of the original volume using sterile or nuclease-free water (*see* **Note 10**). Store the isolated exosomes at –80 °C.

6. Quantify exosomes using Bio-Rad protein assay and Qubit® fluorometric quantitation.

3.5.4 Track Exosomes with Validated Antibody Systems

ExoELISA kit can be used for fast analysis of exosomal protein markers: CD63, CD9, CD81, or Hsp70. The exosome antibody kit allows confirmation of exosomes.

1. Isolate the exosome as described in Subheading 3.5.3 and centrifuge at $1500 \times g$ for 5 min to remove all traces of fluid, and taking care not to disturb the pellet.

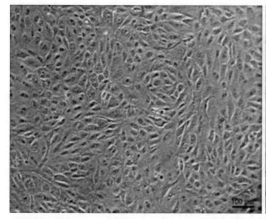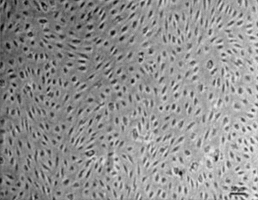

Fig. 1 (**a**) ARPE 19. (**b**) ARPE 19 confluent layer

2. Add 200 μL of RIPA buffer (along with the appropriate protease inhibitor cocktail) to the exosome pellet and vortex for 15 s, and then place at room temperature for 5 min to allow complete lysis. Use a Qubit® assay to determine the yield.

3. Add Laemmli buffer (with beta-mercaptoethanol) and heat the mixture at 95 °C for 5 min, then on ice for 5 min before loading onto the gel. Perform the standard SDS-PAGE electrophoresis and transfer onto PVDF membrane.

4. Block the membrane using blocking buffer for 1 h. Incubate the blot overnight at 4 °C with specific primary antibody (CD63, CD9, CD81, and Hsp70).

5. Wash the blot three times with TBS-T and incubate for 1 h at room temperature in secondary antibody, after which wash the blot three times with TBS-T.

6. Incubate the blot with a chemiluminescent substrate and visualize on LAS-3000 imaging equipment system.

3.6 ARPE-19 Exosome Treatment, Cell Pellet Collection and RNA Extraction

Extract RNA as described in Subheading 3.2.1 to determine the effect of exosomes derived from AMD patients and control, on RPE by using different assays.

1. Seed ARPE-19 cells in 6-well plates at a density of 2×10^5 per well with 3 mL of culture medium. Prepare these in triplicate.

2. The following day, treat the cells with 20 μg serum-derived exosomes from atrophic, neovascular AMD patients and their matched control ($n = 18$). Then incubate the assays for 72 h at 37 °C.

3. At the end of the assay, trypsinize the cells and centrifuge at $500 \times g$ for 5 min to form a pellet.

4. Wash the pellet twice in PBS and process cell pellets for total RNA extraction using GenElute™ Mammalian Total RNA Miniprep Kit.

3.6.1 GenElute™ Mammalian Total RNA Miniprep Protocol

Working in an RNase-free environment is essential when isolating and manipulating RNA. RNA is a relatively fragile molecule, easily degraded by ubiquitous RNase enzymes. RNase may be introduced accidentally into the RNA preparation at any point in the procedure through improper technique (*see* **Note 11**). Thus, stringent measures were required to avoid this potential hazard. Total RNA was isolated from samples using the GenElute Mammalian Total RNA Miniprep Kit, a system that combined organic extraction and centrifuge-based filtration techniques.

1. Vortex cell pellet briefly in order to loosen cells. Add 250 μL of lysis Solution–2-ME mixture and then pipette thoroughly until all clumps are disappeared.

2. Add the lysed cells into a GenElute Filtration Column, centrifuge at maximum speed ($12,000 \times g$) for 2 min, and then discard

the flow through. Add 500 µL of 70% ethanol solution to the filtered lysate and pipette up and down to ensure even mixing.

3. Add 700 µL of the lysate–ethanol mixture into a GenElute Binding Column and centrifuge at maximum speed for 15 s. Retain the collection tube and discard flow-through liquid.

4. Perform a series of wash steps, each of which require the introduction of wash solution to the top of the column, followed by centrifugation at maximum speed for 15 s.

5. Transfer the binding columns to fresh collection tubes, and repeat the process. Again, transfer the binding columns to fresh 2 mL collection tubes, and add 50 µL of the elution solution, before centrifugation at maximum speed for 1 min.

6. Perform elution with a second 50 µL volume of elution solution, with both eluates (same sample) collected in the same tube. Purified RNA was present in the flow-through eluate (~45 or 90 µL total).

7. Store the samples at –80 °C before transcription into complementary DNA (cDNA).

8. RNA yield quantification, Qubit® fluorometric quantitation using 1 µL of RNA sample for each measurement.

3.7 Apoptosis Assay

Cytotoxicity assays for exosomes were performed on RPE-19 cells using the acid phosphatase assay to determine the apoptotic activity of these exosomes.

3.7.1 Cytotoxicity Assays in ARPE-19 Cells Treated with AMD Derived Exosomes

1. Seed RPE-19 cells in 96-well plates at a density of 2×10^3 per well. The following day, treat the with 10 µg serum-derived exosomes from atrophic, neovascular AMD patients and their age- and gender-matched control donors (Fig. 2.9).

2. Incubate the cytotoxicity assays for 72 h, after which, assess the effects of exosomes using the acid phosphatase method. At the end of the assay, remove the media from the plates and wash each well on the plate with 100 µL of PBS.

3. After washing, add 100 µL of freshly prepared phosphatase substrate to each well. Wrap the plates in tinfoil and incubate in the dark at 37 °C for 1–2 h.

4. After incubation, stop the enzymatic reaction by adding 50 µL of 1 M NaOH to each well. Read the plate in a dual beam plate reader at 405 nm with a reference wavelength of 620 nm.

3.7.2 Profiling ARPE-19 Cells Treated with AMD Derived Exosomes

miScript miRNA PCR array

Human Apoptosis miScript miRNA PCR Array profiling was done using ARPE-19 cells treated with AMD derived exosomes. The Human Apoptosis miScript miRNA PCR Array profiles the expression of 84 miRNAs that regulate programmed cell death. A set of controls present on each array enables data analysis using the

$\Delta\Delta$CT method of relative quantification, assessment of reverse transcription performance, and assessment of PCR performance. Using SYBR® Green real-time PCR, the expression of a focused panel of miRNAs related to apoptosis can be easily and reliably analyzed with this iScript miRNA PCR Array.

Layout

The apoptosis miScript miRNA PCR Array layout is as shown in Fig. 2.

The functional gene grouping was as follows:

Anti-apoptotic: miR-106b-5p, miR-141-3p, miR-183-5p, miR-186-3p, miR-210, miR-214-3p, miR-338-3p, miR-378a-3p, miR-98-5p, miR-133a, miR-181a-5p, miR-21-5p, miR-25-3p, miR-30a-5p, miR-30b-5p, miR-30d-5p.

Pro-apoptotic: miR-128, miR-143-3p, miR-144-3p, miR-200c-3p, miR-205-5p, miR-206, miR-212-3p, miR-218-5p, miR-26a-5p, miR-26b-5p, miR-27a-3p, miR-30c-5p, miR-30e-5p, miR-31-5p, miR-365a-3p, miR-409-3p, miR-449a, miR-708-5p, let-7c, let-7 g, miR-1, miR-101-3p, miR-133b, miR-149-3p, miR-153, miR-15b-5p, miR-16-5p, miR-181b-5p, miR-195-5p, miR-203a, miR-204-5p, miR-29a-3p, miR-29c-3p, miR-34a-5p, miR-497-5p, miR-512-5p.

Either anti-apoptotic or pro-apoptotic: let-7e-5p, miR-23a-3p, miR-24-3p, miR-34c-5p, let-7a-5p, miR-29b-3p.

Targets anti-apoptotic genes: let-7c, let-7 g, miR-1, miR-101-3p, miR-122-5p, miR-133a, miR-133b, miR-193b, miR-194-5p, miR-204-5p, miR-491-5p, miR-512-5p, miR-542-3p, miR-7-5p, miR-9-5p.

Targets pro-apoptotic genes: miR-134, miR-221-3p, miR-222-3p, miR-32-5p.

Targets both anti-apoptotic & pro-apoptotic genes: let-7a-5p, miR-125a-5p, miR-125b-5p, miR-1285-3p, miR-145-5p, miR-146a-5p, miR-149-3p, miR-153, miR-15a-5p, miR-15b-5p, miR-16-5p, miR-17-5p, miR-181a-5p, miR-181b-5p, miR-181c-5p, miR-181d, miR-185-5p, miR-192-5p, miR-193a-5p, miR-195-5p, miR-203a, miR-20a-5p, miR-21-5p, miR-25-3p, miR-29a-3p, miR-29b-3p, miR-29c-3p, miR-30a-5p, miR-30b-5p, miR-30d-5p, miR-34a-5p, miR-451a, miR-497-5p, miR-92a-3p.

The miScript PCR system consists of the miScript II RT Kit, miScript miRNA PCR Array, miScript SYBR Green PCR Kit, and miScript miRNA PCR Array data analysis tool. The miScript PCR System allows sensitive and specific detection and quantification of microRNA (miRNA). The miScript PCR System uses total RNA that contains miRNA as the starting material for cDNA synthesis. A single cDNA preparation can be used with a miScript miRNA PCR Array to rapidly profile the expression of mature miRNAs. These PCR arrays were provided in ready-to-use 96-well plate formats with their controls as shown in Table 4. Once raw threshold cycle (CT) data has been uploaded, the tool automatically

	1	2	3	4	5	6	7	8	9	10	11	12
A	hsa-let-7a-5p	hsa-let-7c	hsa-let-7e-5p	hsa-let-7g-5p	hsa-miR-1	hsa-miR-101-3p	hsa-miR-106b-5p	hsa-miR-122-5p	hsa-miR-125a-5p	hsa-miR-125b-5p	hsa-miR-128	hsa-miR-1285-3p
B	hsa-miR-133a	hsa-miR-133b	hsa-miR-134	hsa-miR-141-3p	hsa-miR-143-3p	hsa-miR-144-3p	hsa-miR-145-5p	hsa-miR-146a-5p	hsa-miR-149-3p	hsa-miR-153	hsa-miR-15a-5p	hsa-miR-15b-5p
C	hsa-miR-16-5p	hsa-miR-17-5p	hsa-miR-181a-5p	hsa-miR-181b-5p	hsa-miR-181c-5p	hsa-miR-181d	hsa-miR-183-5p	hsa-miR-185-5p	hsa-miR-186-3p	hsa-miR-192-5p	hsa-miR-193a-5p	hsa-miR-193b-3p
D	hsa-miR-194-5p	hsa-miR-195-5p	hsa-miR-200c-3p	hsa-miR-203a	hsa-miR-204-5p	hsa-miR-205-5p	hsa-miR-206	hsa-miR-20a-5p	hsa-miR-21-5p	hsa-miR-210	hsa-miR-212-3p	hsa-miR-214-3p
E	hsa-miR-218-5p	hsa-miR-221-3p	hsa-miR-222-3p	hsa-miR-23a-3p	hsa-miR-24-3p	hsa-miR-25-3p	hsa-miR-26a-5p	hsa-miR-26b-5p	hsa-miR-27a-3p	hsa-miR-29a-3p	hsa-miR-29b-3p	hsa-miR-29c-3p
F	hsa-miR-30a-5p	hsa-miR-30b-5p	hsa-miR-30c-5p	hsa-miR-30d-5p	hsa-miR-30e-5p	hsa-miR-31-5p	hsa-miR-32-5p	hsa-miR-338-3p	hsa-miR-34a-5p	hsa-miR-34c-5p	hsa-miR-365b-3p	hsa-miR-378a-3p
G	hsa-miR-409-3p	hsa-miR-449a	hsa-miR-451a	hsa-miR-491-5p	hsa-miR-497-5p	hsa-miR-512-5p	hsa-miR-542-3p	hsa-miR-7-5p	hsa-miR-708-5p	hsa-miR-9-5p	hsa-miR-92a-3p	hsa-miR-98-5p
H	cel-miR-39-3p	cel-miR-39-3p	SNORD61	SNORD68	SNORD72	SNORD95	SNORD96A	RNU6-2	miRTC	miRTC	PPC	PPC

Fig. 2 Apoptosis miScript miRNA PCR Array layout

performs all fold-change calculations using the ΔΔCT method of relative quantification, and presents the results in several formats The PCR arrays layout as shown in Fig. 2.

3.7.3 Reverse Transcription for Quantitative Real-Time PCR (qRT-PCR)

For pathway profiling of mature miRNA (pathway-focused miScript miRNA PCR arrays) the recommended RNA input is 125–250 ng/RNA sample.

1. Thaw the template RNA on ice, along with RNase-free water. Thaw 10× miScript Nucleics Mix and 5x miScript HiSpec Buffer at room temperature (15–25 °C). Prepare the reverse-transcription mix was prepared according to the Table 5.

2. Gently mix the reaction components together, and then store on ice. The reverse-transcription master mix contained all components required for first-strand cDNA synthesis, except template RNA.

3. Add the template RNA to each tube containing reverse-transcription master mix. Mix the contents gently, then centrifuge briefly, and then store on ice.

Table 4
Controls in each miScript miRNA PCR array

Control	Purpose
C. elegans miR-39 miScript primer assay	Alternative data normalization using exogenously spiked Syn-cel-miR-39 miScript miRNA Mimic
6 snoRNA/snRNA miScript PCR controls: SNORD61 assay SNORD95 assay SNORD96A assay SNORD68 assay SNORD72 assay RNU6B/RNU6-2 assay	Data normalization using the ΔΔCT method of relative quantification
Positive PCR control (PPC)	Assessment of PCR performance

Table 5
RT reaction mix components

Component	Volume/reaction
5× miScript HiSpec Buffer	4 μL
10× miScript Nucleics Mix	2 μL
RNase-free water	Variable
miScript Reverse Transcriptase Mix	2 μL
Template RNA (added in **step 3**)	Variable

4. Incubate the mix for 60 min at 37 °C (during which time reverse transcription occurred), then incubate for 5 min at 95 °C to inactivate the miScript Reverse Transcriptase enzyme.

5. Place the product again on ice once this step is completed.

6. Dilute the complementary DNA (cDNA) by adding 200 μL RNase-free water to each 20 μL transverse transcription reaction, and then perform real-time PCR.

3.7.4 Real-Time PCR for Mature miRNA Expression Profiling

miScript miRNA PCR arrays in combination with the miScript SYBR Green PCR Kit was used to perform real-time PCR profiling of mature miRNA which contains the miScript Universal Primer (reverse primer) and QuantiTect SYBR Green PCR Master Mix. The standard miScript miRNA PCR array reaction volume is 25 μL per well for a 96-well plate.

1. Thaw 2× QuantiTect SYBR Green PCR Master Mix, 10× miScript Universal Primer, template cDNA, and RNase-free water at room temperature. Then prepare the reaction mix according to Table 6.

2. Add 25 μL of the mixture to each well of the miScript miRNA PCR Array, followed by the real-time PCR cycle conditions as described in Table 7.

Table 6
qPCR reaction mix components

Component	Volume (μL)
2× QuantiTect SYBR Green PCR Master Mix	1100
10× miScript Universal Primer	220
RNase-free water	780
Template cDNA	100
Total volume	2200

Table 7
Thermal cycle conditions

Step	Time	Temperature
PCR Initial activation step	15 min	95 °C
Three-step cycling (40 cycles)		
Denaturation	15 s	94 °C
Annealing	30 s	55 °C
Extension	34 s	70 °C

3.7.5 Data Analysis   Analyze the data using online data analysis software for miScript miRNA PCR Array, available at http://pcrdataanalysis.sabiosciences.com/mirna. Data Analysis Excel® Template can be accessed at the same website. Both tools will automatically perform quantification using the $\Delta\Delta CT$ method of relative quantification. Results are presented in Excel format.

3.8 Angiogenesis Assays on Human Endothelial Cells Treated with AMD Derived Exosomes

Angiogenesis assays were performed using the V2a Kit by TCS-Cellworks as follows:

Day 1

1. Prepare V2a Seeding Medium and pre-equilibrate.
2. Add V2a Co-Culture Cells to Seeding Medium.
3. Add Cells and Medium to 24-well plate cell culture plate Incubate.
4. Culture the human endothelial cells were cultured in a 24-well plate.

Day 2

1. Prepare V2a Growth Medium Dilute control and test compounds as required*.
2. Pre-equilibrate V2a Growth Medium and control/test dilutions.
3. Examine cultures microscopically.
4. Change medium into pre-equilibrated V2a Growth Medium (+/– control or test compounds) as required.

   After 24 h of seeding, cells were treated with VEGF (positive control), Suramin (negative control), and test samples (neovascular, atrophic AMD and control derived exosomes), Experimental layout Fig. 3.

   On days 4, 6, 8, 10, and 12 (i.e., every 48 h), change the medium and treat the cells with the above additions as appropriate until day 14.

Day 4

1. Examine cultures microscopically.
2. Change medium into pre-equilibrated V2a Growth medium (+/– control or test compounds).

Day 6

Repeat Day 4 procedure.

Day 8

Repeat Day 4 procedure.

Day 10

Repeat Day 4 procedure.

Day 12

Repeat Day 4 procedure.

Day 14

1. Examine cultures microscopically.

2. Fix cells and stain tubules.

3. Analyze results either manually or using Cellworks Image Analysis Software, AngioSys 2.0.

---

4   Notes

1. Allow the blood specimens to clot before centrifugation, serum samples need a minimum of 30 min to clot. Keep the tube vertical while clotting.

2. Avoid blood hemolysis to prevent serum cellular contamination. Blood cells have higher miRNA concentration than serum and so cellular RNA from blood cell debris has significant affect on results calculation.

3. Avoid aspirating part of the white interphase (DNA) while removing aqueous supernatant (RNA), always aspirate the aqueous supernatant (RNA) and leave a small amount on top of the white interphase (DNA).

4. Exiqon is based on proprietary Locked Nucleic Acids (LNA™) detection technology, which provide highly sensitive and specific analysis of small RNA targets.

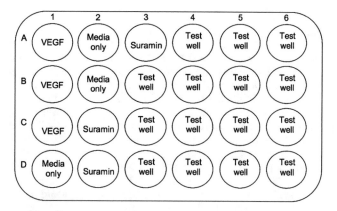

VEGF: Positive control
Media only: Untreated control well.
Suramin: Negative control

Fig. 3 Experimental layout

5. To avoid technical bias, each miRNA was assayed in triplicate by qPCR on the individual the miRNA Ready-to-Use PCR custom Pick-&-Mix panel.

6. The RNA spike-in for quality control of the cDNA synthesis and qPCR experiment provides an internal reference for technical performance of the experiment.

7. It is challenging to normalize serum miRNA qPCR data. Technical biases adjustment (RNA amount, quality, etc.) is required for more precise estimation of biological differences.

8. NormFinder is designed to determine the most stable normalizer (reference genes).

9. Computational and experimental approaches integration expands our understating to the biological and pathological role of miRNAs and their therapeutic potential.

10. The exosome pellet is relatively hard. To resuspend the exosome pellet using sterile or nuclease-free water, we need to pipette the nuclease-free water gently around the pellet until the pellet totally dissolved.

11. For successful RNA extraction, RNase-free environment is essential during isolation and RNA manipulation. Gloves must be worn all the time. Bench area must be cleaned using RNaseZap.

Acknowledgement

This work was supported by Irish Research Council (for Science, Engineering & Technology/EMBARK Initiative), Trinity College Foundation, the Mater Vision Institute, and the Libyan Ministry of Higher Education and Scientific Research.

References

1. Chen Y, Zeng J, Zhao C et al (2011) Assessing susceptibility to age-related macular degeneration with genetic markers and environmental factors. Arch Ophthalmol 129(3):344–351. doi:10.1001/archophthalmol.2011.10

2. Hackler LJ, Wan J, Swaroop A et al (2010) MicroRNA profile of the developing mouse retina. Invest Ophthalmol Visual Sci 51(4):1823–1831, doi:D-NLM:PMC2868396 EDAT- 2009/11/26 06:00 MHDA- 2010/04/27 06:00 CRDT- 2009/11/26 06:00 PHST- 2009/11/20 [aheadofprint] AID - iovs.09-4657 [pii] AID - 10.1167/iovs.09-4657 [doi] PST - ppublish

3. Wang S, Koster KM, He Y et al (2012) miRNAs as potential therapeutic targets for age-related macular degeneration. Future Med Chem 4(3):277–287, doi:D - nlm: nihms364149, D - NLM: PMC3313592 EDAT- 2012/03/08 06:00 MHDA- 2012/07/17 06:00 CRDT- 2012/03/08 06:00 AID - 10.4155/fmc.11.176 [doi] PST - ppublish

4. Keller A, Leidinger P, Lange J et al (2009) Multiple sclerosis: MicroRNA expression profiles accurately differentiate patients with relapsing-remitting disease from healthy controls. PLoS One 4(10), e7440

5. Mar-Aguilar F, Mendoza-Ramirez JA, Malagon-Santiago I et al (2013) Serum circulating microRNA profiling for identification of potential breast cancer biomarkers. Dis Markers 34(3):163–169, doi:D - NLM: PMC3810231 EDAT- 2013/01/22 06:00 MHDA- 2013/07/31 06:00 CRDT- 2013/01/22 06:00 AID - JW81G23204456544 [pii] AID - 10.3233/DMA-120957 [doi] PST - ppublish

6. Li L, Xu J, Yang D et al (2010) Computational approaches for microRNA studies: a review. Mamm Genome 21(1-2):1–12. doi:10.1007/s00335-009-9241-2

7. Deng N, Puetter A, Fau - Zhang K, Zhang K Fau - Johnson K et al. (2011) Isoform-level microRNA-155 target prediction using RNA-seq. (1362-4962 (Electronic)). doi:D - NLM: PMC3089486 EDAT- 2011/02/15 06:00 MHDA- 2011/08/02 06:00 CRDT- 2011/02/15 06:00 PHST- 2011/02/11 [aheadofprint] AID - gkr042 [pii] AID - 10.1093/nar/gkr042 [doi] PST - ppublish

8. Chou CH, Lin Fm Fau - Chou M-T, Chou Mt Fau - Hsu S-D et al. (2013) A computational approach for identifying microRNA-target interactions using high-throughput CLIP and PAR-CLIP sequencing. (1471-2164 (Electronic)). doi:D - NLM: PMC3549799 EDAT- 2013/02/13 06:00 MHDA- 2013/08/13 06:00 CRDT- 2013/02/02 06:00 PHST- 2013/01/21 [aheadofprint] AID - 1471-2164-14-S1-S2 [pii] AID - 10.1186/1471-2164-14-S1-S2 [doi] PST - ppublish

9. Hsu SD, Lin FM, Wu WY et al (2011) miR-TarBase: a database curates experimentally validated microRNA-target interactions. Nucleic Acids Res 39(Database issue):D163–D169. doi:10.1093/nar/gkq1107

10. van Niel G, Porto-Carreiro I, Simoes S et al (2006) Exosomes: a common pathway for a specialized function. J Biochem 140(1):13–21

11. Mathivanan S, Ji H, Simpson RJ (2010) Exosomes: Extracellular organelles important in intercellular communication. J Proteomics 73(10):1907–1920. doi:10.1016/j.jprot.2010.06.006

12. Roccaro AM, Sacco A, Maiso P et al (2013) BM mesenchymal stromal cell-derived exosomes facilitate multiple myeloma progression. J Clin Invest 123(4):1542–1555. doi:10.1172/JCI66517

13. Lin H, Qian J, Castillo AC et al (2011) Effect of miR-23 on oxidant-induced injury in human retinal pigment epithelial cells. Invest Ophthalmol Visual Sci 52(9):6308–6314

14. Wang AL, Lukas TJ, Yuan M et al (2009) Autophagy and exosomes in the aged retinal pigment epithelium: Possible relevance to drusen formation and age-related macular degeneration. PLoS One 4(1), e4160. doi:10.1371/journal.pone.0004160

15. Wang AL, Lukas TJ, Yuan M et al (2009) Autophagy, exosomes and drusen formation in age-related macular degeneration. Autophagy 5(4):563–564

16. Liang Y, Ridzon D, Wong L et al (2007) Characterization of microRNA expression profiles in normal human tissues. BMC Genomics 8:166. doi:10.1186/1471-2164-8-166

17. Ratert N, Meyer HA, Jung M et al (2012) Reference miRNAs for miRNAome analysis of urothelial carcinomas. PLoS One 7(6), e39309. doi:10.1371/journal.pone.0039309

18. Wong L, Lee K, Russell I et al (2010) Endogenous controls for real-time quantitation of miRNA using TaqMan® MicroRNA assays., Applied Biosystems, http://www3.appliedbiosystems.com/cms/groups/mcb_marketing/documents/generaldocuments/cms_044972.pdf

19. Yelamanchili SV, Chaudhuri AD, Chen LN et al (2010) MicroRNA-21 dysregulates the expression of MEF2C in neurons in monkey and human SIV/HIV neurological disease. Cell Death Dis 1, e77

Chapter 11

Profiling the MicroRNA Payload of Exosomes Derived from Ex Vivo Primary Colorectal Fibroblasts

Rahul Bhome, Rebecca Goh, Karen Pickard, Massimiliano Mellone, A. Emre Sayan, and Alex Mirnezami

Abstract

The tumor microenvironment is a heterogeneous and dynamic network that exists between cancer and stroma, playing a critical role in cancer progression. Certain tumorigenic signals such as microRNAs are derived from the stroma and conveyed to cancer cells (and vice versa) in nanoparticles called exosomes. Their identification and characterization is an important step in better understanding cellular cross talk and its consequences. To this end we describe how to culture primary ex vivo derived fibroblasts from colorectal tissue, isolate their exosomes, extract exosomal RNA and perform microRNA profiling.

Key words Tumor microenvironment, Stroma, Fibroblast, Exosome, Colorectal cancer

1 Introduction

It is important to appreciate the tumor microenvironment (TME) as a functional ecosystem that exists between cancer cells and the surrounding stromal milieu. In recent times, there has been increased recognition of the key part played by the microenvironment in the control of both normal physiological processes and development of the malignant phenotype [1]. For example, activated stroma is strongly associated with the acquisition of increased proliferation, invasion and chemoresistance of cancer cells [2]. Consequently, the study of TME methods to delineate the cellular cross talk between different cell types and compartments is of great importance. This will not only enhance our understanding of fundamental biological processes but may pave the way towards more novel therapeutic strategies. Using techniques such as laser capture microdissection and modern single cell isolation methodologies, the stromal and epithelial compartments of a tumor can be separated and subsequently analyzed to determine the origin of deregulated signals [3]. For example, functionally relevant microRNA-21

Sweta Rani (ed.), *MicroRNA Profiling: Methods and Protocols*, Methods in Molecular Biology, vol. 1509,
DOI 10.1007/978-1-4939-6524-3_11, © Springer Science+Business Media New York 2017

originates from stromal myofibroblasts rather than cancer cells in the colorectal setting [4, 5].

MicroRNAs (miRNAs) are small noncoding RNA sequences, which are approximately 20 nucleotides long. Pri-miRNAs are transcribed by RNA polymerase II and undergo enzymatic cleavage within the nucleus (drosha) to form pre-miRNAs and within the cytoplasm (dicer) to form mature miRNAs. The resulting miRNA sequence then binds the 3′ untranslated region of coding mRNAs repressing translation [6]. In this way miRNAs can regulate a number of cellular processes including proliferation, differentiation and apoptosis [7], all of which are relevant to cancer progression.

MiRNAs can be transferred between cells in the TME, allowing one cell to alter protein expression in another [8]. This paracrine signaling is facilitated by nanoparticles called exosomes. Exosomes are extracellular vesicles between 40 and 100 nm in diameter with a lipid bilayer. Unlike shedding vesicles and microparticles, their biosynthesis and secretion is complex and enzyme dependent [9]. Exosomes are secreted by all cellular components of the TME, including cancer cells [10], fibroblasts [11], innate and acquired immune cells [12], and vascular endothelial cells [13]. Moreover, the impact of exosomal transfer on target cells is not momentary but lasts for at least several days [14].

In order to identify stromal microRNA signals in the colorectal cancer setting, we describe how to: (1) culture primary fibroblasts from human colorectal tissue, (2) isolate fibroblast exosomes, (3) label and transfer exosomes from one cell type to another, (4) extract total RNA from exosomes, and (5) perform exosomal miRNA profiling.

2 Materials

2.1 Culture of Primary Fibroblasts

1. 10 cm diameter dish.

2. Scalpel.

3. Forceps (non-toothed).

4. 12-well plate.

5. Phosphate buffered saline (PBS) supplemented with 2% (double-strength) penicillin–streptomycin (Penicillin (200 U/mL)–streptomycin (200 μg/mL; Sigma-Aldrich), and 0.1% (0.25 μg/mL) amphotericin B (Fungizone; Thermo Fisher Scientific) (*see* **Note 1**).

6. Dulbecco's Modified Eagle's Medium (DMEM) supplemented with 20% fetal calf serum (FCS), 2% penicillin–streptomycin and 0.1% amphotericin B.

7. Trypsin–EDTA solution (0.25%; Sigma-Aldrich).

8. Ciprofloxacin (BIOMYC-3 100×; Biological Industries).

2.2 Isolation of Exosomes from Primary Fibroblasts

1. Exosome deplete FCS (produced by collecting the supernatant from FCS which has been centrifuged at $100,000 \times g$ for 16 h).

2. 50 mL polypropylene (Falcon) tubes.

3. 0.22 μm filter with polyethersulfone (PES) membrane (Merck Millipore).

4. 50 mL (Luer lock) syringe.

5. Polycarbonate ultracentrifuge tubes 26.3 mL (Beckman Coulter).

6. Ultracentrifuge with rotor capable of $100,000 \times g$ (e.g., Sorvall Discovery 100 s with titanium rotor TFT 50.38).

7. PBS.

8. Appropriate solvent for further processing of exosomes e.g., Laemmli buffer 2x, Lysis solution (RNAqueous®-Micro Total RNA Isolation Kit, Ambion), sterile water.

2.3 Labeling and Transfer of Exosomes

1. Vybrant Cell Labeling Solution DiO: absorption 484 nm emission 501 nm (Molecular Probes).

2. Laemmli Buffer 2×.

3. Pierce BCA Protein Assay Kit (Thermo Fisher).

2.4 Isolation of Exosomal RNA

1. RNAqueous®-Micro Total RNA Isolation Kit (Ambion).

2. Nuclease-free 1.5–2 mL tubes.

3. 100% ethanol.

4. Nuclease-free water.

2.5 MicroRNA Array

1. Cancer MicroRNA qPCR Array with Quantimir™ (System Biosciences).

2. Primer plate - dried primers for 95 cancer-associated microRNAs (plus U6 for normalization).

3. Power SYBR Green PCR Mastermix (Applied Biosystems).

4. 96-well qPCR reaction plate.

5. Optical adhesive cover (Applied Biosystems).

6. Nuclease-free water.

7. Thermocycler.

8. qPCR instrument e.g., ABI7500 (Applied Biosystems).

3 Methods

3.1 Culture of Primary Colorectal Fibroblasts

1. Collect fresh biopsy (1-2 cm) of malignant and normal colon/rectum (ensuring ethical approval for study and patient consent) in 10 mL PBS supplemented with antimicrobials.

2. Transfer to a 10 cm dish and wash biopsy three times with 10 mL PBS. Do not aspirate PBS after last wash.

3. Divide biopsy into 2–5 mm fragments using sterile scalpel and forceps.

4. Score the bottom of each well in a 12-well plate with a cross ('X').

5. Place the biopsy fragments individually on to the center of each cross allowing them to attach.

6. Add 750 µL medium (DMEM supplemented with 20% FCS and antimicrobials) to each well ensuring that the biopsy fragment is not dislodged.

7. Incubate at 37 °C/5% CO_2.

8. Change medium at 24 h and every 72 h thereafter, checking for outgrowth of fibroblasts and microbial infection at each interval.

9. When fibroblasts are greater than 70% confluent (usually at 4–6 weeks), expand each well into one T25 flask.

10. For expansion: aspirate medium from well, wash twice with PBS, add 500 µL warm trypsin, incubate at 37 °C for 5 min.

11. Then add 1 mL fresh medium, aspirate entire contents of well and transfer to a 15 mL Falcon tube.

12. Centrifuge at $400 \times g$ for 5 min to pellet cells. Discard supernatant.

13. Resuspend cell pellet in 5 mL PBS, centrifuge again at $400 \times g$ for 5 min. Discard supernatant.

14. Resuspend washed cell pellet in 6 mL fresh medium and transfer to a T25 flask.

15. Add 60 µL BIOMYC-3.

16. Incubate at 37 °C/5% CO_2.

17. Expand to T75 and then T175 flasks when cells are 100% confluent using appropriate volumes of trypsin and medium. It is not necessary to use BIOMYC-3 for these expansions.

3.2 Isolation of Exosomes from Primary Colorectal Fibroblasts

1. Primary fibroblasts should be cultured in FCS-deplete medium for 72 h prior to exosome isolation (*see* **Notes 2–4**).

2. Pre-chill ultracentrifuge rotor to 4 °C.

3. Harvest conditioned medium from all flasks and transfer to 50 mL Falcon tubes.

4. Centrifuge at $400 \times g$ for 5 min to pellet out floating cells. It is not necessary to decant supernatant at this step (*see* **Note 5**).

5. Centrifuge at $2000 \times g$ for 10 min to pellet out debris.

6. Attach 0.22 µm filter to 50 mL syringe and remove plunger. Transfer supernatant into the chamber of the syringe. Reattach the plunger and drive supernatant through filter into a fresh 50 mL Falcon tube.

7. Transfer equal volumes of filtered supernatant into ultracentrifuge tubes. Ensure that filled tubes are balanced (to within the manufacturer's recommended limit).

8. Place tubes into ultracentrifuge rotor. Ultracentrifuge at $100,000 \times g$ for 75 min at 4 °C (*see* **Note 6**).

9. The exosome pellet should be visible on the radial aspect of ultracentrifuge tube. Carefully aspirate supernatant without disturbing pellet. (If the pellet is not visible, leave 1 mL at the bottom of the tube and use this when pooling exosomes together - see next step.)

10. Resuspend the exosome pellet in 200 μL PBS. Pool exosomes together into one ultracentrifuge tube. Fill tube to capacity with PBS.

11. Ultracentrifuge again at $100,000 \times g$ for 75 min at 4 °C.

12. Aspirate supernatant as above.

13. Resuspend washed exosome pellet in 200 μL PBS (for cell transfer), 200 μL 2× Laemmli buffer (western blotting), 100 μL Lysis solution (RNA extraction) or 50 μL sterile water (unfixed imaging by transmission electron microscopy) (*see* **Note 7**).

14. Store samples at 4 °C for short term (<1 week) or –80 °C for longer term. Samples for electron microscopy should only be stored at 4 °C (*see* **Note 8**).

3.3 Labeling and Transferring Exosomes

1. Isolate exosomes as above (up to and including **3.2.9**).

2. Resuspend exosome pellet in 200 μL PBS and add 1 μL DiO.

3. Incubate for 20 min at 37 °C.

4. Fill tube to capacity with PBS and ultracentrifuge again at $100,000 \times g$ for 75 min at 4 °C.

5. The washed exosome pellet will be colored with dye. Aspirate supernatant. Resuspend pellet in 200 μL in PBS (*see* **Note 9**).

6. Measure exosomal protein concentration by BCA (or similar) assay as an index of exosome number (*see* **Note 10**).

7. Add the appropriate amount of solubilized exosomes to achieve a concentration of 20-30 μg/mL in the target cell medium. This can be titrated in subsequent experiments.

8. Incubate for 24 h at 37 °C.

9. Visualize using fluorescence microscope with appropriate filter to confirm the presence of fluorescent exosomes within target cells.

3.4 Extraction of Exosomal RNA

1. Resuspend washed exosome pellet in 100 μL Lysis Solution and transfer to a 2 mL nuclease-free tube.

2. Pre-wet the Micro Filter with 30 μL of Lysis Solution.

3. To recover both large and small RNA species add 1.25 volumes of 100% ethanol to the lysate and vortex gently.

4. Load the lysate/ethanol mixture on to the Micro Filter and centrifuge for 1 min at maximum speed to bind the RNA.

5. Add 180 μL of Wash Solution 1 to the filter and centrifuge for 10 s at $16,000 \times g$.

6. Add 180 μL of Wash Solution 2/3 to the filter and centrifuge for 10 s at $16,000 \times g$. Repeat this step once.

7. Remove the Micro Filter cartridge from the collection tube and discard the flow-through. Replace the Micro Filter cartridge into the same collection tube.

8. Centrifuge the Micro Filter cartridge for 1 min at maximum speed to dry the filter.

9. Transfer the Micro Filter cartridge to a clean nuclease-free tube.

10. Elute the RNA in 25 μL of nuclease-free water by centrifuging for 30 s at $16,000 \times g$.

11. Measure the concentration of RNA using a NanoDrop spectrophotometer.

12. Store exosomal RNA at –80 °C.

3.5 Cancer MicroRNA qPCR Array with Quantimir™

1. A minimum amount of 125 ng RNA is required.

2. Set up the Quantimir™ reverse transcription reaction according to the manufacturer's instructions. A total volume of 20.5 μL cDNA is produced.

3. On ice, resuspend forward primers (in the primer plate) with 12.5 μL nuclease-free water per well (see **Note 11**).

4. Load 1 μL primer into each well of the 96-well qPCR reaction plate and cover with adhesive film to prevent evaporation.

5. Combine 2× Power SYBR Green PCR Mastermix, nuclease-free dH_2O and universal reverse primer with 20 μL synthesized cDNA according to the manufacturer's instructions.

6. Load equal volumes of cDNA/Mastermix to each primer in the 96-well qPCR reaction plate.

7. Cover the plate with an optical adhesive cover.

8. Centrifuge plate briefly to bring contents of each well to the bottom.

9. Run real-time qPCR using the following parameters; 50 °C for 2 min, 95 °C for 10 min and 40× cycles of 95 °C for 15 s/60 °C for 1 min.

10. Perform a melt curve after qPCR run to verify specificity of the reaction.

11. Normalize miRNA expression with U6 snRNA CT values (*see* **Note 12**).

12. Calculate fold changes in 95 cancer-associated microRNAs between paired samples, e.g., normal versus cancer-associated exosomes.

4 Notes

1. Penicillin–streptomycin comes as penicillin (10000 U/mL) and streptomycin (10 mg/mL). Fungizone comes as amphotericin B 250 µg/mL. Working concentrations are given in the text as % v/v.

2. Each confluent T175 flask should contain 18 mL medium to concentrate exosomes without depriving cells.

3. 12× T175 flasks of fibroblasts will produce exosomes from which approximately 125–250 ng RNA can be extracted. This is adequate for most downstream analyses.

4. Carcinomatous cells produce approximately three to four times more exosomes than mesenchymal cells as evidenced by total protein and RNA content. A high amount of starting material is therefore required for exosomal protein/RNA analysis from fibroblasts.

5. It is not advised to commence the initial spin at $2000 \times g$ as this may lyse cells releasing organelles into the supernatant.

6. We have found that using an ultracentrifuge with a fixed angle rotor produces a visible exosome pellet (on the radial aspect of the tube) whereas swinging bucket rotors do not.

7. The final exosome pellet is resuspended in whichever solvent is most appropriate for downstream analysis.

8. Samples for electron microscopy should not be frozen as this leads to artifact.

9. Exosome labeling can be incorporated into the routine isolation technique to improve visibility of the pellet.

10. Alternative methods of exosome quantification include lipid assay [15] and NanoSight technology [16].

11. Manufacturer instructions suggest 10 µL of cDNA but 12.5 µL will ensure 10 complete reactions.

12. U6 snRNA was not differentially regulated in our stromal exosome samples, so we use this as an endogenous control. U6 snRNA is also a commonly used endogenous control for normalization of cellular microRNA levels.

References

1. Bhome R, Bullock M, Al Saihati H et al (2015) A top down view of the tumor microenvironment: structure, cells and signaling. Front Cell Dev Biol 3:33

2. Hanahan D, Weinberg RA (2011) Hallmarks of cancer: the next generation. Cell 144: 646–674

3. Emmert-Buck M, Bonner R, Smith P et al (1996) Laser capture microdissection. Science 274:998–1001

4. Bullock MD, Pickard K, Mitter R et al (2015) Stratifying risk of recurrence in stage II colorectal cancer using deregulated stromal and epithelial microRNAs. Oncotarget 6:7262–7279

5. Bullock MD, Pickard KM, Nielsen BS et al (2013) Pleiotropic actions of miR-21 highlight the critical role of deregulated stromal microRNAs during colorectal cancer progression. Cell Death Dis 4, e684

6. Mirnezami A, Pickard K, Zhang L et al (2009) MicroRNAs: key players in carcinogenesis and novel therapeutic targets. Eur J Surg Oncol 35:339–347

7. Esquela-Kerscher A, Slack F (2006) Oncomirs—microRNAs with a role in cancer. Nat Rev Cancer 6:259–269

8. Valadi H, Ekström K, Bossios A et al (2007) Exosome-mediated transfer of mRNAs and microRNAs is a novel mechanism of genetic exchange between cells. Nat Cell Biol 9:654–659

9. Raposo G, Stoorvogel W (2013) Extracellular vesicles: exosomes, microvesicles, and friends. J Cell Biol 200:373–383

10. O'Brien K, Lowry M, Corcoran C et al (2015) miR-134 in extracellular vesicles reduces triple-negative breast cancer aggression and increases drug sensitivity. Oncotarget 6:32774–32789

11. Hu Y, Yan C, Mu L et al (2015) Fibroblast-derived exosomes contribute to chemoresistance through priming cancer stem cells in colorectal cancer. PLoS One 10, e0125625

12. Thery C, Ostrowski M, Segura E (2009) Membrane vesicles as conveyors of immune responses. Nat Rev Immunol 9:581–593

13. van Balkom BW, de Jong OG, Smits M et al (2013) Endothelial cells require miR-214 to secrete exosomes that suppress senescence and induce angiogenesis in human and mouse endothelial cells. Blood 121:3997–4006

14. Lee C, Mitsialis SA, Aslam M et al (2012) Exosomes mediate the cytoprotective action of mesenchymal stromal cells on hypoxia-induced pulmonary hypertension. Circulation 126:2601–2611

15. Osteikoetexea X, Balogh A, Szabo-Taylor K et al (2015) Improved characterization of EV preparations based on protein to lipid ratio and lipid properties. PLoS One 10, e0121184

16. Mehdiani A, Maier A, Pinto A et al (2015) An innovative method for exosome quantification and size measurement. J Vis Exp 95:e50974

Chapter 12

Circulating MicroRNAs in Cancer

Killian P. O'Brien, Eimear Ramphul, Linda Howard, William M. Gallagher, Carmel Malone, Michael J. Kerin, and Róisín M. Dwyer

Abstract

It is believed that microRNAs have potential as circulating biomarkers of disease; however, successful clinical implementation remains a challenge. This chapter highlights broad variations in approaches to microRNA analysis where whole blood, serum and plasma have each been employed as viable sources. Further discrepancies in approaches are seen in endogenous controls and extraction methods utilized. This has resulted in contradictory publications, even when the same microRNA is targeted in the same disease setting.

Analysis of blood samples highlighted the impact of both collection method and storage, on the microRNA profile. Analysis of a panel of microRNAs across whole blood, serum, and plasma originating from the same individual emphasized the impact of starting material on microRNA profile. This is a highly topical field of research with immense potential for translation into the clinical setting. Standardization of sample harvesting, processing and analysis will be key to this translation. Methods of sample harvesting, preservation, and analysis are outlined, with important mitigating factors highlighted.

Key words Circulating microRNAs, Breast Cancer, Whole blood, Serum, Plasma

1 Introduction

1.1 MicroRNAs

Once microRNAs were shown to be detectable in the circulation of patients with cancer, a surge of interest regarding these molecules implementation as biomarkers for the disease quickly ensued. Further research discovered that microRNAs could be protein bound or encapsulated in vesicles in the circulation [1].

In the breast cancer field alone, this breakthrough has resulted in the emergence of a significant number of studies analyzing breast cancer patient blood samples for the possibility of identifying clinically relevant microRNAs. Despite tremendous potential, microRNAs have not yet been implemented in the clinical setting as a biomarker of disease. There is not a standardized approach to investigating these molecules, resulting in many different methods being employed. All three starting materials (whole blood, plasma, or serum) have been analyzed following differing methods of

Sweta Rani (ed.), *MicroRNA Profiling: Methods and Protocols*, Methods in Molecular Biology, vol. 1509,
DOI 10.1007/978-1-4939-6524-3_12, © Springer Science+Business Media New York 2017

extraction (TRIzol or column-based) with data generated being normalized to a large variety of endogenous controls. This variance in approaches to circulating microRNAs has resulted in opposing published results. Contradictory results can be seen in this field even when the same target microRNA is being investigated. For example, in one study circulating levels of miR-10b were found at significantly higher levels in the serum of breast cancer patients when compared to healthy controls, while another study reported no significant difference in the whole blood of patients versus healthy individuals [2, 3]. This pattern was mirrored in other studies where miR-106a and miR-155 were found to be elevated in the serum of patients with breast cancer when compared to healthy individuals [4, 5]. However, when these microRNAs were analyzed in plasma samples by other research groups, no significant change was observed in breast cancer patients compared to healthy controls [4, 5]. miR-145 was also analyzed in the plasma and serum of breast cancer patients and compared to healthy controls by two separate groups [2, 6]. Analyzing miR-145 in the serum suggested a significant increase in the patient cohort, while it was found to be decreased in the plasma of patients when compared to healthy controls [2, 6].

However, separate studies using different source materials can achieve similar results. For example, two separate groups carried out analysis of miR-21 in serum and plasma respectively, and both concluded that it was up-regulated in patients when compared to healthy controls [4, 6].

Variation is not limited to starting material, but is also witnessed in methods of extracting microRNA with some implementing TRIzol based methods, while others opt for column-based approaches on the same source material [7, 8]. Storage and handling of samples vary across the studies also, with some utilizing storage of whole blood at –80 °C in PAXgene™ tubes while others report storage in EDTA tubes at 4 °C [3, 9]. These contrasting approaches to analysis could impact results seen, thus inhibiting publication of consistent findings and preventing the progression of the field into the clinical setting.

1.2 Sample Source

Circulating microRNAs have been analyzed in serum, plasma and whole blood of breast cancer patients and healthy controls. MicroRNAs are found to be relatively stable in these starting materials as well as other fluids such as saliva and urine. This is due to being either protein bound or encapsulated in exosomes; this makes each source material a viable option for analysis [1]. It is imperative for these samples to be stored appropriately. Whichever starting material is routinely collected in the host lab is likely to be the greatest influencing factor for researchers when choosing a starting material. A review of the literature revealed publications using each of these sources, with serum employed in the majority of studies (Table 1).

Table 1
Overview of starting material used in studies analyzing circulating microRNAs in breast cancer

Source of extracted microRNAs	Studies Published to Date	References
Whole Blood	8	[3, 9, 17, 20, 26–29]
Serum	26	[2, 4, 7, 8, 18, 21, 22, 30–48]
Plasma	13	[5, 6, 15, 19, 23, 24, 49–55]

1.3   Whole Blood   Eight papers have published results analyzing circulating microRNAs in the whole blood of patients with breast cancer. This would be an ideal source of identifying and analyzing circulating microRNAs as it could be tested after taking a simple pinprick sample from an individual. While some studies reported use of whole blood collected in standard EDTA tubes, more recently, PAXgene™ tubes have been employed for analysis of whole blood. PAXgene™ tubes contain a blend of proprietary reagents that lyse all cells, allowing immediate stabilization of RNA. This stability is maintained for 3 days when stored at room temperature, and up to 8 years when stored at –80 °C [10]. RNA extracted from whole blood will result in greater amounts of RNA available for downstream analysis when compared to the lower, but adequate, quantity of RNA extracted from serum and plasma.

However, whole blood contains many cellular constituents, which may impact upon levels of microRNAs being detected. The presence of red blood cells can impact particular microRNAs. For example, miR-16 and miR-451 have been found to be at much higher levels on erythrocytes [11]. As a result of the many cellular elements existing in whole blood, a published study took white cell counts, hemoglobin and hematocrit levels into account in order to reduce the likelihood of sample-to-sample variability [3].

An issue when using whole blood as a source of microRNAs is storage of the sample. Samples can be collected in EDTA and PAXgene™ tubes and can then be frozen for long term storage at –80 °C. However, some studies also reported the long term storage of whole blood in EDTA tubes at 4 °C [3]. Stabilizing the RNA in the collected sample is crucial, as it is now understood that certain microRNAs have very short half-lives, some as short as an hour [12]. This highlights the necessity to standardize methods of collecting samples in order to reduce potential variability associated with particular microRNA instability.

1.4   Plasma   As whole blood contains many factors such as erythrocytes that are capable of effecting levels of particular microRNAs, cell-free sources have been employed to analyze circulating microRNAs. There have been 13 published papers that analyzed this source in the breast cancer setting. As with the two other sources of circulating microRNAs, many publications did not provide a rationale as to why plasma was chosen. Plasma is obtained through a centrifugation process and contains certain clotting factors such as fibrinogen, requiring the addition of anticoagulants such as heparin. This addition has been shown to inhibit the downstream process of PCR analysis while citrate and EDTA have been deemed acceptable [13]. Plasma is advantageous when used for retrospective studies as it is routinely stored at –80 °C where it has been reported to remain stable and suitable for subsequent analysis. One study has shown that freeze thawing of plasma samples stored at –80 °C does not affect microRNAs present at high levels [14]. There is a risk of contaminating plasma samples with cells when aspirating the sample as this can subsequently result in detection of cellular based microRNAs as well as increasing levels of certain circulating microRNAs in the extracted RNA [13].

There are certain preanalytic variabilities associated with plasma. The time between sample collection and processing can significantly impact sample quality so it is important to standardize this time for each sample [13]. Differences can also be seen in how samples are centrifuged. Some studies report that samples were spun at $1300 \times g$ for 20 min at 10 °C, and others at $600 \times g$ for 15 min at room temperature [6, 15].

1.5 Serum

The most studied source of circulating microRNAs is serum and this is represented by 26 published studies in breast cancer alone. Serum is also a cell-free source, but unlike plasma, the sample must first undergo the coagulation process prior to centrifugation [13]. Similar to plasma, serum can be stored at –80 °C for long periods of time. A study was carried out where plasma and serum samples from the same group of individuals were compared for certain microRNAs [16]. This study found miR-15b, -16, and -24 to be detected at higher levels in plasma when compared to serum of matched individuals. This study stated that results from serum and plasma samples are not interchangeable when looking at microRNA levels. It states the need for a rigorous protocol for centrifugation to be set in place in order to standardize this method. It was also discovered that hemolysis can lead to the detection of artificially high levels of miR-15b and miR-16 [16].

2 Materials

1. EDTA tubes, serum-separating tubes and PAXgene™ tubes.

2. TRIzol, bromoanisole (BAN), isopropanol, and 75 % ethanol, store at room temperature (RT).

3. PreAnalytix kit (Qiagen/BD).

   (a) RNase-free water

   (b) Buffer BM1

   (c) Buffer BM2

   (d) Buffer BM3 (add 100% ethanol as indicated)

   (e) Buffer BM4 (add 100% ethanol as indicated)

   (f) BR5

   (g) Proteinase K

   (h) DNase 1 stock solution (dissolve in RNase-free water) store at 4 °C

   (i) Buffer RDD

   (j) PAXgene™ shredder spin column

   (k) PAXgene™ RNA spin column

4. miRCURY™ kit (Exiqon):

   (a) Collection tubes

   (b) microRNA mini spin column BF

   (c) Lysis solution BF

   (d) Protein precipitation solution BF

   (e) Wash solution 1 BF

   (f) Wash solution 2 BF (add 100% as outlined)

   (g) RNase-free water

5. Nuclease-free water, store at 4 °C.

6. Isopropanol.

7. NanoDrop-1000 (ND-1000) Spectrophotometer.

8. Deoxynucleotide mix, 10× RT Buffer (100 mM), RNase Inhibitor (20 U/μL), Multiscribe (50 U/μL), Stem loop primer and a Probe (Applied Biosystems), store at –20 °C.

9. GeneAmp PCR system 9700 (Applied Biosystems).

10. TaqMan Fast mix (Applied Biosystems) store at 4 °C.

11. MicroAmp® Fast Optical 96-well Reaction Plate with Barcode (0.1 mL) and a MicroAmp optical adhesive film ·(Applied Biosystems).

12. 7900HT Fast Real Time PCR system (Life Technologies).

13. Shaker-Incubator PHMT (Grant-Bio).

14. 75% Ethanol: 125 mL dH$_2$O and 375 mL 100% Ethanol (make up to 500 mL and store at RT).

15. 100% Ethanol.

3 Methods

3.1 Serum and Plasma Separation

1. Serum: collect whole blood in serum separating tubes and let stand at RT for 30 min for sample to coagulate prior to centrifugation at $3000 \times g$ for 5 min, remove supernatant and subsequently store at -80 °C.

2. Plasma: collect whole blood directly into EDTA tubes in order to prevent coagulation of the sample. Samples are then centrifuged at $3000 \times g$ for 5 min, remove supernatant and store at -80 °C.

3.2 Extraction of RNA

3.2.1 From EDTA Collected Whole Blood Using TRIzol BD [17] Method

1. Collect whole blood directly into an EDTA tube to prevent any coagulation of the sample and store sample at 4 °C as quickly as possible until extraction.

2. Add 3 mL of TRIzol to a 5 mL tube.

3. Add 200 µL of BAN to the TRIzol and the sample is mixed.

4. Add 1 mL of whole blood to the mixture and sample is thoroughly mixed until entire sample is homogenous.

5. Stand samples at RT for 5 min prior to centrifugation at $18,000 \times g$ for 15 min at 4 °C where samples will undergo phase separation leaving a clear aqueous upper phase which contains the required RNA.

6. Remove 1 mL of the aqueous phase without interfering with the middle interphase layer. Discard remaining sample.

7. Add 1 mL of isopropanol to the aqueous phase and stand at RT for 5 min.

8. Spin sample at $18,000 \times g$ for 5 min at 18 °C.

9. Remove supernatant completely from the pellet.

10. Add 1 mL of 75 % ethanol to pellet and mix by vortex.

11. Centrifuge sample at $18,000 \times g$ for 5 min at 18 °C.

12. Remove ethanol without disturbing the pellet and repeat addition of 75 % ethanol and centrifugation step.

13. After removing 75 % ethanol for a second time allow pellet to air-dry at RT for up to 5 min, or until the pellet has dried sufficiently.

14. Add 30 µL of NFW and vortex the sample before leaving it stand at RT for 5 min.

3.2.2 From PAXgene™ Collected Whole Blood

1. Collect whole blood directly into PAXgene™ tube and store at RT for 2 h prior to long term storage at -80 °C (*see* **Note 1**).

2. Thaw sample at RT for at least 1 h prior to extraction.

3. Centrifuge sample at $4500 \times g$ for 10 min.

4. Remove and discard supernatant from pellet.

5. Add 4 mL RNase-free water, seal tube using a new Hemogard closure and vortex sample to suspend pellet.

6. Centrifuge at $4500 \times g$ for 10 min.

7. Remove and discard supernatant; add 350 µL of buffer BM1 and vortex until pellet is dissolved.

8. Transfer sample into 1.5 mL microcentrifuge tube.

9. Add 300 µL buffer BM2 to sample and then 40 µL proteinase K and vortex for 5 s.

10. Incubate sample for 10 min at 55 °C and 900 RPM on shaker-incubator.

11. Pipet sample into PAXgene™ Shredder spin column and centrifuge at $20,000 \times g$ for 3 min.

12. Transfer supernatant to fresh microcentrifuge tube without disrupting pellet.

13. Add 700 µL of isopropanol to supernatant and vortex sample to mix.

14. Pipet 700 µL of sample into PAXgene™ RNA spin column and centrifuge at $20,000 \times g$ for 1 min.

15. Discard flow-through and repeat **Step 14** until entire sample has passed through PAXgene™ RNA spin column.

16. Add 350 µL of buffer BM3 and centrifuge sample at $20,000 \times g$ for 15 s.

17. Add 10 µL DNase 1 stock solution to 70 µL buffer RDD in a separate microcentrifuge tube.

18. Add 80 µL of mixture directly onto PAXgene™ RNA spin column membrane and incubate at RT for 15 min.

19. Add 350 µL of buffer BM3 to column and centrifuge at $20,000 \times g$ for 15 s.

20. Discard flow-through, add 500 µL of buffer BM4 to column and centrifuge at $20,000 \times g$ for 2 min.

21. Repeat **Step 20**.

22. Discard flow-through and centrifuge column at $20,000 \times g$ for 1 min.

23. Place column into fresh collection tube and pipet 40 µL of buffer BR5 directly onto column membrane and centrifuge at $20,000 \times g$ for 1 min.

24. Pipet another 40 µL of buffer BR5 onto column membrane and centrifuge at $20,000 \times g$ for 1 min.

25. Incubate eluate at 65 °C for 5 min in shaker-incubator.

26. Following incubation place sample directly on ice or store at −80 °C for future use.

3.2.3 From Serum and Plasma

1. Allow samples to thaw on ice.

2. Once thawed, centrifuge samples at $3000 \times g$ for 5 min.

3. Transfer 200 μL of sample to microcentrifuge tube and add 60 μL of Lysis solution BF.

4. Vortex for 5 s and incubate for 5 min at RT.

5. Add 20 μL of protein precipitation solution BF and vortex for 5 s.

6. Incubate at RT for 1 min and then centrifuge at $11,000 \times g$ for 3 min.

7. Transfer supernatant to fresh tube without disturbing pellet.

8. Add 270 μL isopropanol to sample and vortex for 5 s.

9. Put microRNA Mini Spin Column BF into a collection tube and add sample to column.

10. Incubate at RT for 2 min and then centrifuge at $11,000 \times g$ for 30 s.

11. Discard flow-through and repeat **Steps 9** and **10** if there is sample remaining.

12. Add 100 μL wash solution 1 BF to column and centrifuge at $11,000 \times g$ for 30 s.

13. Discard flow-through, add 700 μL wash solution 2 BF to column and centrifuge at $11,000 \times g$ for 30 s.

14. Discard flow-through, add 250 μL wash solution 2 BF to column and centrifuge at $11,000 \times g$ for 2 min.

15. Place column in fresh collection tube and add 50 μL RNase-free water directly onto the column membrane.

16. Incubate for 1 min at RT and centrifuge at $11,000 \times g$ for 1 min.

17. Store samples at –80 °C for future use.

3.3 Determining RNA Quality and Quantity

1. Place 1.1 μL of NFW on pedestal of ND-1000 spectrophotometer to act as a blank (*see* **Note 2**).

2. Adjust wavelength to 260 nm for analysis of RNA. Add 1.1 μL of sample onto pedestal and acquire reading to determine quantity and quality of RNA extracted.

3.4 cDNA Synthesis of MicroRNA

1. Appropriate amount of RNA required for cDNA synthesis (25–100 ng) is calculated based on yield following analysis on ND-1000 spectrophotometer.

2. NFW is added to RNA to achieve a final volume of 5μl.

3. A premix of 10 μL is made up for each sample of extracted RNA and each microRNA being reverse transcribed as follows (Table 2):

Table 2
Components of cDNA synthesis premix

Component	Volume (µL)
dNTP mix (100 mM)	0.17
10× RT Buffer	1.65
NFW	4.57
RNase Inhibitor (20 U/µL)	0.21
Multiscribe (50 U/µL)	1.1
Stem Loop Primer	3.1

4. Add components of the premix as outlined in (Table 2).

5. Add 10 µL of premix to 5 µL of RNA. Samples are thoroughly mixed and centrifuged in a microcentrifuge for < 1 min.

6. Place samples into a GeneAmp PCR system 9700 and are set to one cycle of 30 min at 16 °C, 30 min at 42 °C, and 5 min at 4 °C. Samples are then maintained at 4 °C until required.

7. Store samples at −20 °C until further use.

3.5 RQ-PCR Analysis of MicroRNA

1. Make premix up to 9.3 µL for each sample and target microRNA being analyzed, consisting of 5 µL Fast Mastermix, 3.8 µL of NFW and 0.5 µL of microRNA Probe.

2. Add 0.7 µL of cDNA to each well of the 96-well plate.

3. Add the corresponding 9.3 µL of premix to the appropriate cDNA sample where every sample is run in triplicate (*see* **Note 3**).

4. After all samples and premix are added seal the plate with MicroAmp optical adhesive film and centrifuged at $1000 \times g$ for 1 min.

5. Plates are then run on a Thermocycler where cycles of 20 s at 95 °C, 1 s at 95 °C, and 20 s at 60 °C are repeated.

6. Data is collected and analyzed.

3.6 Comparing microRNA Profile in Whole Blood, Serum, and Plasma from Same Individual

Whole blood, plasma, and serum samples, originating from the same patient were collected and subsequently had the microRNA profile analyzed (Fig. 1). Whole blood was collected and stored in PAXgene™ tubes, while plasma samples were collected in EDTA tubes and serum samples were collected in serum separating tubes. Plasma and serum samples were centrifuged at $3000 \times g$ for 5 min. miR-16 was used for this comparison due to its frequent use as an endogenous control.

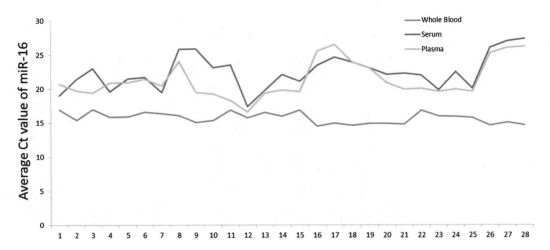

Fig. 1 Comparing levels of miR-16 across whole blood, plasma, and serum from the same individuals

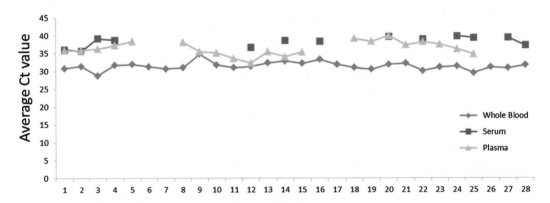

Fig. 2 Comparing levels of miR-504 across whole blood, plasma, and serum from the same individuals

miR-16 was detectable in all samples analyzed (Fig. 1). Different trends in miR-16 levels can be seen across the three sources with similar patterns noticed between certain individuals when analyzing plasma and serum. However, the miR-16 values were clearly more variable in plasma (Ct range: 17–27) and serum (Ct range: 18–26) than in PAXgene™ stabilized blood (Ct range: 14–16) from the same individuals.

Two more microRNAs were also analyzed across these same matching samples, miR-138 and miR-504. Firstly, miR-504 was detected in all whole blood samples. In contrast, it was detected in 46 % of serum samples and 75 % of plasma samples (Fig. 2). This suggests that when analyzing particular microRNAs, source material may be crucial for accurate analysis.

Analysis of miR-138 in the same cohort of samples yielded similar results with the microRNA detectable in every whole blood sample analyzed, while it was detected in only 57 % of serum samples and 68 % of plasma samples (data not shown).

3.7 Impact of Hemolysis

A very important issue to consider when using serum and plasma as a source for microRNA analysis is hemolysis. Hemolysis is the rupturing of erythrocytes and can be measured by quantifying levels of free hemoglobin in the sample (*see* **Note 4**). This is achieved using a spectrophotometer to analyze levels of oxy-hemoglobin, which is detected when peaks at wavelength $\lambda = 414$ are observed indicating that a sample is hemolyzed [11]. Another method of detecting hemolysis is to analyze particular microRNAs that are known to be enriched in erythrocytes, such as miR- 451 and miR-144 [11]. These steps are necessary when determining the quality of the source material as hemolysis does have an effect on the portrait of microRNAs seen in these samples.

Hemolysis is an issue that was ignored at first but as the field has developed it became far too great a problem not to be addressed. It has been shown to effect levels of certain microRNAs, such as miR-16, miR-15b, and miR-24 [11]. As miR-16 has been employed as endogenous control for studies looking at circulating microRNAs in both serum and plasma, it makes the issue of hemolysis a major factor in data analysis and something that cannot be overlooked [18, 19].

3.8 Impact of Variations in Extraction Methods

There is a large variation in extraction methods when looking across all publications regarding circulating microRNAs in breast cancer, with nine different methods employed, eight of which are column-based (Table 3).

As part of the current study, analysis of particular microRNAs in whole blood was carried out on samples stored in EDTA tubes followed by TRIzol BD extraction, as well as microRNAs analyzed

Table 3
Different extraction methods used in analysis of circulating microRNAs in breast cancer. (X indicating at least 1 published use of technique)

Method	Whole Blood	Serum	Plasma
mirVana miRNA isolation kit		X	X
mirVana PARIS kit		X	
miRNeasy mini kit	X	X	X
TRIzol LS method		X	X
TRIzol BD method	X	X	X
BioChain miRNA isolation kit		X	
MagMax viral RNA isolation kit		X	
Norgens RNA purification kit		X	X
Allprep DNA/RNA micro kit	X		

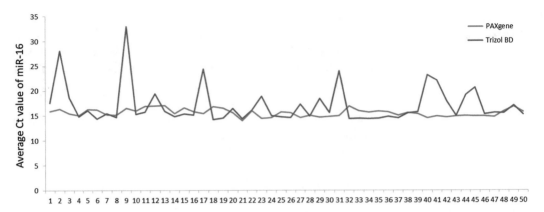

Fig. 3 Comparison of miR-16 levels in whole blood harvested into PAXgene™ tubes followed by PreAnalytix extraction, or EDTA tubes followed by TRIzol BD method respectively

in whole blood samples collected in PAXgene™ tubes followed by extraction using the PreAnalytix kit (Qiagen). Levels of miR-16 were analyzed and detected using RQ-PCR analysis (Fig. 3).

miR-16 was detected at high levels (low Ct value) as it is robustly present in whole blood. Expression was found to be more stable in the PAXgene™ processed samples, with miR-16 ranging from 14 to 16 Ct. In contrast, whole blood collected in EDTA tubes with subsequent TRIzol extraction was found to be much less stable, with miR-16 ranging from 14 to 34 Ct. In samples collected, stored and extracted in this manner, miR-16 would not be deemed a suitable endogenous control.

3.9 Impact of Endogenous Controls

Following a similar pattern, there is also inconsistency in relation to which endogenous controls are employed for the analysis of circulating microRNAs in breast cancer, with 12 different endogenous controls used for analysis of serum microRNAs alone (Table 4). An endogenous control would ideally be stably expressed across all samples used for analysis so that sample-to-sample variability can be accounted for, as well as variations in template loading and varying efficiencies of reaction.

These endogenous controls range from microRNAs to ribosomal RNAs, to spiked in controls. Entire studies are carried out to establish appropriate endogenous controls for analysis of blood [20]. Many published studies determine suitability of endogenous control across a range of samples to ensure that it is stably expressed prior to employment [21].

miR-16 is seen as an appropriate endogenous control for each source material and one that has featured in several publications [7, 9, 18–20, 22–24]. There has also been work stating that miR-16 along with other microRNAs are impacted by blood cells and hemolysis [25]. As shown in Fig. 3, miR-16 can fluctuate depending on storage and extraction method. In our hands it was found to be robust and stable in PAXgene™ collected whole blood.

Table 4
Variation in endogenous controls used in literature of circulating microRNAs in breast cancer

Endogenous Control	Whole Blood	Serum	Plasma
5 s rRNA		X	
18S rRNA		X	
cel-miR-39		X	X
miR-16	X	X	X
GAPDH		X	
miR-1825		X	
U6 snRNA		X	
RNU6B		X	X
miR-191		X	
miR-484		X	
SNORD44		X	
miR-192		X	
U6			X
miR-92			X

One study chose to normalize the data to the mean and median of all microRNAs measured in a sample [26]. As endogenous controls heavily influence data analysis it is crucial that there is not a large degree of variability seen in this sector of the field. Standardization of starting material, methods of harvesting, storage and extraction will impact endogenous controls.

3.10   Conclusion

This chapter highlights a number of issues that have a significant impact on the outcome of circulating microRNA studies. This in turn is preventing the realization of the full potential of microRNAs as biomarkers of disease. Standardization of approaches to analyzing microRNAs in the circulation could help establishment of these molecules as clinically relevant biomarkers.

Whole blood, plasma, and serum have all been shown to be appropriate for analyzing circulating microRNAs, and each with varying methods of sample collection and storage. This shows that there are many ways of analyzing microRNAs and that overall, no one method is necessarily superior to another. The issue is reproducibility, and that the different starting materials are not suitable for comparison. Consistency is required to support reliable comparison of data generated by different groups. Until the factors influencing microRNA presence, stability and detection in the circulation are clearly defined it is imperative that there is an attempt at standardization.

Understanding and addressing the mitigating factors that can negatively impact upon a study, such as hemolysis, is critical in achieving standardization across this field and resulting in more consistent and reproducible findings. If achieved, this may allow microRNAs to fulfill their potential as circulating biomarkers of many diseases.

3.11 Outcome

If using whole blood, authors recommend collection in PAXgene™ tubes where the collection and storage guidelines are strictly adhered to. For plasma and serum collection it is crucial that samples are handled carefully and guidelines for temperature, time and centrifugation are followed rigidly. It is necessary to check and compensate for hemolysis in both plasma and serum samples. It is important to note that each starting material is a viable source; however, certain microRNAs are not present at sufficiently high levels to be detected in particular fractions. Therefore, it is necessary to carry out preliminary analysis prior to commencing a large study analyzing a particular microRNA in the circulation.

4 Notes

1. When collecting whole blood into PAXgene™ tubes it is important for samples to be incubated for 2 h at RT in order to allow the reagents in the tube to lyse the whole blood sample.

2. When analyzing samples on the ND-1000 it is important to pay particular attention to both the 260/230 nm and 260/280 nm ratios. If ratios are not in the required range of 1.8–2.1 for samples analyzed, it could impact subsequent RQ-PCR analysis.

3. For RQ-PCR analysis keep mixtures containing the probe in opaque tubes in order to prevent any photo-bleaching of the fluorophore which may impact analysis.

4. When harvesting serum and plasma, care in handling is critical in order to prevent hemolysis of the sample. When carrying out analysis on a patient cohort it is important to take hemolysis into consideration. As hemolysis is not always readily detectable through visual analysis, it is important to analyze samples by means mentioned previously in this chapter.

Acknowledgements

This material is based upon works supported by the Irish Cancer Society collaborative cancer research centre BREAST-PREDICT Grant CCRC13GAL and funding agency "Breast Cancer Research".

References

1. Chen X, Liang H, Zhang J et al (2012) Secreted microRNAs: a new form of intercellular communication. Trends Cell Biol 22(3):125–132. doi:10.1016/j.tcb.2011.12.001, doi:S0962-8924(11)00238-8 [pii]

2. Mar-Aguilar F, Mendoza-Ramirez JA, Malagon-Santiago I et al (2013) Serum circulating microRNA profiling for identification of potential breast cancer biomarkers. Dis Markers 34(3):163–169. doi:10.3233/Dma-120957

3. Heneghan HM, Miller N, Kelly R et al (2010) Systemic miRNA-195 differentiates breast cancer from other malignancies and is a potential biomarker for detecting noninvasive and early stage disease. Oncologist 15(7):673–682. doi:10.1634/theoncologist.2010-0103, doi:theoncologist.2010-0103 [pii]

4. Wang F, Zheng Z, Guo J et al (2010) Correlation and quantitation of microRNA aberrant expression in tissues and sera from patients with breast tumor. Gynecol Oncol 119(3):586–593. doi:10.1016/j.ygyno.2010.07.021, S0090-8258(10)00550-0 [pii]

5. Cookson VJ, Bentley MA, Hogan BV et al (2012) Circulating microRNA profiles reflect the presence of breast tumours but not the profiles of microRNAs within the tumours. Cell Oncol (Dordr) 35(4):301–308. doi:10.1007/s13402-012-0089-1

6. Ng EKO, Li RFN, Shin VY et al (2013) Circulating microRNAs as specific biomarkers for breast cancer detection. PLoS One 8(1), e53141, doi:ARTN e53141. DOI 10.1371/journal.pone.0053141

7. Wu XW, Somlo G, Yu Y et al (2012) De novo sequencing of circulating miRNAs identifies novel markers predicting clinical outcome of locally advanced breast cancer. J Transl Med 10:42. doi:10.1186/1479-5876-10-42

8. Schwarzenbach H, Milde-Langosch K, Steinbach B et al (2012) Diagnostic potential of PTEN-targeting miR-214 in the blood of breast cancer patients. Breast Cancer Res Treat 134(3):933–941. doi:10.1007/s10549-012-1988-6

9. Schrauder MG, Strick R, Schulz-Wendtland R et al (2012) Circulating micro-RNAs as potential blood-based markers for early stage breast cancer detection. PLoS One 7(1), e29770. doi:10.1371/journal.pone.0029770, PONE-D-11-17907 [pii]

10. Shaffer J (2012) miRNA profiling from blood — challenges and recommendations. Qiagen

11. Kirschner MB, Kao SC, Edelman JJ et al (2011) Haemolysis during sample preparation alters microRNA content of plasma. PLoS One 6(9), e24145. doi:10.1371/journal.pone.0024145

12. Sethi P, Lukiw WJ (2009) Micro-RNA abundance and stability in human brain: specific alterations in Alzheimer's disease temporal lobe neocortex. Neurosci Lett 459(2):100–104. doi:10.1016/j.neulet.2009.04.052

13. Kroh EM, Parkin RK, Mitchell PS et al (2010) Analysis of circulating microRNA biomarkers in plasma and serum using quantitative reverse transcription-PCR (qRT-PCR). Methods 50(4):298–301. doi:10.1016/j.ymeth.2010.01.032

14. Mitchell PS, Parkin RK, Kroh EM et al (2008) Circulating microRNAs as stable blood-based markers for cancer detection. Proc Natl Acad Sci U S A 105(30):10513–10518. doi:10.1073/pnas.0804549105, 0804549105 [pii]

15. Leidner RS, Li L, Thompson CL (2013) Dampening enthusiasm for circulating MicroRNA in breast cancer. PLoS One 8(3), e57841. doi:10.1371/journal.pone.0057841

16. McDonald JS, Milosevic D, Reddi HV et al (2011) Analysis of circulating microRNA: preanalytical and analytical challenges. Clin Chem 57(6):833–840. doi:10.1373/clinchem.2010.157198

17. Heneghan HM, Miller N, Lowery AJ et al (2010) Circulating microRNAs as novel minimally invasive biomarkers for breast cancer. Ann Surg 251(3):499–505. doi:10.1097/Sla.0b013e3181cc939f

18. Si HY, Sun XM, Chen YJ et al (2013) Circulating microRNA-92a and microRNA-21 as novel minimally invasive biomarkers for primary breast cancer. J Cancer Res Clin 139(2):223–229. doi:10.1007/s00432-012-1315-y

19. Zeng RC, Zhang W, Yan XQ et al (2013) Down-regulation of miRNA-30a in human plasma is a novel marker for breast cancer. Med Oncol 30(1):477. doi:10.1007/S12032-013-0477-Z

20. McDermott AM, Kerin MJ, Miller N (2013) Identification and validation of miRNAs as endogenous controls for RQ-PCR in blood specimens for breast cancer studies. PLoS One 8(12), e83718. doi:10.1371/journal.pone.0083718

21. Anfossi S, Giordano A, Gao H et al (2014) High serum miR-19a levels Are associated with inflammatory breast cancer and Are predictive of favorable clinical outcome in patients with metastatic HER2(+) inflammatory breast cancer. PLoS One 9(1), e83113. doi:10.1371/journal.pone.0083113

22. Wang HJ, Tan G, Dong L et al (2012) Circulating MiR-125b as a marker predicting

chemoresistance in breast cancer. PLoS One 7(4), e34210. doi:10.1371/journal.pone.0034210

23. Chen W, Cai F, Zhang B et al (2013) The level of circulating miRNA-10b and miRNA-373 in detecting lymph node metastasis of breast cancer: potential biomarkers. Tumour Biol 34(1):455–462. doi:10.1007/s13277-012-0570-5

24. Kumar S, Keerthana R, Pazhanimuthu A et al (2013) Overexpression of circulating miRNA-21 and miRNA-146a in plasma samples of breast cancer patients. Indian J Biochem Biophys 50(3):210–214

25. Pritchard CC, Kroh E, Wood B et al (2012) Blood cell origin of circulating microRNAs: a cautionary note for cancer biomarker studies. Cancer Prev Res (Phila) 5(3):492–497. doi:10.1158/1940-6207.CAPR-11-0370

26. Sieuwerts AM, Mostert B, Bolt-de Vries J et al (2011) mRNA and microRNA expression profiles in circulating tumor cells and primary tumors of metastatic breast cancer patients. Clin Cancer Res 17(11):3600–3618. doi:10.1158/1078-0432.CCR-11-0255

27. Khan S, Brougham CL, Ryan J et al (2013) miR-379 regulates cyclin B1 expression and is decreased in breast cancer. PLoS One 8(7):e68753. doi:10.1371/journal.pone.0068753

28. Waters PS, Dwyer RM, Brougham C et al (2014) Impact of tumour epithelial subtype on circulating microRNAs in breast cancer patients. PLoS One 9(3), e90605. doi:10.1371/journal.pone.0090605

29. Waters PS, McDermott AM, Wall D et al (2012) Relationship between circulating and tissue microRNAs in a murine model of breast cancer. PLoS One 7(11), e50459. doi:10.1371/journal.pone.0050459

30. Wang PY, Gong HT, Li BF et al (2013) Higher expression of circulating miR-182 as a novel biomarker for breast cancer. Oncol Lett 6(6):1681–1686. doi:10.3892/Ol.2013.1593

31. Eichelser C, Flesch-Janys D, Chang-Claude J et al (2013) Deregulated serum concentrations of circulating cell-free MicroRNAs miR-17, miR-34a, miR-155, and miR-373 in human breast cancer development and progression. Clin Chem 59(10):1489–1496. doi:10.1373/clinchem.2013.205161

32. Sun Y, Wang MJ, Lin GG et al (2012) Serum MicroRNA-155 as a potential biomarker to track disease in breast cancer. PLoS One 7(10), e47003. doi:10.1371/journal.pone.0047003

33. van Schooneveld E, Wouters MCA, Van der Auwera I et al (2012) Expression profiling of cancerous and normal breast tissues identifies microRNAs that are differentially expressed in serum from patients with (metastatic) breast cancer and healthy volunteers. Breast Cancer Res 14(1):R34. doi:10.1186/Bcr3127

34. Asaga S, Kuo C, Nguyen T et al (2011) Direct serum assay for MicroRNA-21 concentrations in early and advanced breast cancer. Clin Chem 57(1):84–91. doi:10.1373/clinchem.2010.151845

35. Zhu W, Qin W, Atasoy U et al (2009) Circulating microRNAs in breast cancer and healthy subjects. BMC Res Notes 2:89. doi:10.1186/1756-0500-2-89

36. Li J, Zhang Y, Zhang W et al (2013) Genetic heterogeneity of breast cancer metastasis may be related to miR-21 regulation of TIMP-3 in translation. Int J Surg Oncol 2013:875078. doi:10.1155/2013/875078

37. Godfrey AC, Xu Z, Weinberg CR et al (2013) Serum microRNA expression as an early marker for breast cancer risk in prospectively collected samples from the Sister Study cohort. Breast Cancer Res 15(3):R42. doi:10.1186/bcr3428

38. Tang D, Zhang Q, Zhao S et al (2013) The expression and clinical significance of microRNA-1258 and heparanase in human breast cancer. Clin Biochem 46(10-11):926–932. doi:10.1016/j.clinbiochem.2013.01.027

39. Zhao FL, Hu GD, Wang XF et al (2012) Serum overexpression of microRNA-10b in patients with bone metastatic primary breast cancer. J Int Med Res 40(3):859–866

40. Guo LJ, Zhang QY (2012) Decreased serum miR-181a is a potential new tool for breast cancer screening. Int J Mol Med 30(3):680–686. doi:10.3892/ijmm.2012.1021

41. Wang X, Wu X, Yan L et al (2012) Serum miR-103 as a potential diagnostic biomarker for breast cancer. Nan Fang Yi Ke Da Xue Xue Bao 32(5):631–634

42. Wu Q, Wang C, Lu Z et al (2012) Analysis of serum genome-wide microRNAs for breast cancer detection. Clin Chim Acta 413(13-14):1058–1065. doi:10.1016/j.cca.2012.02.016

43. Hu Z, Dong J, Wang LE et al (2012) Serum microRNA profiling and breast cancer risk: the use of miR-484/191 as endogenous controls. Carcinogenesis 33(4):828–834. doi:10.1093/carcin/bgs030, doi:bgs030 [pii]

44. Appaiah HN, Goswami CP, Mina LA et al (2011) Persistent upregulation of U6:SNORD44 small RNA ratio in the serum of breast cancer patients. Breast Cancer Res 13(5):R86. doi:10.1186/bcr2943

45. Wu Q, Lu Z, Li H et al (2011) Next-generation sequencing of microRNAs for breast cancer

detection. J Biomed Biotechnol 2011:597145. doi:10.1155/2011/597145

46. Gotte M (2010) MicroRNAs in breast cancer pathogenesis. Minerva Ginecol 62(6):559–571

47. Roth C, Rack B, Muller V et al (2010) Circulating microRNAs as blood-based markers for patients with primary and metastatic breast cancer. Breast Cancer Res 12(6):R90. doi:10.1186/bcr2766, doi:bcr2766 [pii]

48. Guo L, Zhao Y, Yang S et al (2013) Genome-wide screen for aberrantly expressed miRNAs reveals miRNA profile signature in breast cancer. Mol Biol Rep 40(3):2175–2186. doi:10.1007/s11033-012-2277-5

49. Jung EJ, Santarpia L, Kim J et al (2012) Plasma microRNA 210 levels correlate with sensitivity to trastuzumab and tumor presence in breast cancer patients. Cancer 118(10):2603–2614. doi:10.1002/cncr.26565

50. Cuk K, Zucknick M, Madhavan D et al (2013) Plasma microRNA panel for minimally invasive detection of breast cancer. PLoS One 8(10), e76729. doi:10.1371/journal.pone.0076729

51. Liu JJ, Mao QX, Liu Y et al (2013) Analysis of miR-205 and miR-155 expression in the blood of breast cancer patients. Chin J Cancer Res 25(1):46–54. doi:10.3978/j.issn.1000-9604.2012.11.04

52. Madhavan D, Zucknick M, Wallwiener M et al (2012) Circulating miRNAs as Surrogate Markers for Circulating Tumor Cells and Prognostic Markers in Metastatic Breast Cancer. Clin Cancer Res 18(21):5972–5982. doi:10.1158/1078-0432.Ccr-12-1407

53. Zhao RH, Wu JN, Jia WJ et al (2011) Plasma miR-221 as a Predictive Biomarker for Chemoresistance in Breast Cancer Patients who Previously Received Neoadjuvant Chemotherapy. Onkologie 34(12):675–680. doi:10.1159/000334552

54. Zhao H, Shen J, Medico L et al (2010) A Pilot Study of Circulating miRNAs as Potential Biomarkers of Early Stage Breast Cancer. PLoS One 5(10), e13735. doi:10.1371/journal.pone.0013735

55. Tjensvoll K, Svendsen KN, Reuben JM et al (2012) miRNA expression profiling for identification of potential breast cancer biomarkers. Biomarkers 17(5):463–470. doi:10.3109/1354750X.2012.686061

Profiling Circulating miRNAs from the Plasma of Individuals with Metabolic Syndrome

Sadhbh O'Neill and Lorraine O'Driscoll

Abstract

The technique of RT-qPCR (real time-quantitative polymerase chain reaction) is invaluable in miRNA research both at the profiling and individual RT-qPCR stages. At the profiling stage, numerous miRNAs are looked at in the plasma of numerous individuals from two or more cohorts (*i.e.*, control vs. case). The miRNAs of interest would be either upregulated or downregulated by more than twofold in the case cohort compared to the control cohort. Profiling human specimens for miRNA biomarkers has exploded over the last decade, with researchers profiling plasma, serum, urine, and also the miRNA content of extracellular vesicles, which are also isolated from human specimens. RT-qPCR is a relatively easy technique; however, sample preparation from plasma to RNA to RNA input in RT reaction requires accuracy and precision.

Key words Metabolic syndrome, Blood plasma, RNA isolation, miRNA profiling, RT-qPCR

1 Introduction

Metabolic syndrome (MetS) is the culmination of a number of components, *i.e.*, hypertension, dyslipidemia, abdominal obesity and insulin resistance, resulting in an increased risk of type 2 diabetes mellitus (T2DM), cardiovascular disease (CVD), and cancer [1]. Obesity is reaching epidemic proportions world-wide and therefore; the rate of MetS is steadily increasing alongside obesity. There is call for a novel method for diagnosis of MetS to subsequently reduce the risk of T2DM, CVD and cancer, which are among the leading causes of death globally [1].

microRNAs (miRNA) are small, approximately 22 nucleotide long noncoding RNA molecules found in animals, plants, and numerous viruses. miRNAs regulate gene expression via their association with target sites on mRNAs and association with effector complexes [2]. Their function is posttranscriptional gene regulation, primarily downregulation of the target protein through translational repression (binding or cleavage) of the target mRNA untranslated regions. However, recent studies have shown

Sweta Rani (ed.), *MicroRNA Profiling: Methods and Protocols*, Methods in Molecular Biology, vol. 1509,
DOI 10.1007/978-1-4939-6524-3_13, © Springer Science+Business Media New York 2017

miRNAs can function to posttranscriptionally stimulate gene expression, by working in concert with their associated proteins, microribonucleoproteins by a direct or indirect mechanism [2]. It is therefore, not surprising that aberrant miRNA expression is associated with numerous disorders, including obesity [3, 4], diabetes [4], and various cancer subtypes [5, 6].

In recent years, miRNA profiling has developed as the preferred method over traditional gene expression profiling due to (1) the stability of miRNAs, this is due to their short length, (2) high sensitivity, (3) reliable as diagnostic tools, and (4) the origin of cancer at a metastatic site can be determined [5]. Additionally, miRNAs are easily assessed in body fluids, *i.e.*, serum and plasma; therefore, they are minimally invasive biomarkers. However, they can also be assessed in tumor or tissue specimens. In this method plasma miRNAs from obese individuals and individuals diagnosed with MetS according to the International Diabetes Federation were analyzed.

Numerous high-throughput miRNA profiling technologies exist, including, Quantitative reverse Transcription PCR (RT-qPCR), miRNA microarray, and RNA sequencing, either smaller scale or high-throughput [5]. In this chapter we discuss the use of the miR-CURY LNA™ Universal RT miRNA qPCR Panels. This method was selected as (1) the RT reaction is universal and so supplies templates for all miRNAs in the qPCR reaction and (2) both the reverse and forward amplification primers are specific to the miRNA of interest providing notable sensitivity and specificity.

Blood plasma is a pale yellow liquid and acts as the extracellular matrix of blood cells. It accounts for 55 % of the body's total blood volume. In this method, plasma was chosen for further miRNA analysis as the preparation of plasma is less complex than that for serum. Preparation of plasma involves centrifugation of whole blood to remove white blood cells and red blood cells; however, serum requires blood clotting followed by centrifugation. Plasma isolated from EDTA tubes was, therefore, used to reduce the procedural variation resulting from differences in clotting and subsequent serum collection.

2 Materials

2.1 RNA Isolation and Quality Control

1. TRIReagent™, should be used in the fume hood: store at 4 °C.

2. Chloroform, should be used in the fume hood: store at 4 °C.

3. 120 μg/mL of glycogen: store at –20 °C for up to 1 year.

4. Isopropanol: store at 4 °C.

5. Ethanol: prepare 75 % using ddH$_2$O and store at room temperature.

6. RNase-free water: store at room temperature.

2.2 Agilent Pico and Small RNA Kits	1. Chips: store at room temperature.
	2. Gel matrix, dye concentrate, conditioning medium, and marker (provided with the kit): store at 4 °C.
	3. Ladder (provided with the kit): store at –20 °C.
2.3 Reverse Transcription	1. 5× reaction buffer: store at –20 °C.
	2. Enzyme mix: store at –20 °C.
	3. Spike in RNA (UniSP6) (*see* **Note 1**): store at –20 °C.
	4. Nuclease-free water: store at –20 °C.
	5. RNA template: store at –80 °C.
2.4 PCR Analysis	1. SYBR Green master mix: store at –20 °C.
	2. Profiling plates and individual primer: store at –20 °C.
	3. cDNA store at –20 °C.
2.5 Required Equipment	1. NanoDrop.
	2. BioAnalyzer.
	3. Thermal cycler.
	4. Real-time PCR instrument.

3 Methods

3.1 RNA Isolation and Quantification

RNA from plasma is isolated using TRIReagent™ and the resulting RNA is quantified using the NanoDrop. Care is needed when isolating RNA, as RNase enzymes easily degrade RNA. Therefore, benches should be wiped with RNaseZap and 70% ethanol. Eppendorfs and RT-qPCR plates should be RNase-free, RNase-free filter tips should be used and all reagents should be molecular grade.

1. Plasma specimens are procured by standard collection protocols. Specifically, whole blood is procured in EDTA vials and mixed by inversion of the tube (8–10 times). Specimens are immediately centrifuged at $2000 \times g$ at room temperature (RT) for 15 min. Following centrifugation the top yellowish layer is collected and stored in 1 mL aliquots in cryovials at –80 °C until required.

2. Plasma specimens are thawed slowly on ice, 250 μL is transferred to an Eppendorf and plasma specimens are returned to –80 °C. 250 μL of plasma and 750 μL of TRIReagent™ (*see* **Note 2**) are combined, mixed, and incubated at RT for 10 min.

3. To this, 200 μL of chloroform is added, mixed vigorously for 15 s and incubated at RT for 10 min.

4. After incubation the resulting mixture is centrifuged at $13,200 \times g$ at 4 °C for 15 min to separate the RNA, DNA, and protein layers.

5. The upper colorless aqueous phase is transferred to a fresh Eppendorf tube.

6. To the aqueous phase 1.2 μL of glycogen and 500 μL of ice-cold isopropanol is added, mixed and incubated at RT for 10 min. Samples are then stored at –20 °C overnight to allow maximum precipitation of the RNA.

7. The precipitated RNA is subsequently pelleted by centrifugation at $13,200 \times g$ at 4 °C for 30 min.

8. The supernatant is discarded and the pellet is washed with 75 % ethanol and vortexed. The pellet is then centrifuged at $7500 \times g$ at 4 °C for 5 min.

9. **Step 8** is repeated, however, centrifuged at $13,200 \times g$.

10. The RNA pellet is then allowed to air dry until translucent and resuspended in 10 μL of RNase-free water. The resuspended RNA pellet is incubated on ice for 30 min to allow complete dissolution.

11. Store RNA at –80 °C (*see* **Notes 3** and **4**).

12. Quantification of the RNA is performed using the NanoDrop, with readings taken at 260, 280 and 230 nm (*see* **Notes 2** and **3**).

3.2 Quality Assessment: Agilent Chips (See Notes 4 and 5)

1. Agilent small RNA chips are used to assess the quality and percentage of miRNAs present in the total RNA sample.

2. The chip is placed on the priming station and 9 μL of gel matrix with dye concentrate is added to the appropriate well (Fig. 1a).

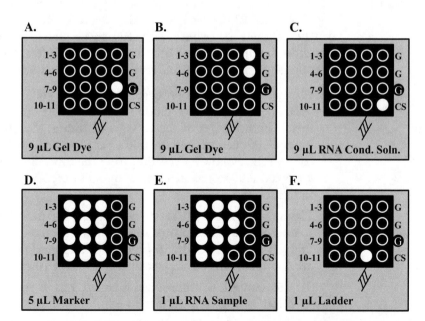

Fig. 1 Diagram of the addition of reagents and samples to the Agilent Small RNA chip for RNA characterization

3. The chip priming station is closed and the syringe plunger pressed until held by the clip for 60 s.

4. The plunger is released and moved to the 1 mL mark.

5. The priming station is opened and 9 μL of gel matrix is added to two additional wells (Fig. 1b).

6. 9 μL of conditioning solution is added to the appropriate well (Fig. 1c).

7. To all sample wells and the ladder well, 5 μL of marker is added (Fig. 1d).

8. Finally, 1 μL of denatured RNA sample is added to wells numbered 1–11 (Fig. 1e).

9. To the ladder well, 1 μL of ladder solution is added (Fig. 1f).

10. The chip is then placed in the IKA vortex for 1 min at 2400 rpm.

11. Subsequently the chip is placed in the BioAnalyzer (*see* **Notes 4** and **5**) and results visualized on an electropherogram (Fig. 2).

3.3 MicroRNA Profiling (Discovery Phase)

There are many techniques available for miRNA profiling as is described in the introduction. Here, we will provide the protocol for the use of miRCURY LNA™ Universal RT miRNA qPCR panels for use with serum/plasma. Under this category of miRNA profiling there are a number of options available to the researcher, *i.e.*, miRNome panels, focus panels and pick and mix custom panels. The basic principal of the RT-qPCR is the same for all options; the choice of panel depends on the researchers focus.

3.3.1 First Strand cDNA Synthesis (RT Reaction) (See Note 6)

Although quantification of the RNA is performed using the NanoDrop, the amount of RNA present in a plasma specimen cannot be accurately determined due to phenol contamination from the TRIReagent™. Therefore, an input volume of RNA rather than an input concentration is the preferred option. Performing a serial dilution of RNA input volumes will determine the correct

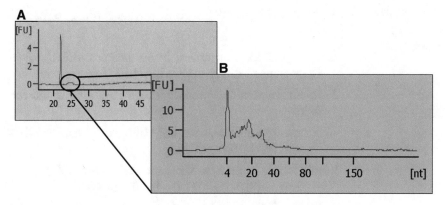

Fig. 2 Agilent electropherograms. A. RNA 6000 Pico kit electropherogram illustrating a peak of small RNAs at ~25 s. B. Small RNA kit illustrating miRNA content (22–26 nt) in the total RNA

RNA input volume to avoid inhibitors of the RT reaction (*see* **Note 7**). Exiqon have recommended the use of 5 potential endogenous control genes (miR-103, 191, 423-5p, 93, 425). miR-93 and miR-425 are usually stably expressed in serum/plasma. One of these miRNAs may be used for determining the input volume for the RT reaction. miR-451 and miR-16 may also be used as controls for hemolysis.

1. From serial dilutions (*see* **Note 7**) 1.6 µL of input RNA was determined as the optimum input volume for our specimens.

2. In an Eppendorf, the RT master mix is set up as follows (volume for one sample):

5× Reaction buffer	2 µL
Enzyme mix	1 µL
Spike ins (optional - *see* **Note 1**)	0.5 µL
Nuclease-free water	4.9 µL

3. Combine all reagents, mix by flicking and centrifuge briefly to bring all reagents to bottom of tube. Place on ice.

4. In a 96-well fast optical reaction plate pipette 8.4 µL of master mix to each well (1 well per RNA sample).

5. Add 1.6 µL of RNA to the appropriate well in the 96-well fast optical plate.

6. Seal the plate with optical sealing film and briefly centrifuge to bring reagents to bottom of plate.

7. Place plate in thermocycler and run the following cycle:
   (a) 42 °C for 60 min.
   (b) 95 °C for 5 min.
   (c) Cool to 4 °C.

8. The cDNA is then stored at −20 °C, until required.

3.3.2   PCR Amplification: miCURY LNA Profiling Panels (See Note 6)

Real-time PCR (qPCR) is performed according to manufacturer's protocol.

1. Thaw cDNA synthesized in Subheading 3.3.1 slowly on ice. Once thawed dilute cDNA 50× in RNase-free water.

2. In an Eppendorf prepare the SYBR Green master mix as follows:

   Serum/plasma focus panels: 1000 µL 2× master mix + 980 µL ddH$_2$O + 20 µL cDNA.

   miRNome human, mouse, and rat panels: 2000 µL 2× master mix + 1940 µL ddH$_2$0 + 40 µL cDNA.

3. Mix by flicking and spin down to bring contents to bottom of tube.

4. Place solution in a trough and using a multichannel pipette 10 μL into each well of the 384-well plates.

5. Seal the plate and centrifuge for 1 min at 1200×*g* to bring contents to bottom of well (*see* **Note 8**).

6. Place plate in real-time PCR machine and run the following cycle:

(a) Hold Stage - 95 °C for 10 min.

(b) PCR Stage (×40 cycles).

- 95 °C for 10 s.
- 60 °C for 1 min.

(c) Melt Stage.

- 95 °C for 15 s.
- 60 °C for 1 min.
- 95 °C for 15 s.

3.4 Individual RT-qPCR Validation Stage

miRNAs identified as upregulated or downregulated from the miRNA profiling need to be validated in a separate cohort of specimens. The method involves the synthesis of cDNA and qPCR analysis similar to the miRNA profiling, discovery phase.

3.4.1 First Strand cDNA Synthesis

First strand cDNA synthesis is performed as per Subheading 3.3.1 (Fig. 3).

3.4.2 PCR Amplification: Individual Assay (See Note 6) (Fig. 3)

1. Thaw cDNA synthesized in Subheading 3.4.1 slowly on ice. Once thawed, dilute cDNA 40× in RNase-free water.

2. In an Eppendorf prepare the SYBR Green master mix as follows (volume for one reaction):

SYBR Green PCR Master Mix	5 μL
miRNA Primer	1 μL

3. Place 6 μL of the SYBR Green master mix in each well of a 96-well fast optical PCR plate.

4. Add 4 μL of cDNA to each well (in triplicate for each sample) of the 96-well plate.

5. Seal the plate and centrifuge for 1 min at 1200×*g* to bring contents to bottom of well (*see* **Note 8**).

6. Place plate in real-time PCR machine and run the following cycle:

(a) Hold Stage - 95 °C for 10 min.

(b) PCR Stage (×40 cycles).

- 95 °C for 10 s.
- 60 °C for 1 min.

Step 1: Reverse Transcription

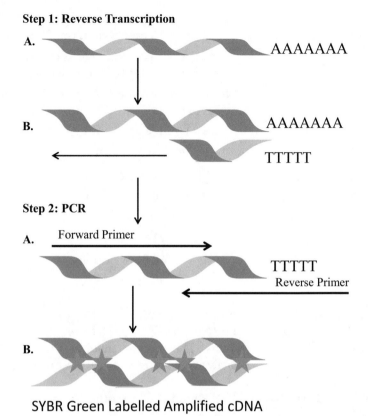

SYBR Green Labelled Amplified cDNA

Fig. 3 RT-qPCR Amplification. Step 1 A: a poly-A tail is added to the mature miRNA. Step 1 B: cDNA is synthesized using a poly-T primer with a 5′ universal tag. Step 2 A: The cDNA template is then amplified using forward and reverse primers. Step 2 B: SYBR Green is used for detection of the amplified cDNA

(c) Melt Stage.
- 95 °C for 15 s.
- 60 °C for 1 min.
- 95 °C for 15 s.

3.5 Data Analysis   Each plate contains a plate calibrator UniSp3IPC. The raw C_T values are calibrated for differences between plates using the UniSp3IPC CT values. Specifically,

C_T *of sample-*(C_T *of UniSp3IPC on plate*)*-*(*average of UniSp3 IPC for all plates*).

Following calibration miRNA profiling data is analyzed using the $2^{(-\Delta\Delta C_T)}$ method. Specifically:

1. $\Delta C_T = C_T$ value of sample – C_T value (mean C_T value) of endogenous control gene(s).

2. $\Delta\Delta C_T = \Delta C_T$ case sample – ΔC_T of control sample.

3. Fold change = $\Delta\Delta C_T$ value input into formula $2^{(-\Delta\Delta C_T)}$.

4   Notes

1. RNA spike-ins, such as UniSp6 may be used in the RT reaction and PCR stages to ensure the RT reaction was successful and undetermined values in the PCR are not due to poorly synthesized cDNA.

2. When isolating using TRIReagent™ or TRIzol contamination with phenol may result. Therefore, NanoDrop readings may be inaccurate and RNA input volume may be superior to input concentration in the RT reaction.

3. RNA input volume should be determined by serial dilution, in order to ensure there are no RT reaction inhibitors in the plasma specimens.

4. Isolated RNA should be stored at −80 °C no longer than 30 min after reconstitution in order to ensure integrity of RNA for subsequent RT reaction.

5. Plasma RNA will not show the 18S rRNA or 28S rRNA when using the Agilent Pico kit. Plasma will also only show the miRNA content when using the Agilent Small RNA kit.

6. Use of Agilent BioAnalyzer should be restricted to areas where other instruments are not being used, as vibrations from other instruments may skew results.

7. Setting up of RT and PCR reactions should be done extremely carefully to avoid as much as possible pipetting error.

8. Premade PCR reaction plates may be stored for 24 h at 4 °C.

Acknowledgements

Danish Strategic Research Council and HEA PRTLI Cycle 5 funding of TBSI.

References

1. O'Neill S, O'Driscoll L (2015) Metabolic syndrome: a closer look at the growing epidemic and its associated pathologies. Obesity Rev 16(1):1–12. doi:10.1111/obr.12229

2. Vasudevan S (2012) Posttranscriptional upregulation by microRNAs. Wiley Interdiscip Rev RNA 3(3):311–330. doi:10.1002/wrna.121

3. Williams MD, Mitchell GM (2012) MicroRNAs in insulin resistance and obesity. Exp Diabetes Res 2012:484696. doi:10.1155/2012/484696

4. Pescador N, Perez-Barba M, Ibarra JM et al (2013) Serum circulating microRNA profiling for identification of potential type 2 diabetes and obesity biomarkers. PLoS One 8(10):e77251. doi:10.1371/journal.pone.0077251

5. Di Leva G, Croce CM (2013) miRNA profiling of cancer. Curr Opin Genet Dev 23(1):3–11. doi:10.1016/j.gde.2013.01.004

6. Blenkiron C, Goldstein LD, Thorne NP et al (2007) MicroRNA expression profiling of human breast cancer identifies new markers of tumor subtype. Genome Biol 8(10):R214. doi:10.1186/gb-2007-8-10-r214

Chapter 14

Manipulating MiRNA Expression to Uncover Hidden Functions

Sinéad T. Aherne and Nga T. Lao

Abstract

There are a numerous target prediction algorithms that allow users to identify putative targets of their microRNAs (miRNAs) of interest. Although these tools are useful to gain insight into the potential role of miRNAs in regulating cellular processes, physical manipulation of the expression of the miRNA is the most superior way to truly determine the function of the miRNA in the system of interest. This chapter outlines methods to reveal miRNA function by modulating miRNA expression by transient transfection of miRNA mimics and inhibitors, and stable overexpression and reduction of miRNA expression using plasmid overexpression and sponge vectors.

Key words miRNA-Target, Transfection, Cloning, Ligation

1 Introduction

There are a numerous target prediction algorithms such as Miranda, PicTar, and TargetScan that allow users to identify putative targets of their miRNA of interest. Most algorithms utilize the principles by which miRNAs identify their target sites in the mRNA code. One such principle is the conserved Watson–Crick pairing of the mRNA target with the miRNA "seed region," generally defined as nucleotides 2–7 in the 5′ region of the miRNA. The type of miRNA target site is also important for prediction. There are several types of target sites, the first category, "5′ dominant" sites, includes targets that base-pair well to the 5′ end of the miRNA. There is also an element of 3′ pairing in this group so it is subdivided into two subtypes; "canonical" sites, which pair well at both the 5′ and 3′ ends of the miRNA, and "seed" sites, which require little or no 3′ pairing support but show continuous pairing of at least 7 bp at the 5′ end. The second target site category, titled "3′ compensatory" sites, shows weak base-pairing to the 5′ end of the miRNA (with seeds of 4–6 bp, or seeds of 7–8 bp including bulges, mismatches and G:U pairs) and relies heavily on compensatory pairing to the

Sweta Rani (ed.), *MicroRNA Profiling: Methods and Protocols*, Methods in Molecular Biology, vol. 1509,
DOI 10.1007/978-1-4939-6524-3_14, © Springer Science+Business Media New York 2017

3' region of the miRNA. The final feature considered by most algorithms is that highly conserved miRNAs have many conserved targets [1]. In addition, some algorithms consider the thermodynamic stability of the putative miRNA-target duplex.

Although these tools are no doubt useful in one's quest to discover the function and relevance of one's miRNA of interest, physical manipulation of the expression of the miRNA is the most superior way to truly determine the function of the miRNA in the system of interest. There are several ways to manipulate miRNA expression in vitro and in vivo, some transient and others stably modifying the expression of the transcript. Each method has its own benefits and drawbacks and choosing the most appropriate approach depends on the overall goal of the experiment. The transient methods are quicker, but also more expensive than the more reproducible stable modification techniques.

Several companies offer miRNA mimics and inhibitors for transient overexpression or knockdown of miRNA expression, respectively. Mimics are synthetic "copies" of miRNAs that can be transfected into cells and incorporated into the RISC complex to mediate miRNA induced expression repression. miRNA inhibitors (Anti-miRs) work in the opposite manner—sequestering the endogenous miRNAs from entering the RISC complex (Fig. 1). Various types of vectors can be utilized for the stable overexpression or knockdown of miRNA expression. These vectors can be lentiviral, adenoviral or plasmid in structure and usually include a reporter gene (e.g., Green, Red or Yellow Fluorescent Protein for easy assessment) [2]. Downregulation vectors (often referred to as sponges) allow not only the reduction in expression of one particular miRNA but also a family of miRNAs with similar seed preferences to be targeted simultaneously [3, 4]. To generate miRNA vectors, long oligos are phosphorylated, denatured at high temperature and slowly annealed to allow the binding of the two oligos. The annealed oligos are then ligated to digested vectors [5]. Alternatively the SanDI restriction enzyme can be employed to rapidly generate sponges with multiple binding sites (MBS) of target miRNAs [3]. The most effective sponges have been determined to contain multiple antisense MBS with imperfect complementary to sequester miRNAs and impair functions.

For the purposes of this chapter, methods to transiently manipulate miRNA expression using mimics and inhibitors, and stably manipulate miRNA expression using plasmid overexpression and sponge vectors are outlined.

2 Materials

2.1 Transient Transfections

1. Cell line.
2. Tissue culture media.

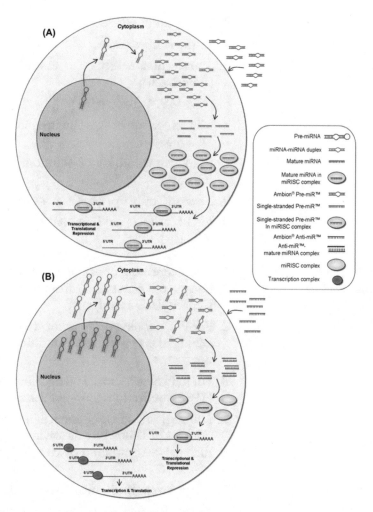

Fig. 1 miRNA mimics and inhibitors functioning in cell lines. (**a**) Illustrates mimics mimicking endogenous miRNA expression. Mimics can be used when there is a low expression of a particular miRNA in the cell (i.e., a tumor suppressor miRNA). The endogenous black pre-miRNA are transported from the nucleus and cleaved into a mature miRNA. This would then be taken into an miRISC complex, and as there is low miRNA expression, a low level of transcriptional and translational repression would result. When the red mimics are transfected into the cell, the correct strand representing the mature miRNA is taken into the miRISC complex. This will cause an increase in the transcriptional and translational repression of the miRNA target genes. (**b**) Illustrates miRNA inhibitors decreasing miRNA expression. Anti-miRs can be used when there is high expression of a particular miRNA in the cell (i.e., an oncogenic miRNA). In this part of the diagram several pre-miRNAs are synthesized and transported into the cytoplasm of the cell. These are then cleaved into many mature miRNAs. However, when the anti-miRs are introduced into the cell, they bind to the single-stranded mature miRNAs. This sequesters them and prevents them from being taken up into the miRISC complex and thus allows transcription and translation of the miRNA target genes to continue

3. Tissue culture flasks.

4. Tissue culture plates.

5. Transfection reagent, for example Lipofectamine RNAiMax (Invitrogen).

6. Opti-MEM (Invitrogen).

7. Mimics or inhibitors (Invitrogen or Qiagen or Exiquon or Dharmacon).

8. RNA extraction kit or solution, e.g., TRIzol or MiRNeasy (Qiagen).

9. Reverse Transcription Kit, e.g., MiScript II RT Kit (Qiagen).

10. qPCR primers and master mix, e.g., the MiScript system (Qiagen).

2.2 Stable Transfections

1. Overexpression or sponge vector: vectors can be made in-house or purchased from several companies including Genecopia and Addgene.

2. For PCR cloning order primers for your region of interest containing the appropriate restriction sites for the vector being used.

3. For long oligos above 100 nucleotides, purchase from Eurofins, HPSF purification, 0.05 μmol scale.

4. 100 mg/mL stock of ampicillin sodium salt: Make 100 mg/mL stock (1000×) by dissolving 1 g of ampicillin in water to the final concentration of 10 mL. Store aliquots of 1 mL each at −20 °C.

5. Hygromycin B (50 mg/mL) or other selection antobiotic.

6. Restriction enzymes: Fast digest enzymes (Fisher Scientific), store at −20 °C.

7. Fast Alkaline Phosphatase (Fisher Scientific).

8. T4 Polynucleotide Kinase (NEB).

9. T4 ligase (Roche).

10. 10× T4 Ligation Buffer (NEB).

11. Competent cells, e.g., MAX Efficiency DH5α Competent Cells (Invitrogen).

12. SOC media (Invitrogen).

13. LB Broth: Dissolve 2 g of LB Broth in 100 mL water, sterilize by autoclaving. Allow to cool before adding antibiotics.

14. LB Agar: Use the same recipe as LB Broth and add 1.5 g Agar.

15. Petri Dishes.

16. Plasmid Mini-prep kit (e.g., Qiagen).

17. 50× Tris–Acetate–EDTA (TEA): For routine electrophoresis, dilute 10 mL with 490 mL water (1× TEA).

18. Agarose Gel; for a 0.8% gel mix 0.8 g of agarose powder with 100 mL of 1× TEA buffer. Microwave for 1–2 min. Cool down the solution for 5 min and add ethidium bromide or 8 μL Safe View Nucleic Stain (NBS Biologicals). Pour solution into the gel casting tray and insert comb. Allow the gel to solidify.

19. DNA Gel Loading Dye (6×).

20. GeneRuler DNA Ladder (Thermo Fisher).

21. QiaQuick Gel Extraction Kit (Qiagen).

22. Heat block.

23. Water bath.

24. PCR machine.

25. Orbital shaker.

26. Incubator.

27. Gel running unit.

28. Transilluminator.

3 Methods

3.1 For Examination of Short-Term Modulations of miRNA Expression

The number of cells transfected, miRNA mimic or Anti-miR concentration, and transfection reagent volume vary depending on the cells being transfected and the culture dish being used. It is recommended in most cases to optimize the optimal conditions for the cell line of interest in a 24-well plate. Appropriate positive, negative, mock and untransfected controls should always be used, and transfection efficiency should be monitored using qPCR for both the miRNA of interest and a known validated target of the miRNA. Western blot to assess alterations of a validated protein target of the miRNA can also be used for validation.

3.1.1 Preparation of Transfectants (Volumes Outlined Are for 1 Well of a 24-Well Dish)

1. Dilute miRNA mimics or Anti-miRs to appropriate concentration in 50 μL Opti-MEM serum-free media (see Note 1).

2. Dilute Lipofectamine in 50 μL Opti-MEM serum-free media.

3. Incubate for 5 min to allow lipid complexes to form.

4. Add 50 μL of the inhibitor/mimic complex and 50 μL of the Lipofectamine complex to wells.

5. Gently mix a little by pipetting up and down and incubate for 20 min at room temperature.

6. Add media to untransfected wells and Opti-MEM to mock-transfected control wells.

3.1.2 Transfection

1. Trypsinize and count cells.

2. Dilute them to the appropriate concentration in media without antibiotics.

3. Slowly add 500 μL of cell solution to each well.

4. Mix the cell and lipid solutions by gently tilting the plate to and fro to avoid cells clumping in the center of the wells, do not swirl the dish as this will cause cells to clump in the center of the wells.

5. Incubate the transfections for 24–72 h.

6. Assess transfection efficiency by performing RNA extraction and real-time PCR for the miRNA and validated targets of interest.

3.2 Method for Generation of Stable Cell Populations Using Overexpression or Knockdown Vectors

For all stable manipulations, appropriate control vectors should also be used to control for off target effects and background fluorescence. Expand plasmid copy number of the backbone vector by transforming plasmids into *E. coli* competent cells and preparing plasmid DNA (*see* **Note 2**).

3.2.1 Transforming Plasmids

1. Thaw competent cells on wet ice.

2. Add 10 μL competent cells and 1 μL (10 ng/μL) DNA to a 1.5 mL tube. Mix and incubate for 30 min on ice (*see* **Note 3**).

3. Heat-shock the cells in a water bath at 42 °C for 45 s. Do not shake.

4. Place on ice for 2 min.

5. Add 100 μL of SOC medium.

6. Incubate at 37 °C on an orbital shaker at 225 rpm for 1 h.

7. While the cells are incubating pour LB petri plates.

8. If concentration is required centrifuge the tube at $6000 \times g$ for 3 min. Remove the majority of the supernatant leaving approx. 40 μL.

9. Mix the cells and spread the mixture onto the LB plates containing 100 μg/mL ampicillin.

10. Incubate overnight upside down at 37 °C.

11. Colonies should form overnight. Using a pipette tip, pick single colonies and add the tip into LB broth.

12. Incubate at 37 °C on an orbital shaker at 225 rpm for overnight.

13. The following day, perform 1–2 mini-preps using a mini-prep kit of choice.

14. Quantify the plasmid using a NanoDrop spectrophotometer.

*3.2.2   Cloning of miR
Duplex or miR-MBS
into Backbone Vectors
(Fig. 2)*

Digest Backbone Vector
and Treat with Alkaline
Phosphatase

1. Set up digest.

   - 3 μg DNA.
   - 10 μL Fast digest buffer ×10.
   - 3 μL Fast digest Enzyme 1 (30 U).
   - 3 μL Fast digest Enzyme 2 (30 U).
   - 3 μL Fast alkaline phosphatase (1 U/μL).
   - H_2O to 100 μL.

2. Mix well by gently pipetting.

3. Incubate at 37 °C for 1 h.

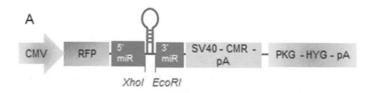

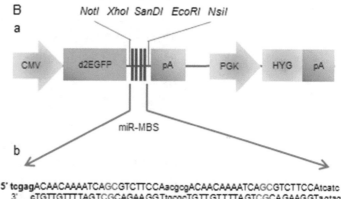

Fig. 2 Maps of miR overexpression (**A**) and sponge vectors (**B**). Part (**B**) of the figure illustrates the sponge vector (a) and an example of an oligo duplex with four binding sites (*capital letters*) for human miR-7 is shown (b). Overhang bases in the duplex for cloning into vectors, in this example using *XhoI* and *EcoRI* sites, are highlighted in *bold text*, and the spacer sequences between each binding site are *small letters*. The *red letters* in (b) and (c) are bulged sequence for imperfect pairing of an miRNA and the miR sponge

4. To ensure the plasmid was successfully digested, add 1.5 µL of 6× DNA loading buffer to 10 µL of digest solution.

5. Mix by pipetting and load the solution onto an agarose gel, beside a DNA ladder.

6. Electrophorese at 100 V for 30 min and visualize gel on a transilluminator.

7. If the digestion has been successful, run the remainder of the digestion reaction in two or three wells of another gel to gel purify the vector if necessary (e.g., if the vector is not a unique fragment). Otherwise, the rest of the vector digest can be purified using PCR purification kit according to the manufacturer's instructions.

8. Once the gel has run, cut the band out using a scalpel and purify the DNA using the QiaQuick Gel Extraction kit according to the manufacturers' instructions.

9. Elute in 30–35 µL of elution buffer and store at –20 °C.

Phosphorylate and Anneal Each Pair of Oligos

1. Turn on a heat block to 99 °C 45 min before use. Use a thermometer to check the temperature.

2. Set up the reaction as follows and add the largest volume first. Mix by swirling as pipetting may damage oligos.
   - 1 µL oligo 1 (100 µM).
   - 1 µL oligo 2 (100 µM).
   - 1 µL 10× T4 ligase buffer.
   - µL H2O.
   - 0.5 µL T4PNK.
   - 10 µL total volume.

3. Incubate at 37 °C for 30 min and centrifuge briefly to collect the solution at the bottom of the tube.

4. Load tubes into the preheated heating block and incubate at 100 °C for 5 min and centrifuge.

5. Turn off the heat block and return to heat block for 3 h or until the temperature returns to ~40 °C.

6. Allow the samples to then return to room temperature for 10 min.

7. Store at –20 °C.

8. Before use for ligation, make a 1:250-fold dilution for routine cloning of oligos of up to 110 nucleotides. For cloning into a sponge vector at a SanDI restriction enzyme site a 1:3 dilution of the oligo stock is used to give approximately 300–400 ng/µL when measured using the NanoDrop.

Set up Ligation

- 1 µL digested and purified vector (50 ng).
- 1 µL diluted oligo duplex.

- 1 μL 10× T4 Ligation Buffer.
- 1 μL T4 Ligase.
- 6 μL nuclease-free water.
- 10 μL Reaction Volume.
  - Incubate at –16 °C for at least 2 h before transformation.
  - Store the rest of the ligation mixture at –20 °C.

Perform Transformation

Transformation is carried out as described in Subheading 3.2.1, with 50 μL competent cells and 5 μL ligation reaction. After heat shock, 500 μL SOC is added, bacteria are grown, colonies picked and expanded, and the DNA is prepped as previously described.

Verify the Transformant Clones

Digest 200–300 ng of the DNA mini-prep with suitable restriction enzymes and verify that each clone contains an insert on a 0.8 % agarose gel. Those clones with insert of expected size are then verified by sequencing using sequencing service companies. If the efficiency of transformant clones with correct insert is low, the identification of positive transformant clones can be carried out first by PCR screening before preparing DNA miniprep as follows:

1. Pick a colony with a pipette tip and suspend cells in 2 μL ddH$_2$O.
2. Prepare a PCR master mix.
3. Add 18 μL PCR master mix into 2 μL cell suspension.
4. Perform the PCR according to the conditions specified by the primers.
5. Determine whether the PCR product is of the correct size by running 5 μL of the PCR reaction on a gel.

3.2.3 Isolating Pure Populations of Stably Transfected Cells

The plasmid can now be transfected into the cells of interest. Transfected cells can then be grown under the selective antibiotics (i.e., puromycin or hygromycin growth conditions) to produce stably transfected cell populations. Flow cytometry for green or red fluorescent proteins can then be used to further select mix-cell populations of a certain level of expression of the candidate miRNA or MiR-MBS for further characterization. Single cell clones can be isolated using the same procedure.

3.3 Assessment of miRNA Driven Changes Following Expression Manipulation

Once the expression of the miRNA of interest is significantly up-regulated or down-regulated either transiently or stably, a plethora of subsequent experiments can be performed to investigate the impact and importance of the miRNA. Global unbiased omics experiments determining altered mRNAs and proteins can be explored in addition to a wide variety of phenotypic assays such as proliferation, migration, invasion, *anoikis*, and colony formation.

4   Notes

1. All transfection conditions require optimization as optimal conditions depend on the cell line of interest. The most important factors to consider are cell density, transfection reagent volume, and mimic/inhibitor/vector concentration. For transient transfections, all steps should be performed under sterile conditions.

2. For cloning and bacterial work, benchtop aseptic conditions should be followed using a Bunsen burner for flaming to reduce contamination. Handle restriction enzymes with care; only remove them from the freezer when required, keep them on ice at all times, and return them to the freezer as soon as possible.

3. DO NOT pipet up and down; gently swirl the solution using a pipette tip after adding the DNA.

Acknowledgements

This work was supported by the ELEVATE: Irish Research Council International Career Development Fellowship—cofunded by Marie Cure Actions and Scientific Foundation of Ireland (SFI) grant number 13/IA/1963.

References

1. Bartel DP (2009) MicroRNAs: target recognition and regulatory functions. Cell 136(2): 215–233

2. Kotal J, Chivukula RR, O'Donnell KA et al (2009) Therapeutic delivery of miR-26a inhibits cancer cell proliferation and induces tumor-specific apoptosis. Cell 137(6):1005–1017

3. Ebert MS, Neilson JR, Sharp PA (2007) MicroRNA sponges: competitive inhibitors of small RNAs in mammalian cells. Nat Methods 4(9):721–7264

4. Kluiver J, Gibcus JH, Hettinga C et al (2012) Rapid generation of MicroRNA sponges for MicroRNA inhibition. PLoS One 7(1):e29275

5. Sanchez N, Kelly P, Gallagher C (2014) CHO cell culture longevity and recombinant protein yield are enhanced by depletion of miR-7 activity via sponge decoy vectors. Biotechnol J 9:396–404

Chapter 15

Analysis of the Distribution Profiles of Circulating MicroRNAs by Asymmetrical Flow Field Flow Fractionation

Kenneth Flack, Luis A. Jimenez, and Wenwan Zhong

Abstract

MicroRNAs (miRNAs) are stably present in circulatory systems. They are bound to various carriers like proteins, lipoprotein particles, and exosomes. Investigating the process of miRNA distribution among these carriers will help improve our understanding of their functions in the extracellular environment and their potential relationship with diseases. Here, we describe how to obtain the distribution profiles of circulating miRNAs by separation of different miRNA carriers in human serum with asymmetrical flow field flow fractionation (AF4), and detection of the miRNAs in the eluted fractions that enrich particular types of carriers with RT-qPCR.

Key words Fractionation, Exosomes, Lipoprotein, Cancer biomarkers, Circulating microRNA, Extracellular miRNA carriers

1 Introduction

MicroRNAs (miRNAs) are promising biomarkers for diagnosis and prognosis of diseases including diabetes, drug-resistant epilepsy, liver disease, coronary artery disease, and Alzheimer disease. MiRNAs have been found to be more closely related to disease stages and subtype and are more tissue specific than messenger RNAs [1–4]. Moreover, miRNAs can be released into the circulatory system and are stably present at levels detectible by sensitive techniques like RT-qPCR [5–8]. Owing to their appealing features - disease specificity, stably present at significant levels in circulatory system, mature detection methods, etc. - circulating miRNAs have attracted great research efforts to study their expression profiles, as well as to discover and validate their relationship with diseases [9–11]. Circulating miRNAs are protected from the abundant ribonucleases in the extracellular environment by various types of carriers [12, 13] including proteins, lipoprotein complexes, and microvesicles. Their carriers could reflect on how they are secreted and transported in between cells [14].

Sweta Rani (ed.), *MicroRNA Profiling: Methods and Protocols*, Methods in Molecular Biology, vol. 1509,
DOI 10.1007/978-1-4939-6524-3_15, © Springer Science+Business Media New York 2017

Therefore, it is more informative to present the relative levels of miRNAs with correlation to their carriers, in comparison to simply quantifying their overall quantities in the extracellular fluid.

Compared to the conventional techniques used in separation of miRNA carriers, i.e., size-exclusion chromatography (SEC) and ultracentrifugation, asymmetrical flow field flow fractionation (AF4) is gentler because of its unpacked separation channel and the low shear, liquid flow-based separation force [15–18], both of which avoids the disruption of the native structure of biovesicles and protects the non-covalent binding between miRNAs and their non-vesicle carriers [15]. AF4 can isolate intact macromolecular complexes formed between nucleic acid and protein, antibody and antigen, and ligand and receptor [19–21]. Therefore, AF4 is the method of choice for separation of different miRNA carriers based on their hydrodynamic sizes, enabling screening of miRNA distribution among all potential carriers. We have demonstrated the ability of AF4 to rapidly and reproducibly separate serum into fractions, thereby enriching various types of miRNA carriers. After recovering the miRNAs from the collected fractions, and quantifying them through RT-qPCR, we profiled the extracellular miRNAs associated with various carriers in serum. We also explored whether such a profile could help us better understand the relation between extracellular miRNAs and cancer development, by analyzing a number of serum samples collected from cancer patients and healthy individuals [22]. We did find that the quantity of some miRNAs in particular fractions exhibited more distinct differences between healthy individuals and breast cancer patients compared to overall quantity. More studies are needed to reveal the fundamentals behind differential secretion of the miRNA markers by cancer cells and their transportation pathways in the circulation system.

2 Materials

All solutions should be prepared with ultrapure water and analytical or biological grade reagents.

2.1 AF4 Buffer Solution

Running Buffer: 1× Phosphate Buffered Saline (PBS), pH 7.4. The following reagents should be weighed and transferred to a 1-L graduated container: 1.44 g Na_2HPO_4, 0.24 g KH_2PO_4, 8.0 g NaCl, 0.2 g KCl. Add water to bring the volume to 900 mL and mix to dissolve salts (*see* **Note 1**). Adjust the pH as necessary with NaOH or HCl (*see* **Note 2**). Bring volume to 1.0 L with water. Filter solution through a 0.22 μm filter. Store at room temperature.

2.2   AF4 Instrumentation and Components

1. AF2000 MultiFlow FFF: equipped with an Analytical Asymmetrical FFF channel (tip-to-tip length of 275 mm, with an inlet triangle width of 20 mm and an outlet width of 5 mm), a 350-μm channel spacer, a regenerated cellulose membrane (294 mm × 30 mm, with the molecular weight cut-off value of 10 kDa), and a 20-μL injection loop (Postnova Analytics Inc, Salt Lake City, UT, USA).

2. UV–Vis absorbance (SPD-20, Shimadzu, Kyoto, Japan) and fluorescence (480 nm/510 nm ex/em, Waters, Milford, MA, USA) detectors.

3. Automated Fraction Collector Model 2110 (Bio-Rad, Hercules, CA, USA).

4. DiO (3,3′-dioctadecyloxacarbocyanine perchlorate) lipophilic dye (Invitrogen, Carlsbad, CA).

2.3   Total RNA Chemical Extraction

1. Concentrated guanidine isothiocyanate-phenol (TRIzol LS Reagent, Ambion, USA).

2. Molecular biology grade chloroform, isopropanol, and 200-proof ethanol.

3. RNA grade glycogen.

4. RNase-free ultrapure water.

2.4   RT-qPCR

1. TaqMan MicroRNA Assay kits (Applied Biosystems, Foster City, CA, USA).

2. TaqMan MicroRNA Reverse Transcription kit (Applied Biosystems, Foster City, CA, USA) containing 10× RT buffer, dNTPs (100 mM total), RNase inhibitor (20 U/μL), and MultiScribe MuLV RT enzyme.

3. Taq 5× Master Mix (New England Biolabs, Ipswich, MA, USA).

4. Molecular biology grade dimethyl sulfoxide (DMSO) and ethylene glycol.

5. Real-time PCR detection system.

3   Methods

All procedures are to be carried out at room temperature unless specified differently.

3.1   AF4 Separation

1. System equilibration: The separation system should be equilibrated with the 1× PBS running buffer for one hour prior to sample injection. For the first 30 min all the pumps are set to run at 2.00 mL/min with the flow exiting through the channel into waste. For the second 30 min only the tip flow pump is set

to 0.30 mL/min (cross flow and focus flow at zero) and the flow exits to the detectors.

2. Sample injection: Using a 20 µL injection loop, a whole serum sample is injected onto the channel. For fluorescence detection the sample should be stained with DiO lipophilic dye (*see* **Note 3**).

3. Separation: The following focusing and elution method should be employed for serum separations using the 1× PBS running buffer. An initial focusing step of 8 min with the cross flow set at 3.00 mL/min, tip flow at 0.30 mL/min, and the focus flow at 3.00 mL/min. After the focusing step, the tip flow is increased to 3.30 mL/min and the focus flow is reduced to zero during a 1 min transition period. Afterwards, the tip flow is kept at 3.30 mL/min with the cross flow at 3.00 mL/min for 5 min. Then the tip flow and cross flow are reduced to 0.30 mL/min and 0.00 mL/min, respectively over the course of 15 min (decreased at a constant rate) (*see* **Note 3**). The cross flow is adjusted to keep the detector flow (the channel outlet flow) at 0.30 mL/min during the course of the separation.

4. Fraction collection: A fraction collector is used to perform stepwise collections of the eluent in 1 min intervals into the 2-mL microcentrifuge tubes. These collections are combined into six fractions corresponding to the eluted carriers based on absorbance and fluorescence fractogram traces: with fraction 1 (F1) collected from 6 to 9 min, F2 from 9 to 13 min, F3 from 13 to 16 min, F4 from 16 to 19 min, F5 from 19 to 23 min, and F6 from 23 to 28 min (*see* **Note 4**). F1 contains the protein carriers, F2–F3 contains mainly high-density lipoproteins; F4-F5 enriches the low-density lipoproteins, and F6 contains mainly exosomes.

3.2 MiRNA Extraction from Carrier Fractions

1. Immediately after collection of the six fractions, exogenous control (miRNA from *Caenorhabditis elegans* are good choices) should be added to each tube and mixed (*see* **Note 5**). Subsequently TRIzol LS reagent should be added (in the ratio of 1.00 mL TRIzol LS per 0.3 mL collected eluent), mixed and incubated for 5 min.

2. Following the incubation, add 0.30 mL of chloroform to each tube for every 1.0 mL of TRIzol LS. Mix the solution and incubate for 5 min.

3. Centrifuge the sample for 15 min at $12,000 \times g$ at 4 °C.

4. The upper aqueous phase exclusively containing RNA should be transferred to a fresh tube by carefully pipetting, avoiding the organic phase or interphase (*see* **Note 6**).

5. Add 20 µg of glycogen to each tube to keep the final concentration to ≤ 4 µg/µL in the RNA resuspension (*see* **Note 7**).

6. Add 0.8 mL of 100% isopropanol per 1.0 mL of TRIzol initially used.

7. Incubate overnight (~8 h) at –20 °C (*see* **Note 8**).

8. Centrifuge at $15,000 \times g$ for 15 min at 4 °C.

9. Remove and dispose the supernatant, with caution not to disturb the RNA pellet (*see* **Note 9**).

10. Wash the RNA pellet with 1.0 mL of 80% ethanol per 1.0 mL of TRIzol initially used.

11. Mix and incubate at –20 °C for a minimum of 4 h (*see* **Note 8**).

12. Centrifuge at $15,000 \times g$ for 15 min at 4 °C.

13. Remove and dispose the supernatant, with caution not to disturb the RNA pellet (*see* **Note 9**).

14. Dry the RNA pellet by vacuum.

15. Resuspend the RNA in RNase-free ultrapure water (20–50 μL) and incubate in a water bath at 50–60 °C for 5–10 min to ensure the pellet is completely dissolved. Mix and centrifuge briefly.

16. The RNA solution can then be used, stored at –20 °C for short-term storage, or stored at –80 °C for long-term storage.

3.3 RT-qPCR

1. Mix 1.1 μL nuclease-free water, 1.0 μL of 10× RT buffer, 0.13 μL of RNase inhibitor, 0.1 μL of dNTP mix, and 0.67 μL of reverse transcriptase (*see* **Note 10**).

2. Add 5.0 μL RNA (sample extract) and 2.0 μL of the target specific 5× TaqMan RT primer.

3. Centrifuge mixture briefly and incubate on ice for 5 min.

4. Place on thermocycler and run the following temperature program: 30 min at 16 °C, 32 min at 42 °C, then 5 min at 85 °C. Store the solutions (the RT products from miRNAs) at –20 °C until further use.

5. Prepare a qPCR master mix for each target containing the following per reaction: 4.9 μL nuclease-free water, 1.0 μL ethylene glycol, 0.1 μL DMSO, 0.5 μL 25 mM magnesium chloride, 2.0 μL Taq 5× Master Mix, and 0.5 μL of the specific 20× qPCR primer mix (*see* **Note 10**).

6. On a PCR plate, add 1 μL of RT product and 9 μL of the corresponding qPCR master mix in each well. MiRNA standards (10 zmol to 10 fmol) for each target should be run on each qPCR plate in addition to the targets in the sample and the exogenous control for accurate quantification.

7. Place plate on the real-time PCR system with the following temperature cycles; initial denaturation/activation at 95 °C for 90 s and then annealing at 59 °C for 50 s, followed by 40 cycles of; 95 °C for 30 s and then 53 °C for 70 s, measuring the plate fluorescence at the end of each cycle.

8. MiRNA content can then be calculated from the constructed standard curves, using the quantification of the exogenous control for miRNA recovery adjustment (the calculated absolute concentration in sample divided by the relative recovery fraction).

9. Correlation of the miRNA content associated with each collected fraction can then be used for profiling the miRNA based on the carrier species.

4   Notes

1. The salts will take time to dissolve and adequate mixing will speed up the process. Ensure the salts are fully dissolved before adjusting the pH.

2. Concentrated NaOH or HCl (12 N) can be used for larger adjustments and 1 N solution can be used for finer pH adjustment. The concentrated acid and base are corrosive and should handle with caution.

3. This flow profile allows for elution of small species and the gradual elution of larger species over a large size range. The actual flow rates should be optimized using standard HDL, LDL, and the isolated exosomes. These standards can be stained with the lipid-sensitive dyes like DiO (3 μg of DiO in 24 μL of serum and incubated for 20 min). The optimized flow rates should separate HDL and LDL well, and LDL and exosome could have some overlap (Fig. 1a).

4. The time windows for fraction collection should also be determined by spiking these standards into serum and fractionating the spiked serum using the optimized flow rates. The peaks from the standards spiked in the serum can then determine the elution window(s) for each carrier (Fig. 1b).

5. MiRNA from *C. elegans* are ideal, as many of these do not have analogs with human miRNA. Typically used analogs are cel-miR-39, -54, or -67.

6. There should be two distinct layers, a lower organic phase (pink) and upper aqueous phase (colorless) with an interphase between the two layers. The top phase can be isolated by pipetting carefully. Holding the microcentrifuge tube at a 45° angle can help maximize removal.

7. Over 4 mg/mL of glycogen can have potential PCR inhibition effects.

8. Low temperature and long incubations increase miRNA recovery due to their slight solubility in alcohol solutions at higher temperatures.

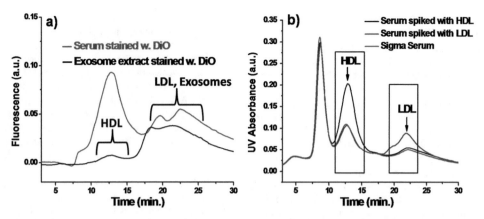

Fig. 1 (**a**) Separation of pooled healthy male AB serum and exosome extract stained with DiO for fluorescence detection of lipophilic species; (**b**) Separation of pooled serum and pooled serum spiked with HDL or LDL with absorbance detection at 260 nm

9. The RNA pellet is usually invisible but forms on the bottom side of the tube.

10. Mix solutions gently by hand inversion to prevent denaturation of enzymes.

References

1. Hagen JW, Lai EC (2008) microRNA control of cell-cell signaling during development and disease. Cell Cycle 7:2327–2332

2. Nicoloso MS, Spizzo R, Shimizu M, Rossi S, Calin GA (2009) MicroRNAs—the micro steering wheel of tumour metastases. Nat Rev Cancer 9:293–302. doi:10.1038/nrc2619

3. Shi M, Liu D, Duan H, Shen B, Guo N (2010) Metastasis-related miRNAs, active players in breast cancer invasion, and metastasis. Cancer Metastasis Rev 29:785–799. doi:10.1007/s10555-010-9265-9

4. Volinia S, Galasso M, Costinean S, Tagliavini L, Gamberoni G, Drusco A, Marchesini J, Mascellani N, Sana ME, Abu Jarour R, Desponts C, Teitell M, Baffa R, Aqeilan R, Iorio MV, Taccioli C, Garzon R, Di Leva G, Fabbri M, Catozzi M, Previati M, Ambs S, Palumbo T, Garofalo M, Veronese A, Bottoni A, Gasparini P, Harris CC, Visone R, Pekarsky Y, de la Chapelle A, Bloomston M, Dillhoff M, Rassenti LZ, Kipps TJ, Huebner K, Pichiorri F, Lenze D, Cairo S, Buendia M-A, Pineau P, Dejean A, Zanesi N, Rossi S, Calin GA, Liu C-G, Palatini J, Negrini M, Vecchione A, Rosenberg A, Croce CM (2010) Reprogramming of miRNA networks in cancer and leukemia. Genome Res 20:589–599. doi:10.1101/gr.098046.109

5. Dontu G, de Rinaldis E (2010) MicroRNAs: shortcuts in dealing with molecular complexity? Breast Cancer Res 12:301. doi:10.1186/bcr2455

6. Ma L, Weinberg RA (2008) Micromanagers of malignancy: role of microRNAs in regulating metastasis. Trends Genet 24:448–456. doi:10.1016/j.tig.2008.06.004

7. Ventura A, Jacks T (2009) MicroRNAs and cancer: short RNAs go a long way. Cell 136:586–591. doi:10.1016/j.cell.2009.02.005

8. Creemers EE, Tijsen AJ, Pinto YM (2012) Circulating microRNAs: novel biomarkers and extracellular communicators in cardiovascular disease? Circ Res 110:483–495. doi:10.1161/CIRCRESAHA.111.247452

9. Laganà A, Russo F, Veneziano D, Bella SD, Giugno R, Pulvirenti A, Croce CM, Ferro A (2013) Extracellular circulating viral microRNAs: current knowledge and perspectives. Front Genet. doi:10.3389/fgene.2013.00120

10. Olivieri F, Rippo MR, Procopio AD, Fazioli F (2013) Circulating inflamma-miRs in aging and age-related diseases. Front Genet 4:121. doi:10.3389/fgene.2013.00121

11. Rykova EY, Laktionov PP, Vlassov VV (2010) Circulating nucleic acids in health and disease. In: Kikuchi Y, Rykova EY (eds) Extracellular

nucleic acids. Springer, Berlin, Heidelberg, pp 93–128

12. Etheridge A, Lee I, Hood L, Galas D, Wang K (2011) Extracellular microRNA: a new source of biomarkers. Mutat Res 717:85–90. doi:10.1016/j.mrfmmm.2011.03.004

13. Turchinovich A, Weiz L, Burwinkel B (2012) Extracellular miRNAs: the mystery of their origin and function. Trends Biochem Sci 37:460–465. doi:10.1016/j.tibs.2012.08.003

14. Wang K, Zhang S, Weber J, Baxter D, Galas DJ (2010) Export of microRNAs and microRNA-protective protein by mammalian cells. Nucleic Acids Res gkq601. doi: 10.1093/nar/gkq601

15. Wahlund KG, Giddings JC (1987) Properties of an asymmetrical flow field-flow fractionation channel having one permeable wall. Anal Chem 59:1332–1339. doi:10.1021/ac00136a016

16. Kim KH, Moon MH (2011) Chip-type asymmetrical flow field-flow fractionation channel coupled with mass spectrometry for top-down protein identification. Anal Chem 83:8652–8658. doi:10.1021/ac202098b

17. Oh S, Kang D, Ahn S-M, Simpson RJ, Lee B-H, Moon MH (2007) Miniaturized asymmetrical flow field-flow fractionation: application to biological vesicles. J Sep Sci 30:1082–1087

18. Kim KH, Lee JY, Lim S, Moon MH (2013) Top-down lipidomic analysis of human lipoproteins by chip-type asymmetrical flow field-flow fractionation-electrospray ionization-tandem mass spectrometry. J Chromatogr A 1280:92–97. doi:10.1016/j.chroma.2013.01.025

19. Madörin M, van Hoogevest P, Hilfiker R, Langwost B, Kresbach GM, Ehrat M, Leuenberger H (1997) Analysis of drug/plasma protein interactions by means of asymmetrical flow field-flow fractionation. Pharm Res 14:1706–1712

20. Pollastrini J, Dillon TM, Bondarenko P, Chou RY-T (2011) Field flow fractionation for assessing neonatal Fc receptor and Fcγ receptor binding to monoclonal antibodies in solution. Anal Biochem 414:88–98. doi:10.1016/j.ab.2011.03.001

21. Schachermeyer S, Ashby J, Zhong W (2013) Aptamer-protein binding detected by asymmetric flow field flow fractionation. J Chromatogr A 1295:107–113. doi:10.1016/j.chroma.2013.04.063

22. Ashby J, Flack K, Jimenez LA, Duan Y, Khatib A-K, Somlo G, Wang SE, Cui X, Zhong W (2014) Distribution profiling of circulating microRNAs in serum. Anal Chem 86:9343–9349. doi:10.1021/ac5028929

Chapter 16

MicroRNA Expression Profiling Using Agilent One-Color Microarray

Carmela Dell'Aversana, Cristina Giorgio, and Lucia Altucci

Abstract

MicroRNA (miRNA) expression profiling is an important tool to identify miRNA regulation in physiological or pathological states. This technique has a large number of molecular diagnostic applications, including in cancer, cardiovascular and autoimmune diseases, and forensics. To date, a multitude of high-throughput genomic approaches have been developed. Here, we focus on miRNA expression profiling by microarray using SurePrint technology, providing a description of both the workflow and methods for expression profiling by Agilent One-Color Microarray.

Key words Expression profile, miRNA, Microarray, Platform, Slide

1 Introduction

MicroRNAs (miRNAs) are a class of noncoding RNAs that regulate gene expression at posttranscriptional and translational levels. Strong and converging evidence indicates an important role for miRNAs in wide range of fundamental biological processes, including development, cell proliferation and differentiation [1, 2]. Dysregulation of tightly controlled miRNA expression, processing and functional activity characterizes many disease states, including cancer [3]. The significance of miRNAs in diagnostic and prognostic determination as well as for potential therapeutic intervention has also been reported [4].

Given the importance of regulating gene expression, the advent of miRNA research has led to the development of ever more widely used molecular and biological technologies, such as microarray [5]. Microarray technology applied to miRNA profiling is a promising high-throughput tool able to identify and monitor miRNA expression in both normal and abnormal states. In particular, it can define specific signatures linked to prognosis, diagnosis, and response to treatment in many pathologies [6].

Sweta Rani (ed.), *MicroRNA Profiling: Methods and Protocols*, Methods in Molecular Biology, vol. 1509,
DOI 10.1007/978-1-4939-6524-3_16, © Springer Science+Business Media New York 2017

One major advantage of the microarray approach is its ability to detect small amounts of miRNAs, quickly and simultaneously screening up to thousands of miRNA genes in a single experiment and in a cost-effective manner [7].

The choice of platform depends on key features that may arise from capture probe design spotted on a slide or on beads that influence the improvement of sensitivity, detection of labeled individual miRNAs, miRBase content, species coverage, extraction of intensity signals, and successive and accessible data analyses.

Currently, a wide range of commercial platforms based on different technologies are available for global miRNA expression profiling, such as oligonucleotide microarray, LNA (locked nucleic acid) arrays (Exiqon), bead-based technology (Illumina), and microfluidic system (Agilent, LC Biosciences) [8, 9] (Table 1).

This chapter focuses on miRNA expression profiling using Agilent Microarray SurePrint technology. Specifically, the SurePrint platform has a higher throughput with eight arrays on a single slide, assuring a comprehensive coverage of updated miRBase content. This high-throughput system combines a unique probe design and an optimized direct labeling method with SurePrint inkjet technology, where 40–60-mer oligonucleotide probes are directly synthesized on the array. The powerful outcome is a result of the high-fidelity of probes, reproducibility, optimal sensitivity and specificity for both sequence and size discrimination. The superior performance of SurePrint technology lies in the low input of total RNA requirement (about 100 ng) and in the possibility to omit fractionation or amplification steps and thus eliminate any resulting bias. Finally, Agilent's miRNA microarray platform supplies different types of catalogue kits and custom array designs for human, mouse, and rat. This chapter provides a detailed description of the workflow and methods for microarray miRNA profiling (Fig. 1).

Table 1
Schematic comparison of microRNA microarray platforms. List of aspects of RNA amount and hybridization and probe features

	Exiqon	Agilent	Illumina	LC Biosciences	Reference
Platform	miRCURY LNA microRNA arrays	Agilent 60-mer SurePrint technology	Sentrix® Array Matrix and BeadChips	µParaFlo™ Biochip Array	[8]
Channels	Dual	Single	Single	Dual	
Labeling	Hy3	Cy3	Cy3	Cy3/Cy5	
Input total RNA	1000 ng	100 ng	200 ng	1000–3000 ng	
miRBase version	19	21	12	20	

Total RNA, including miRNAs (100 ng) + Labeling Spike-In (optional)

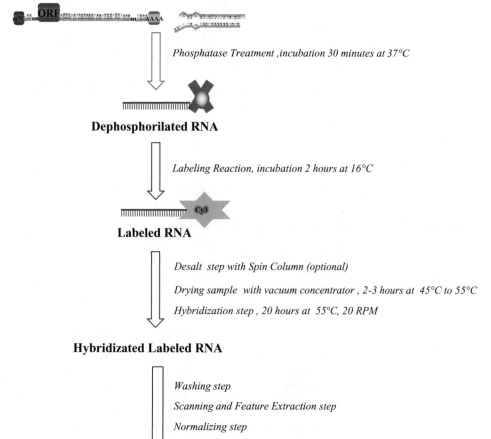

Phosphatase Treatment ,incubation 30 minutes at 37°C

Dephosphorilated RNA

Labeling Reaction, incubation 2 hours at 16°C

Labeled RNA

Desalt step with Spin Column (optional)

Drying sample with vacuum concentrator , 2-3 hours at 45°C to 55°C

Hybridization step , 20 hours at 55°C, 20 RPM

Hybridizated Labeled RNA

Washing step

Scanning and Feature Extraction step

Normalizing step

miRNA profile

Fig. 1 Workflow for sample preparation and array processing

2   Materials

Prepare a clean work area. To prevent contamination of reagents by nucleases, always wear powder-free laboratory gloves, and use dedicated solutions and pipettors with nuclease-free aerosol-resistant tips.

2.1   Required Equipment

1. Platform. G4871A Custom G3 miRNA Microarray, 8 × 60 K or G4474A Custom HD miRNA Microarray, 8 × 15 K.

2. Agilent Microarray Scanner (Agilent p/n G4900DA, G2565CA or G2565BA).

3. Hybridization Chamber, stainless Agilent p/n G2534A.

4. Hybridization gasket slides eight microarrays/slide, five slides/ Agilent p/n G2534-60014.

5. Hybridization oven; temperature set at 55 °C Agilent p/n G2545A.

6. Hybridization oven rotator for Agilent Microarray Hybridization Chambers Agilent p/n G2530-60029.

7. 2100 Bioanalyzer Agilent p/n G2939AA.

8. Ozone-Barrier Slide Cover (Agilent p/n G2505-60550).

9. Micro Bio-Spin P-6 Gel Column Bio-Rad p/n 732-6221.

10. Dye filter Sigma p/n Z361569 thermal cycler.

2.2 Required Reagents

1. Gene Expression wash buffers.
   Add 0.005% Triton X-102 (10%) to Gene Expression wash buffers 1 and 2 (Agilent p/n 5188–5327) to reduce the possibility of array wash artifacts.

2. miRNA Complete Labeling and Hyb Kit Agilent p/n 5190–0456.

3. Stabilization and Drying Solution Agilent p/n 5185–5979.

4. MicroRNA Spike-In Kit Agilent p/n 5190–1934.

5. RNA 6000 Nano Assay Kit (RNA Series II Kit) Agilent p/n 5067–1511 or RNA 6000 Pico Kit Agilent p/n 5067–1513 or Small RNA Kit Agilent p/n 5067–1548.

6. MicroRNA Spike-In Kit Agilent p/n 5190–1934.

7. 1× tris EDTA pH 7.5.

8. Acetonitrile Sigma p/n 271004-1 L.

2.3 Reagent Required for miRNA Isolation

1. TRIzol.

2. 2-bromo-3-chloropropane.

3. Isopropyl alcohol.

4. 70% ethanol.

5. NanoDrop 1000 spectrophotometer (Thermo Scientific).

6. Agilent 2100 Bioanalyzer.

7. RNA 6000 Nano Kit Agilent p/n 5067–1511; RNA 6000 Pico Kit Agilent p/n 5067–1513; Small RNA it Agilent p/n 5067-1548.

3 Methods

Carry out all procedures at controlled temperature as specifically indicated.

3.1 Total RNA, Including miRNA, Isolation

1. Resuspend the cells, collected by centrifugation, in 1 mL TRIzol reagent, shake vigorously and store at –20 °C overnight.

2. The following day, add 100 μL 2-bromo-3-chloropropane to the samples, shake gently and incubate for 15 min at RT.

3. After centrifugation at $18,900 \times g$ for 15 min at 4 °C, put the supernatants in a fresh tube and add with 500 μl cold isopropyl alcohol.

4. Carry out the RNA precipitation reaction for 30 min at –80 °C, followed by centrifugation at $18,900 \times g$ for 30 min at 4 °C.

5. Resuspend pellet in 1 ml cold 70% ethanol and centrifuge again at $5974 \times g$ for 10 min at 4 °C.

6. Dry the pellet at 42 °C for a few minutes and resuspend in DEPC-treated H_2O.

7. Quantify RNA extract with a NanoDrop 1000 spectrophotometer.

8. Prior to use, determine the integrity of the input RNA using the Agilent 2100 Bioanalyzer (*see* **Note 1**).

9. The RNA 6000 Nano Kit Agilent can be used. For low concentration samples, use the RNA 6000 Pico Kit Agilent. To better characterize the small RNA content of which a fraction is miRNA, use the Small RNA it Agilent.

3.2 Sample Preparation and Labeling

This step is performed using the miRNA Complete Labeling and Hyb Kit to generate Cyanine 3-pCp RNA molecules at the 3′ end, with greater than 90% efficiency and with a sample input of 100 ng of total RNA.

3.2.1 Prepare Spike-In Solutions (Optional)

1. Prepare the first Dilution Labeling Spike-In solution mixing 198 μL of the Dilution Buffer and 2 μL of the Labeling Spike-In solution.

2. Prepare the first Dilution Hyb Spike-In solution mixing 198 μL of the Dilution Buffer and 2 μL of the Hyb Spike-In solution.

3. Mix well and briefly spin tubes.

4. Prepare the second Dilution Spike-In solutions (second Dilution Labeling Spike-In solution and second Dilution Hyb Spike-In solution) mixing 2 μL of 1st Dilution Labeling Spike-In solution or 2 μL of 1st Dilution Hyb Spike-In solution with 198 μL of nuclease-free water.

5. Mix well and briefly spin tubes.

6. Prepare the third Dilution Spike-In solutions (third Dilution Labeling Spike-In solution and third Dilution Hyb Spike-In solution) mixing 2 μL of second Dilution Labeling Spike-In solution or 2 μL of second Dilution Hyb Spike-In solution with 198 μL of nuclease-free water.

7. Discard the second Dilution Spike-In solutions and third Dilution Spike-In solutions after use.

8. Store first Dilution Spike-In solutions at −80 °C (*see* **Note 2**).

3.2.2 Dephosphorylate the Sample

1. Dilute total RNA sample to 50 ng/μL in 1× tris EDTA pH 7.5 or DNase/RNase-free distilled water.

2. Add 2 μL (100 ng) of the diluted total RNA to a nuclease-free 1.5 mL microfuge tube and maintain on ice.

3. Immediately prior to use, add the components in the order indicated in Table 2 to create the Calf Intestinal Phosphatase (CIP) Master Mix. Maintain on ice.

4. Add 2 μL of the CIP Master Mix to each sample tube for a total reaction volume of 4 μL. Gently mix by pipetting.

5. Incubate the reaction at 37 °C in a circulating water bath or heat block for 30 min.

3.2.3 Denature the Sample

1. Add 2.8 μL of DMSO to each sample.

2. Incubate samples at 100 °C in a circulating water bath or heat block for 5–10 min.

3.2.4 Ligate the Sample

1. Warm the 10× T4 RNA Ligase Buffer at 37 °C and mix on a vortex mixer until all precipitate is dissolved.

2. Immediately prior to use, prepare the Ligation Master Mix. Gently mix the components listed in Table 3 and maintain on ice.

3. Immediately add 4.5 μL of the Ligation Master Mix to each sample tube for a total reaction volume of 11.3 μL. Gently mix by pipetting and gently spin down (*see* **Note 3**).

4. Incubate at 16 °C in a circulating water bath or cool block for 2 h. The sample can be stored at −80 °C, if needed.

3.2.5 Purify the Labeled RNA (Optional)

This step removes DMSO and free Cyanine 3-pCp with Micro Bio-Spin P-6 Gel Column (*see* **Note 4**).

Table 2
Preparation of dephosphorylation mix

CIP master mix	Volume (μL) for reaction
10× Calf intestinal phosphatase buffer	0.4
Third dilution labeling spike-in solution or nuclease-free water	1.1
Calf intestinal phosphatase	0.5
Total volume	2.0

Table 3
Preparation of labeling mix

Ligation master mix	Volume (μL) for reaction
10× T4 RNA ligase buffer	1.0
Cyanine 3-pCp	3.0
T4 RNA ligase	0.5
Total volume	4.5

1. Invert the Micro Bio-Spin P-6 Gel Column sharply several times to resuspend the settled gel and to remove any air bubbles.

2. Snap off the tip and place into a 2-mL collection tube supplied with the Micro Bio-Spin P-6 Gel Column.

3. Remove the green cap from the Micro Bio-Spin P-6 Gel Column. If the buffer does not drip into the 2-mL collection tube, press the green cap back onto the Micro Bio-Spin P-6 Gel Column and remove it again. Let the buffer drain for about 2 min.

4. Check to make sure that all columns are evenly drained.

5. Discard the drained buffer from the 2-mL collection tube and then place the Micro Bio-Spin P-6 Gel Column back into the tube.

6. Spin the microcentrifuge tube containing the Micro Bio-Spin P-6 Gel Column for 2 min at $1000 \times g$ in a centrifuge.

7. Remove the Micro Bio-Spin P-6 Gel Column from the 2-mL collection tube and place it into a clean nuclease-free 1.5 mL microfuge tube. Discard the 2-mL collection tube. The sample can be stored at −80 °C, if needed.

8. Add 38.7 μL of 1× tris EDTA pH 7.5 or DNase/RNase-free distilled water to the labeled sample for a total volume of 50 μL. Without disturbing the gel bed, use a pipette to transfer the 50 μL sample onto the gel bed from step above.

9. Spin the microcentrifuge tubes that contain the columns for 4 min at $1000 \times g$ in a centrifuge to elute the purified sample. Discard the columns and keep on ice the flow-through that contains the miRNA sample. Check that the final flow-through is translucent and slightly pink. The flow-through volume needs to be uniform across the samples and close to 50 μL.

3.3 Dry the Sample

After the 16 °C labeling reaction or sample purification, completely dry the samples. Use a vacuum concentrator with heater at 45–55 °C or on the medium–high heat setting (*see* **Note 5**).

3.4 Hybridization

3.4.1 Prepare the 10×
Blocking Agent

1. Add 125 µL of nuclease-free water to the vial containing lyophilized 10× Gene Expression Blocking Agent supplied with the miRNA Complete Labeling and Hyb Kit.

2. Gently mix on a vortex mixer. If the pellet does not go into solution completely, heat the mix for 4–5 min at 37 °C.

3.4.2 Prepare
Hybridization Samples

1. Equilibrate water bath or heat block to 100 °C.

2. Resuspend the dried sample in 17 µL of nuclease-free water when the Hyb Spike-In solution is used and 18 µL when the Hyb Spike-In solution is not used.

3. For each microarray, add each of the components as indicated in Tables 4 or 5 to a 1.5 mL nuclease-free microfuge tube. Mix well but gently on a vortex mixer. Incubate at 100 °C for 5 min.

4. Immediately transfer to an ice water bath for 5 min.

5. Quickly spin in a centrifuge to collect any condensation at the bottom of the tube. Immediately proceed to following step.

3.4.3 Prepare
the Hybridization Assembly

1. Load a clean gasket slide into the Agilent SureHyb chamber base with the label facing up and aligned with the rectangular section of the chamber base.

2. Slowly dispense all of the volume of hybridization sample onto the gasket well in a "drag and dispense" manner.

Table 4
Preparation of hybridization mix with Hyb Spike-In solution

Hybridization mix for miRNA microarrays with Hyb Spike-In solution	Volume (µL) for reaction
Labeled miRNA sample	17
3rd Dilution Hyb Spike-In solution	1.0
10× Gene expression blocking agent	4.5
2× Hi-RPM hybridization buffer	22.5
Total volume	45

Table 5
Preparation of Hybridization mix without Hyb Spike-In solution

Hybridization mix for miRNA microarrays without Hyb Spike-In solution	Volume (µL) for reaction
Labeled miRNA sample	18
10× Gene Expression Blocking Agent	4.5
2× Hi-RPM hybridization buffer	22.5
Total volume	45

3. Avoid the introduction of air bubbles to the gasket wells (*see* **Note 6**). If you have any wells unused (*see* **Note 7**).

4. Grip the slide on either end and slowly put the slide "active side" down, parallel to the SureHyb gasket slide, so that the "Agilent"-labeled barcode is facing down and the numeric barcode is facing up.

5. Make sure that the sandwich-pair is properly aligned.

6. Put the SureHyb chamber cover onto the sandwiched slides and slide the clamp assembly onto both pieces.

7. Firmly hand-tighten the clamp onto the chamber. Vertically rotate the assembled chamber to wet the gasket and assess the mobility of the bubbles. If necessary, tap the assembly on a hard surface to move stationary bubbles.

3.4.4 Hybridize

1. Load each assembled chamber into the oven rotator rack.

2. Hybridize at 55 °C for 20 h with rotation at 20 rpm.

3.5 Microarray Wash

This step is optional but highly recommended.

1. Prewarm 1000 mL of Gene Expression Wash Buffer 2 and slide-staining dish directly into a sterile storage bottle by storing overnight in an incubator set to 37 °C. Wash staining dishes, racks and stir bars with 100% acetonitrile or isopropyl alcohol for 5 min. Air-dry the staining dish in the vented fume hood. Wash all dishes, racks, and stir bars with Milli-Q water.

2. Disassemble the hybridization chamber. Remove the array-gasket sandwich from the chamber base by grabbing the slides from their ends. Submerge the array-gasket sandwich into the slide-staining dish containing Gene Expression Wash Buffer 1 at room temperature. Remove the cover slide and keep the microarray slide with numeric barcode.

3. Perform 1st wash with Gene Expression Wash Buffer 1 at room temperature for 5 min.

4. Transfer microarray slide into Gene Expression Prewarm Wash Buffer 2 at 37 °C. Wash slide for 5 min using stir bar at moderate speed setting.

5. Slowly remove the slide rack minimizing droplets on the slides (*see* **Note 8**).

6. Discard used Gene Expression Wash Buffer 1 and 2.

7. Put the slides in a slide holder.
For SureScan microarray scanner: Carefully put the end of the slide without the barcode label onto the slide ledge. Gently lower the microarray slide into the slide holder. Make sure that the active microarray surface (with "Agilent"-labeled barcode) faces up, towards the slide cover. Close the plastic slide cover, pushing on the tab end until you hear it click (*see* **Note 9**).

For Agilent Scanner C only: In environments in which the ozone level exceeds 50 ppb, immediately put the slides with active microarray surface (with "Agilent"-labeled barcode) facing up in a slide holder. Make sure that the slide is not caught up on any corner. Put an ozone-barrier slide cover on top of the array.

8. Scan slides immediately to minimize the impact of environmental oxidants on signal intensities (*see* **Note 10**).

3.6 Scanning and Feature Extraction

This section describes how to scan and extract data from miRNA microarrays (*see* **Note 11**).

3.6.1 A. Slide Scan

For Agilent SureScan Microarray Scanner

1. Put assembled slide holders into the scanner cassette.

2. Select the appropriate scanner protocol: AgilentG3_miRNA (for G3 format)/AgilentHD_miRNA (for HD format).

3. Verify that the Scanner status in the main window says Scanner Ready.

4. Click Start Scan.

For Agilent C Scanner Settings

1. Put assembled slide holders with or without the ozone-barrier slide cover into scanner carousel.

2. Select Start Slot *m* End Slot *n* where the letter *m* represents the Start slot where the first slide is located and the letter *n* represents the End slot where the last slide is located.

3. Select AgilentG3_miRNA (for SurePrint G3 formats) or AgilentHD_miRNA (for SurePrint HD formats).

4. Verify scan settings for -colour scans (Table 6).

5. Verify that Output Path Browse is set for desired location.

6. Verify that the Scanner status in the main window says Scanner Ready.

Table 6
Agilent C microarray scanner setting

C Scanner scan settings	For HD microarray formats	For G3 microarray formats
Dye channel	G (*green*)	G (*green*)
Scan region	Agilent HD (61×21.6 mm)	Agilent HD (61×21.6 mm)
Scan resolution	5 µm	3 µm
TIFF file dynamic range	20 bit	20 bit
Green PMT gain	100%	100%

7. Click Scan Slot *m-n* on the Scan Control main window where the letter *m* represents the Start slot where the first slide is located and the letter *n* represents the End slot where the last slide is located.

For Agilent B Scanner Settings

1. Put slide into slide holder, with or without the ozone-barrier slide cover, with Agilent barcode facing up.

2. Put assembled slide holders into scanner carousel.

3. Change scan settings -colour scans (Table 7).

4. Select settings for the automatic file naming (*see* **Note 12**).
   - Prefix1 is set to Instrument Serial Number.
   - Prefix2 is set to Array Barcode.

5. Verify that the Scanner status in the main window says Scanner Ready.

6. Click Scan Slot *m-n* on the Scan Control main window where the letter *m* represents the Start slot where the first slide is located and the letter *n* represents the End slot where the last slide is located.

3.6.2 B. Extract Data Using Agilent Feature Extraction Software

Feature Extraction is the process by which information from probe features is extracted from microarray scan data, allowing researchers to measure miRNA expression in their experiments (*see* **Note 13**).

1. Open the Agilent Feature Extraction (FE) program (*see* **Note 14**).

2. Add the images (.tif) to be extracted to the FE Project.
   (a) Click Add New Extraction Set(s) icon on the toolbar or right-click the Project Explorer and select Add Extraction…

Table 7
Agilent B microarray scanner setting

B Scanner scan settings	For all formats
Scan region	Scan Area (61 × 21.6 mm)
Scan resolution (μm)	5
5 μm scanning mode	Single Pass
eXtended Dynamic range	(selected)
Dye channel	Green
Green PMT	XDR Hi 100 % XDR Lo 5 %

(b) Browse to the location of the .tif files, select the .tif file(s) and click Open. To select multiple files, use the Shift or Ctrl key when selecting.

The FE program automatically assigns a default grid template and protocol for each extraction set, if the following conditions are met:

1. For auto assignment of the grid template, the image must be generated from the Agilent scanner and have an Agilent barcode.

2. For auto assignment of the -Colour miRNA FE protocol, the default miRNA protocol must be specified in the FE Grid Template properties.

To access the FE Grid Template properties, double-click on the grid template in the Grid Template Browser.

Set FE Project Properties.

(a) Select the Project Properties tab.

(b) In the General section, enter your name in the Operator text box.

(c) In the Input section, verify the default settings.

(d) For versions of FE earlier than 10.7.3, in the Other section, from the QC Metric Set drop-down list, select miRNA_QCMT_Jan09.

1. Check the Extraction Set Configuration.

(a) Select the Extraction Set Configuration tab.

(b) Verify that the correct grid template is assigned to each extraction set in the Grid Name column. To assign a different grid template to an extraction set, select one from the pull down menu.

(c) Verify that the correct protocol is assigned to each extraction set in the Protocol Name column. For Agilent miRNA microarrays, select miRNA_107_Sept09.

2. Save the FE Project (.fep) by selecting File > Save As and browse for desired location.

3. Verify that the icons for the image files in the FE Project Window no longer have a red X through them. A red X through the icon indicates that an extraction protocol was not selected. If needed, reselect the extraction protocol for that image file.

4. Select Project > Start Extracting.

5. After the extraction is completed successfully, view the QC report for each extraction (Fig. 2) set by double-clicking the QC Report link in the Summary Report tab.

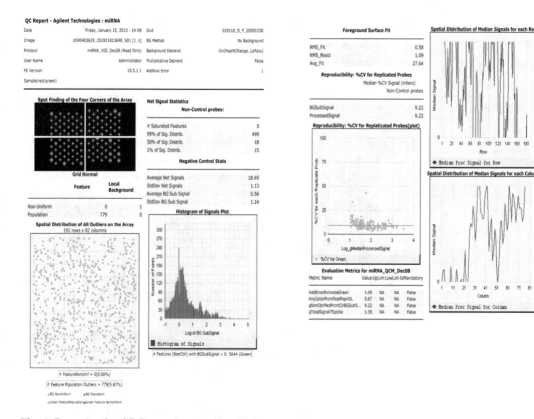

Fig. 2 Example of a QC Report for 8x15K miRNA microarray, generated Agilent Feature Extraction Software Version 10.5.1.1 (FE 10.5.1) without Spike-in miRNA

3.7 Normalizing Agilent One-Color Microarray Data

It is recommended to use the signal value of the 90th percentile of all of non-control probes on the microarray as a start. GeneSpring GX 11.5 or later (*see* **Note 12**) or Feature Extraction software may be used.

3.7.1 To Use Feature Extraction

To normalize Agilent one-color microarray data without the GeneSpring program, use the 90th percentile value for each microarray assay in the Agilent Feature Extraction text file.

1. Generate a Feature Extraction text file.

2. Find the "STATS Table" in the middle section of the text file. This section describes the results from the array-wide statistical calculations.

3. Find the 90th percentile value of the non-control signals under the column with the heading gPercentileIntensityProcessedSignal.

4. Divide each of the green processed signals (gProcessedSignal) by the 90th percentile signal (gPercentileIntensityProcessed-Signal) to generate the 90th percentile normalized microarray processed signals.

5. You can further scale the resulting 90th percentile-normalized signals by a constant, such as the average of the 90th percentile signals of the arrays in the experiment.

4 Notes

1. This step is important to increase the likelihood of a successful experiment. Valuate the presence of contaminants by 260/230 nm value. This ratio should be greater than 1.8. If the ratio is less than 1.8, then the sample needs to be further purified by performing additional extractions with chloroform, followed by an ethanol precipitation. Furthermore, the Agilent 2100 Expert Software automatically provides an RNA Integrity Number (RIN). The ideal RIN value should be 8–10.

2. Do not freeze/thaw the original or 1st Dilutions Spike-In solutions more than twice. Prepare aliquots when thawed the first time for subsequent use.

3. From this step, it is very important to protect the samples from direct light by use of wrapped aluminum foil.

4. The use of the column reduces the necessary drying time in Subheading 3.3.

5. This step can take up to 1 h after column purification and up to 3 h without column purification. Check the samples after 30 min. Continue vacuum concentration until they are dry. To check for sample dryness, flick hard on the tube and make sure that the pellets do not move or spread.

6. Air bubbles can affect the final sample volume and can cause leakage from the gasket well.

7. Make a 1× solution of the 2× Hi-RPM Hybridization Buffer and add an equal amount of the sample volume to each unused well. Empty wells can cause failure in hybridization (e.g., gridding errors in Feature Extraction).

8. Remove the slide rack in 5 to 10 s to minimize scratch or droplets on the slide, which may disturb the signal scanning.

9. For more detailed instructions, refer to the Agilent G4900DA SureScan Microarray Scanner System User Guide.

10. If necessary, store slides in orange slide boxes in a nitrogen purge box, in the dark.

11. In Slide Scan step, the use of Agilent Scan Control software v7.0. is recommended for 5 μm scans of SurePrint HD formats.

12. The Agilent B Scanner does not support G3 microarrays. For G3 microarrays, use the Agilent C Scanner or SureScan microarray scanner.

13. To get the most recent Feature Extraction software for gene expression, go to the Agilent web site at www.agilent.com/chem/fe. To get the most recent Feature Extraction protocols for gene expression, go to www.agilent.com/chem/feprotocols.

14. For more information on the GeneSpring GX program, go to http://www.agilent.com/chem/genespring.

Acknowledgements

We thank C. Fisher for linguistic editing. This work was supported by: Blueprint (282510); EPIGEN (MIUR-CNR); MIUR (PRIN-2012ZHN9YH).

References

1. Subramanian S, Steer CJ (2010) MicroRNAs as gatekeepers of apoptosis. J Cell Physiol 223(2):289–298. doi:10.1002/jcp.22066

2. Fabbri M, Croce CM, Calin GA (2008) MicroRNAs. Cancer J 14(1):1–6. doi:10.1097/PPO.0b013e318164145e

3. Hata A, Lieberman J (2015) Dysregulation of microRNA biogenesis and gene silencing in cancer. Science signaling 8(368):re3. doi:10.1126/scisignal.2005825

4. Wahid F, Khan T, Kim YY (2014) MicroRNA and diseases: therapeutic potential as new generation of drugs. Biochimie 104:12–26. doi:10.1016/j.biochi.2014.05.004

5. Pritchard CC, Cheng HH, Tewari M (2012) MicroRNA profiling: approaches and considerations. Nat Rev Genet 13(5):358–369. doi:10.1038/nrg3198

6. Croce CM (2008) Oncogenes and cancer. N Engl J Med 358(5):502–511. doi:10.1056/NEJMra072367

7. Mestdagh P, Feys T, Bernard N et al (2008) High-throughput stem-loop RT-qPCR miRNA expression profiling using minute amounts of input RNA. Nucleic Acids Res 36(21), e143. doi:10.1093/nar/gkn725

8. Kolbert CP, Feddersen RM, Rakhshan F et al (2013) Multi-platform analysis of microRNA expression measurements in RNA from fresh frozen and FFPE tissues. PLoS One 8(1):e52517. doi:10.1371/journal.pone.0052517

9. Keller P, Gburcik V, Petrovic N et al (2011) Gene-chip studies of adipogenesis-regulated microRNAs in mouse primary adipocytes and human obesity. BMC Endocr Disord 11:7. doi:10.1186/1472-6823-11-7

Chapter 17

A Multiplex Ligation Assay for miRNA Copy Number Profiling

Duncan Kilburn, Yunke Song, Tza-Huei Wang, and Kelvin J. Liu

Abstract

Ligo-miR is an assay technology that can perform multiplexed detection of miRNAs from a wide range of biological sources. At its core are two sequential ligation steps. First in the capture ligation, template molecules are created by ligating a DNA adapter to the 3′ end of all miRNA molecules. Then in the coding ligation these templates are used to generate, linearly amplified, DNA products encoded by length. The resultant number of each DNA product is proportional to the original number of miRNA molecules. The products and their corresponding miRNA can be identified and quantified using common DNA sizing methods such as electrophoresis.

Key words miRNA, Quantification assay, Multiplex, Profiling, Ligation, Copy number

1 Introduction

We have developed a rapid and easy-to-use multiplex assay that can accurately determine miRNA copy number called Ligo-miR. Ligo-miR uses a multiplex, two-step ligation process to generate length-coded, fluorescently labeled DNA products in direct proportion to the initial number of miRNA molecules. Length coding allows the DNA products to be separated and quantified using DNA sizing methods such as polyacrylamide gel electrophoresis (PAGE), capillary electrophoresis (CE) and single molecule separation [1]. Ligo-miR forms the core of a flexible three part workflow consisting of: (1) miRNA isolation, (2) Ligo-miR assay, and (3) data analysis. The core Ligo-miR assay can be customized for sensitivity, multiplex capability, and sample throughput based on application requirements and detection methodology.

Herein, we describe Ligo-miR with PAGE analysis to perform 18-plex miRNA profiling in an implementation called Ligo-miR EZ. This simple assay is unique in requiring only common laboratory equipment including a thermal cycler, PAGE system, and gel scanner to analyze up to 96 samples per day at 20 copies per cell

Sweta Rani (ed.), *MicroRNA Profiling: Methods and Protocols*, Methods in Molecular Biology, vol. 1509,
DOI 10.1007/978-1-4939-6524-3_17, © Springer Science+Business Media New York 2017

sensitivity. Due to its high sample throughput and high quantification accuracy, Ligo-miR EZ is ideally suited to targeted profiling of cells and tissues and validation of miRNA panels.

The carefully designed two-step ligation mechanism ensures high linearity across 4.5 orders of magnitude, high reproducibility, and low expression bias. Specificity studies using panels of closely related family members demonstrate high specificity discrimination of single nucleotide differences and perfect identification of precursor vs. mature miRNA. Analysis of mock expression panels demonstrates that differential sensitivity as low as <1.2 fold is reliably achieved. In direct comparisons to microarray and qRT-PCR, Ligo-miR EZ shows high correlations ($R^2 > 0.9$). Furthermore, Ligo-miR EZ can be used to transform relative and differential expression profiles into absolute miRNA copy number profiles by simply integrating the included spike-in controls and running 4 additional reference sample reactions. This system enables direct comparison of copy number expression profiles against relative expression profiles, increasing the breadth of analysis that can be performed and reducing dependence on biological controls.

2   Materials

2.1   Buffers Required

1. Gel Loading Buffer: 95 % formamide, 18 mM EDTA, 0.25 % SDS. For normal assay protocol, mix gel loading buffer with 4 % bromophenol blue dye.

2. Gel Running Buffer: 1× TBE buffer. 89 mM Tris base, 89 mM boric acid, 2 mM EDTA, pH = 8 at 25 °C.

2.2   Circulomics Provided Components

1. Capture Ligase.

2. Coding Ligase.

3. Capture Ligation Master Mix. Includes capture ligation buffer and adenylated adapter oligomer. Supplied as 5/3× concentration.

4. Coding Ligation Master Mix. Includes coding ligation buffer, fluorophore-labeled common probe, and 13-plex core panel discrimination probe mix. Supplied as 10× concentration.

5. 1-plex Custom Discrimination Probes. Individually supplied at 325 nM.

6. Post-isolation Spike-In Control S_1. Contains Crc1. Supplied at 1 μM.

7. Pre-isolation Spike-In Control S_2. Contains Crc2. Supplied at 1 μM.

8. 11-plex Core Panel Synthetic miRNA Target Mix. Synthetic target miRNA are supplied as master stock at concentrations of

1 μM. These can be further diluted using water and stored at concentrations no lower than 20 nM in –80 °C freezer. All lower concentrations are made just prior to use and discarded immediately after.

9. 1-plex Custom Synthetic miRNA Targets. Individually supplied at 1 μM. Handle as with miRNA Target Mix (**item 8** of Subheading 2.2).

10. HandyBand Software.

2.3 Equipment and Commercially Available Kits Required

1. GE Typhoon 9410 variable mode imager or equivalent confocal gel imager with 633 nm laser.

2. Qiagen miRNeasy kit (*see* **Note 1**).

3. PAGE apparatus and 15% denaturing urea PAGE gels. We typically use pre-cast Bio-Rad Mini-PROTEAN and ThermoFisher Novex gels.

4. Thermal cycler.

3 Methods

Keep all reagents on ice during protocol.

3.1 Spiking and Total RNA Isolation

1. This protocol is for 1×10^6 cultured cells (*see* **Notes 2** and **3**) and uses the Qiagen miRNeasy kit (*see* **Note 1**).

2. Dilute spike-in controls S_1 and S_2 to 10 nM with water.

3. Pellet the cell suspension as described in the Qiagen protocol.

4. Isolate total RNA using Qiagen miRNeasy kit. During protocol, spike 4 μL of S_2 into cells resuspended in Qiazol Lysis Reagent.

5. Elute total RNA from kit using 43 μL of water.

6. Transfer 38.7 μL of this resuspended stock to new tube.

7. Spike 1.80 μL of S_1 into transferred stock from **step 6** of Subheading 3.1

8. The final stock has total volume $V_F = 40.5$ μL. For different pellet sizes and different final miRNA and spike-in control concentrations, use the equations in **Note 2** to calculate new volumes for the isolation protocol.

9. The spiked total RNA is ready to use. Measure the isolated total RNA concentration, C_{RNA} (ng/μL). The effective cell concentration of the eluate above is 1×10^6 cells $\times (1/43) \times (38.7/40.5) = 22222$ cells/μL. The user now has an equivalence between RNA concentration and effective cell concentration. Literature values of the mass of RNA per cell are around 15 pg/cell, so for an RNA extraction of 22222 cells/μL we

would expect to measure 333 ng/μL. For specific cells the mass of RNA per cell can be calculated using: C_{RNA}/C_{cell} and may differ depending on cell type and experimental conditions. This stock can be used directly in the assay or diluted to the desired concentration. If total RNA is being used we recommend not exceeding 75 ng input for the assay or 1.5 μL of 50 ng/μL. These numbers can be used to back-calculate miRNA expression per cell when combined with data from the calibration curves (*see* next section).

10. Make the synthetic RNA samples for reference curves. Remove 20 nM 11-plex RNA stocks from −80 freezer. Combine with Crc1 and Crc2 spiking targets and appropriate 1-plex RNA stocks and dilute to 1 nM, 100 pM, 10 pM and 1 pM. 1.5 μL of these dilutions gives 1500, 150, 15, and 1.5 attomoles per miRNA input for the assay (*see* **Notes 4** and **5**). A gel image for a synthetic titration is shown in Fig. 1.

3.2 Capture Ligation

1. Combine:

Capture ligation master mix	3 μL
Sample	1.5 μL
Capture ligase	0.5 μL

Mix thoroughly by pipetting. Pipette slowly to avoid bubbles as the mixture is very viscous. Leave tip submerged under the surface of the solution for 10 s after the plunger has reached its maximum extension—this will allow the correct volume of

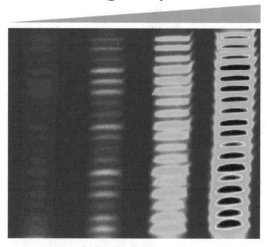

Fig. 1 Gel image of titration response curves for Ligo-miR EZ. Synthetic 18-plex targets were diluted in steps of 10 over 3 orders of magnitude from 1500 attomoles (*right*) to 1.5 attomoles (*left*)

solution to equilibrate properly (*see* **Notes 6** and **7**). If performing n assays, mix $n \times 3$ µL Capture Ligation Master Mix $+ n \times 0.5$ µL Capture Ligase in 1.5 mL tube and aliquot 3.5 µL into each PCR tube before adding 1.5 µL of sample. We recommend preparing 115% of master mix + ligase to account for pipetting error.

2. Incubate in a thermal cycler using the following steps:

I. Ligation: 25 °C for 1 h.

II. Enzyme deactivation: 65 °C for 25 min.

III. Program the thermal cycler to hold at 4 °C after enzyme deactivation to keep the sample cool until the Coding Ligation step.

3.3 Prepare Coding Ligation Reaction Mix

Combine:

Coding ligation master mix	1.3 µL
5 × 1-plex discrimination probe mixes (1 µL each)	5 µL
Water	0.7 µL

Mix thoroughly by pipetting. If performing n assays, mix required $n \times 1.3$ µL Coding Ligation Master Mix $+ n \times 1$ µL of each 1-plex discrimination probe mix (5 in total) $+ n \times 0.7$ µL water in 1.5 mL tube to use in next step. We recommend preparing 115% of master mix to account for pipetting error.

3.4 Coding Ligation

1. Combine:

Capture ligation product (from Subheading 3.2):	5 µL
Coding ligation reaction mix (from Subheading 3.3)	7 µL
Coding ligase	1 µL

Mix thoroughly by pipetting slowly. If performing n assays, mix required $n \times 7$ µL Coding Ligation Reaction Mix $+ n \times 1$ µL Coding Ligase in a 1.5 mL tube and aliquot 8 µL into the PCR tubes from Subheading 3.2 that contain the 5 µL Capture Ligation product. We recommend preparing 115% of master mix + enzyme to account for pipetting error.

2. Incubate in a thermal cycler using the following steps:

1. Denaturation: 95 °C for 30 s.

II. Hybridization: 30 °C for 15 s.

III. Ligation: 61 °C for 5 min.

IV. Cycle through **steps I–III** 50 times.

V. Program the thermal cycler to hold at 4 °C after 50 cycles is completed to keep the sample cool until DNA sizing analysis.

3.5 DNA Sizing Analysis by Denaturing PAGE

1. The final product from the Coding Ligation step (from Subheading 3.4) contains single stranded DNA species, whose lengths encode specific miRNA. These lengths vary between approximately 50 nt and 200 nt. The number of copies of each DNA species is directly proportional to the original miRNA sample copy number and can be quantified using various DNA sizing methods including denaturing PAGE.

2. Denaturing PAGE gel. We recommend using 15 % TBE-Urea Gels and 1× TBE running buffer. Pre-run the gel for 20 min at 300 V (usually equilibrates at approximately 15–20 mA per gel). Clean the accumulated urea out of the wells directly before loading sample by pipetting running buffer into wells several times. The accumulated urea should be visible as it is flushed out of the wells.

3. Add 7 μL gel loading buffer to 13 μL Coding Ligation product (from Subheading 3.4).

4. Vortex to mix. Spin down on benchtop centrifuge.

5. Denature at 95 °C for 5 min. Vortex and spin down.

6. Load 14 μL into gel. Run for 1.8 times the time it takes for the loading dye to run off the gel, usually 55–60 min at 300 V. If multiple gels are run simultaneously within the same cell, the gels and running buffer will get warmer and the DNA will run faster. Therefore, it may be necessary to decrease the running time.

7. Remove the gel and scan promptly. We have scanned gels after 30 min with no adverse effects.

3.6 Fluorescent Gel Scanning

1. The confocal gel imager should be set to measure using the 633 nm laser excitation and emission detector filter set to 670 nm. The GE Typhoon 9410 variable mode imager has these settings as standard for Cy5 dye detection. We typically use a photomultiplier tube (PMT) voltage of 600 V; experimenters should test a range of voltages between 400 and 600 V to ensure they measure in the linear range of their imager's PMT. We recommend scanning with a pixel size of 50 μm, focused at the platen, and normal sensitivity. These settings should be used as a baseline and optimized by the experimenter as necessary. Before loading the gel onto the scanner, lightly wet the surface of the platen with water before laying the gel down. This will help the gel lay flat on the surface and improve fluorescence reproducibility. Remove the gel from its running case and lay down carefully to prevent formation of air bubbles between the gel and platen. Do not use the scanner's option to press the gel down. Scan.

3.7 Gel Image Analysis

1. The scanner generates an image file with the extension *.gel*, which can be analyzed using the HandyBand software provided with the assay kit (*see* **Note 8**).

2. Starting the program will open a Load_gel window. First, click on the "Load gel file button" and select the .gel file to analyze. This will open a window with a grey scale image of the gel. If the lanes are not visible, try adjusting the contrast and/or color scheme. Do this via: Edit > Colormap.

3. Next, select the area on the gel to be analysed: left-click vertices of a square enclosing the area of interest—make sure the last point, forming the square is directly over the first point—the cursor will become a circle to indicate this is the case; right-click inside the area and select "Create mask".

4. The selected area then appears in a new window. Adjust the color scheme again using Edit > Colormap. It is particularly useful to adjust the color data min and max.

5. Once the bands are clear, count the number of bands in each lane. Then, in the first Load_gel window enter the number of lanes into the drop-down box "Number of lanes" (maximum = 12). This will unblock the correct number of drop-down boxes under "Lanes".

6. Using the drop-down boxes enter the number of bands in each lane (maximum = 26 per lane).

7. Choose the method for analysis. "Gradient cutoff" sums the area under each peak, where the edge of each peak is defined by the point, at which the gradient falls below a certain value. "Fit to Gaussian peaks" fits each band to a Gaussian peak and returns the fitted area under each peak.

8. Once the above choices are made, press any button. This will reopen a new window with the same color scheme as optimized before. Enlarge the window.

9. Left-click on the middle of each peak. After each click a red cross will appear. Continue until all peaks are selected (number of peaks defined as number of lanes × number of rows in Load_gel window).

10. After the last peak is selected, peak areas are calculated. They are returned in Peak_area file (Peak_area.txt).

4 Notes

1. We have used total RNA extracted using TRIzol and Qiagen RNeasy. We have used small RNA fractions isolated using Sigma mirPremier, Qiagen miRNeasy, and Ambion mirVana. Ligo-miR can be used with either total RNA or small RNA as

input, and there are advantages to either. Background RNA molecules (i.e., non-microRNA molecules that make up the majority of molecules in a total RNA sample) reduce the linear amplification ligation efficiency and, therefore, reduce overall fluorescent signal intensity slightly. For example, the presence of 50 ng total RNA reduces the signal by an average of 50 %. On the other hand, we have found that the small RNA fraction extraction kits are less reproducible than the total RNA equivalent, and the concentration of the small RNA fraction is more challenging to quantify than total RNA.

2. The procedure and volumes in this paper are for a pellet of one million cells as starting material. For pellets with different amounts of cells users can calculate the volumes using the following equations (numbers used to give volumes in protocol are in italics):

   N = number of cells in pellet ($N = 1 \times 10^6$). This should be accurately determined by counting.

   C_{s1}, C_{s2} = stock concentrations of spike-in controls ($C_{s1} = 10$ nM, $C_{s2} = 10 \ nM$).

   M_{s1}, M_{s2} = number of moles of spiking controls desired in final assay ($M_{s1} = 666 \ attomoles$, $M_{s2} = 1333 \ attomoles$).

   N_{assay} = number of cells' input desired in final assay ($N_{assay} = 33333$ $cells$).

   V_{assay} = Volume of isolated RNA sample used in assay (Subheading 3.2) ($V_{assay} = 1.5 \ \mu L$).

   α = fraction of elution buffer used (*see* **Note 3**) ($\alpha = 0.9$).

   Volume for pre-isolation spike-in. $V_{s2} = (M_{s2} \times N)/(N_{assay} \times C_{s2})$.

   Volume for post-isolation spike-in. $V_{s1} = (M_{s1} \times \alpha \times N)/(N_{assay} \times C_{s1})$.

   Final volume. $V_F = (V_{assay} \times \alpha \times N)/N_{assay}$.

   Resuspension volume. $V_R = (V_F - V_{s1})/\alpha$.

3. When using column-based RNA isolation kits we have found that the volume of elution buffer recovered is less than the amount of elution buffer applied to the column (i.e., a small amount of buffer is retained within the column). We account for this by purposely only using a fraction of the eluate (e.g., $\alpha = 90 \%$). This ensures that all concentrations of spiking miRNA downstream are accurate. If the RNA isolation method allows perfect recovery of all eluate, use $\alpha = 1$.

4. Use DNA Lobind microcentrifuge tubes (Eppendorf #925000064) for all synthetic RNA dilutions. This is most important for the lowest two synthetic RNA concentrations. We observed significant differences between fluorescence measured at the end of the assay for 10 and 1 pM solutions when

using LoBind vs. other tubes. We routinely use Lobind tubes for all preparations.

5. 1.5 attomoles of synthetic RNA input is approximately 3× the lowest detectable levels of RNA using this assay, and signals should be readily quantifiable for all the miRNA. The detection threshold is approximately 500 zeptomoles or 300,000 molecules.

6. Use PCR tubes and caps that can reseal tightly with no loss of volume during thermal cycling. The Coding Ligation step is long and performed using resealed PCR tubes. In our experience, resealing with the same PCR tube caps does not form an adequate seal and evaporation is a significant problem. We use RNase-free 8-strip PCR tubes and cap strips from ThermoFisher Scientific (Catalog # AM12230) for the Capture Ligation step and then replace with new cap strips for the coding ligation step using Eppendorf MasterClear cap strips (Catalog # 951022089). We have seen reduced signal intensity due to adsorption when using other brands of PCR tubes though not with the recommended tubes.

7. After every instance of mixing by pipetting, spin the samples down using a bench-top centrifuge.

8. Experimenters may wish to use their own analysis programs for the gels. The .gel file is similar to a .tif file but uses a nonlinear pixel intensity coding. The pixel values in the .gel file must be squared to be obtain the proper linear fluorescent intensity ($FI = 1/26055 *$ pixel value^2).

Reference

1. Liu KJ, Rane TD, Zhang Y, Wang TH (2011) Single-molecule analysis enables free solution hydrodynamic separation using yoctomole levels of DNA. J Am Chem Soc 133:6898

Chapter 18

Practical Bioinformatics Analysis of MiRNA Data Using Online Tools

James A.L. Brown and Emer Bourke

Abstract

The purpose of this chapter is to provide a starting point for the analysis of miRNA array data, using freely available online suites of tools. This chapter does not describe how to perform analysis of primary array data, rather how to use the top differentially regulated miRNA (returned from comparing one miRNA group to another) as the starting point for further practical analysis.

Here we describe the methods and tools required to identify targets worthy of additional investigation, using the identified miRNA as a starting point. Importantly, this additional information (pathways targeted, gene expression, mRNA targets, miRNA families) can be used to positively inform any project.

Key words microRNA, miRNA, Bioinformatics, miRBase, DAVID, miRandola, PicTar, DIANA, microT-CDS

1 Introduction

The process of collecting samples, isolating miRNA and determining their levels is only the starting point of a project. Once the miRNA array is completed, the expression profile of each individual miRNA is defined, ranked and compared. Relative expression of each miRNA is compared and the most differentially expressed miRNA (between samples) revealed. Often these ranked miRNA become the targets of further validation, frequently by RQ-PCR in additional samples. In addition to the physical validation using independent samples and techniques, this ranked list of differentially expressed miRNA can itself be used for analysis. This bioinformatics analysis can provide further insights into the underlying molecular mechanisms, signaling, and pathways that are altered [1, 2]. This type of bioinformatics analysis can also lead to the identification of complementary or redundant mechanisms and novel pathways not immediately apparent, which would benefit from additional investigation.

Sweta Rani (ed.), *MicroRNA Profiling: Methods and Protocols*, Methods in Molecular Biology, vol. 1509,
DOI 10.1007/978-1-4939-6524-3_18, © Springer Science+Business Media New York 2017

Currently, a number of highly regarded online suites of tools exist which can be used to analyze the lists of differentially expressed miRNA revealed by arrays [3]. Here, we have chosen to discuss and describe the use of four regularly updated, reliable, commonly utilized suites of tools: DNA Intelligent Analysis (DIANA) [4–8], miRBase [9–12], PicTar [13] and microRNA.org [14–16]. These particular suites have been selected due to their ease of use, size of their databases, quality of returned results and because, more importantly, these tools have undergone peer-review (through descriptive publication of their tools/databases).

Here, we detail suggested strategies and the methods for extracting useful information from each of the different complimentary software suites, which can be used to inform further research activities.

2   Materials

The basic materials required are:

1. Computer.

2. Internet connection and browser (Firefox or Chrome recommended).

3. List of target miRNA differentially expressed in a specific tissue, a disease, or following a treatment. Preferentially the list should be ranked in order of the most to least differentially expressed.

   In all cases the Homo sapiens databases/sequences/pathways will be the default setting.

3   Methods

3.1   DNA Intelligent Analysis (DIANA), miRPath

(http://diana.imis.athena-innovation.gr/DianaTools/index.php?r=mirpath)

The suite of DIANA tools is best utilized by accessing it from within your own individual user account. This allows the user to save experiments and will allow the software suite to suggest customized relevant publications.

miRPath V.3 [17] allows a user to input a number of miRNA and determine if any common genes or pathways are targeted by the entered miRNA and to what degree [4]. There are four distinct options for viewing how the entered miRNA interact: genes union, genes intersection, and pathways union, pathways intersection. The protocol for use of the software is as follows:

1. Choose the species of interest from the drop-down menu (Fig. 1A).

2. Set database to search against: either TarBase (a manually curated collection of experimentally supported microRNA targets) or microT-CDS (microRNA target prediction database) from the drop-down menu (Fig. 1B).

3. Enter the miRNA identifier (Fig. 1C) and use the plus (+) button to add the miRNA [if only a number is entered (i.e., without the hsa-mir-prefix) a list of matching miRNA returned will be available for selection (Fig. 1D)].

4. Continue to add miRNA until the desired list is generated. The results will automatically update each time a new miRNA is added.

5. Select the desired P-value threshold (defaults to 0.05) and MicroT threshold (default 0.8) (Fig. 1E).

6. Select the way to merge results: there are four distinct result sets that can be displayed via the hyperlinked text (Fig. 1F). Results displayed: KEGG pathway affected, p-value, number of genes in the pathway targeted and the number of selected miRNA targeting the pathway.

   (a) *Genes union*
       Provides information on the number of genes targeted by the indicated number of miRNA. All genes targeted by at least one selected miRNA.

   (b) *Genes intersection*
       Genes targeted by all selected miRNA. The minimum number of miRNA required to target a gene could be set using the box to the right of the genes intersection selection link.

   (c) *Pathways union*
       Identifies all pathways that are significantly targeted by the indicated miRNAs.

   (d) *Pathways intersection*

       Only pathways that are significantly targeted by all the selected miRNA are displayed.

7. Select either: the Significance Clusters/Heatmap or Targeted Pathways Clusters/Heatmap and then choose either the "Show Heatmap" or "Show microRNA/Pathway Clusters" hyperlinks to produce downloadable images (in a new browser tab) that are excellent for illustration purposes (Fig. 1G).

8. For each option returned the KEGG pathway, p-value, number of genes (#genes), and number of miRNA (#miRNA) are displayed (Fig. 1H).

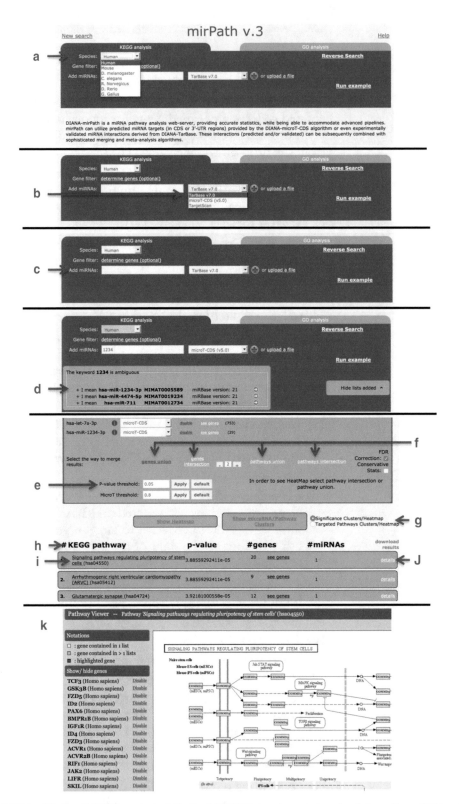

Fig. 1 DIANA mirPath v.3-KEGG analysis (http://snf-515788.vm.okeanos.grnet.gr/) An online miRNA pathway analysis tool hosted by Web Services at DIANA-LAB (http://snf-515788.vm.okeanos.grnet.gr/index.php?r=site/page&view=software)

9. The indicated KEGG pathway targeted (in order of significance) is accessed through the hyperlinked pathway name [4] (Fig. 1I).

10. In addition for each specific pathway/gene list returned, the details can be displayed through the "details" link (Fig. 1J).

11. Three distinct labeling mechanisms are displayed for ease of reference (Fig. 1K): (a) Yellow, indicates gene targeted by one selected miRNA; (b) Orange, indicates gene targeted by >1 selected miRNAs and (c) Red, user chosen gene. Each displayed gene can individually be enabled/disabled to display or hide the gene in the pathway. Hovering over a target gene (using the mouse) will display information regarding the source of the data for the interaction (TarBase or DIANA-microT-CDS) and display the miRNA indicated to be involved. Any pathway component can be selected, taking users to the KEGG entry.

3.1.2 GO (Gene ontology) Analysis geneontology.org/

1. Choose the GO tab (Fig. 2A).

2. Choose the Subcategories (Fig. 2B).

3. Choose the Species (Fig. 2C).

4. If required, a gene filter list can be uploaded (Fig. 2D).

5. Set database to search against: either TarBase (a manually curated collection of experimentally supported microRNA targets) or microT-CDS (microRNA target prediction database) from the drop-down menu (Fig. 2E).

6. Enter the miRNA identifier (Fig. 2F) and use the plus (+) button to add the miRNA [if only a number is entered (i.e., without the hsa-mir-prefix) a list of matching miRNA returned will be available for selection (Fig. 2G)].

7. Continue to add miRNA until the desired list is generated. The results will automatically update each time a new miRNA is added.

8. Select the desired *P*-value threshold (defaults to 0.05) and MicroT threshold (default 0.8) (Fig. 2H).

9. Select the way to merge results: there are four distinct result sets that can be displayed via the hyperlinked text (Fig. 2I). Results displayed: GO Category, p-value, number of genes in the pathway targeted, and the number of selected miRNA targeting the pathway.

   (a) *Genes union*
   Provides information on the number of genes targeted by the indicated number of miRNA. All genes targeted by at least one selected miRNA.

   (b) *Genes intersection*
   Genes targeted by all selected miRNA. The minimum number of miRNA required to target a gene could be set using the box to the right of the genes intersection selection link.

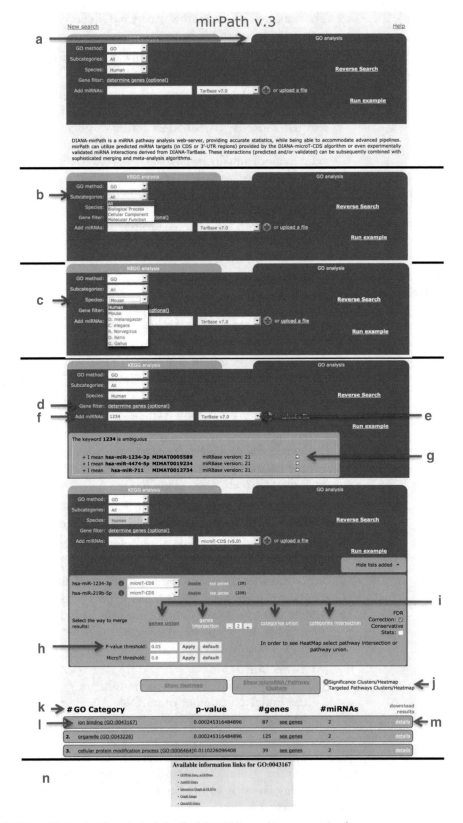

Fig. 2 DIANA mirPath v.3-GO analysis (http://snf-515788.vm.okeanos.grnet.gr/)

(c) *Categories union*

Identifies all pathways that are significantly targeted by the indicated miRNAs.

(d) *Categories intersection*

Only pathways that are significantly targeted by all the selected miRNA are displayed.

10. Select either: the Significance Clusters/Heatmap or Targeted Pathways Clusters/Heatmap and then choose either the "Show Heatmap" or "Show microRNA/Pathway Clusters" hyperlinks to produce downloadable images (in a new browser tab) that are excellent for illustration purposes (Fig. 2J).

11. For each option returned the GO Categories, p-value, number of genes (#genes), and number of miRNA (#miRNA) are displayed (Fig. 2K).

12. The indicated GO pathway targeted (in order of significance) is accessed through the hyperlinked pathway name (Fig. 2L).

13. In addition for each specific pathway/gene list returned, the details can be displayed through the "details" link (Fig. 2M).

14. Following the GO pathway link will present you with a page (N) with links to related data from the following sources: GOWiki Entry at GONuts, AmiGO Entry, Interactive Graph at OLSVis, Graph Image, or the QuickGO Entry.

3.2 miRBase (www. mirbase.org)

The current version of miRBase [9] (V21, 2014) contains information from over >2500 mature human miRNA entries (from >1800 annotated miRNA loci) and additionally miRNA data from 206 species. This simple to use database provides key information related to individual miRNA (such as structure, sequence, and genomic location).

The search page of miRBase (Fig. 3A) allows a number of different searches to be performed.

1. Enter the miRNA identifier (either mir number alone or correct nomenclature: hsa-mir-####) or a keyword and submit query (Fig. 3B).

2. The results returned containing the search term are displayed in a table, with the section, description and number of hits (in each section) displayed (Fig. 3C).

3. If a unique hsa-mir-#### was not used, below this, another table containing unique miR is displayed. Hyperlinks of the accession of ID (miR) can be selected.

4. ID (miR) will lead to a page displaying information related to the selected miR. Information displayed includes:

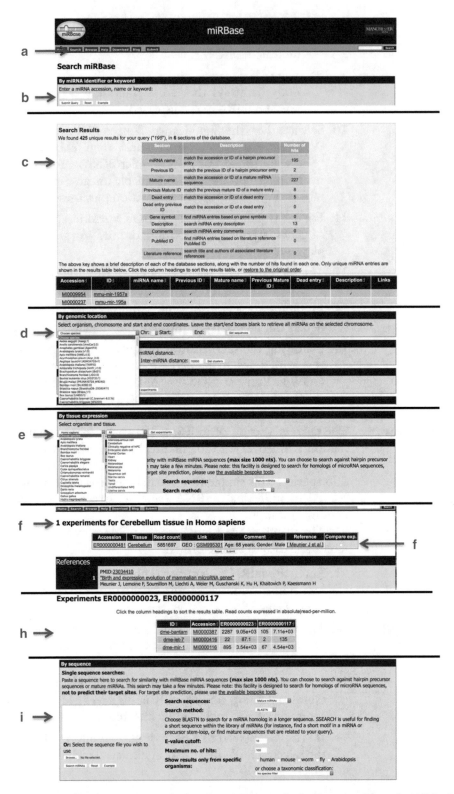

Fig. 3 miRBase (http://www.mirbase.org/). A online database of allowing searching of published miRNA sequences and annotations

(a) *Stem-loop sequence*

The stem-loop structure is displayed and can be downloaded. Deep sequencing related data is shown as well as the genome context. In addition, users can leave feedback on the confidence (by voting), with current results displayed. Links to additional databases are provided (miR-Base-Tracker, Entrezgene, and Hugo Gene Nomenclature Committee (HGNC)).

(b) *Mature sequence*

The mature miRNA sequence is provided (and can be downloaded). Referenced evidence (either experimental or not) and the confidence for existence of the mature miR are shown.

(c) *References*

References containing the chosen miR are listed (including direct links to PubMed or the specific article).

5. Additionally, published miRNA data [including all published miRNA data (EMBL format) or by genome coordinates] can be downloaded for further analysis (either directly using the links or using FTP page).

6. Identification of miRNAs at a specific genomic location can also be performed (Fig. 3D). Select the search species, chromosome number, and start and end site of search (leave these blank to search for all miRNAs on the selected chromosome).

7. miRNAs expressed in specific tissues of a particular species can also be found within the tissue expression menus (Fig. 3E).

8. Select "Get experiments" and the resulting references, including the publication details (at the bottom of the page) will be displayed (Fig. 3F). The details returned are: Accession (hyperlinked to specific experiment details), Tissue, Read count, Link [hyperlinked to Gene Expression Omnibus (GEO) details of specific experimental data set], Comment, Reference (hyperlinked), and Compare exp.

9. If multiple experiments are displayed, checking the "compare exp" box (Fig. 3G) of multiple experimental data sets and selecting submit button (at the bottom of the list) will allow comparison of selected data sets. The results will be returned in a new page (Fig. 3H) including hyperlinked: ID (mirR), Accession (Mir), and the expression values in the selected experiments. Following the hyperlinks will display the relevant miR specific mirBase data page.

10. To search for homologues of a specific sequence within the miRNA database (not miRNA target sequences), enter the base sequence into the "by sequence" menu (Fig. 3I). Using the search options the search can be against precursor hairpin sequences or mature miRNAs.

**3.3 PicTar (pictar.
mdc-berlin.de)**

The PicTar site allows the identification of targets of individual miRNA. At the bottom of the PicTar homepage are links (buttons) for predictions in vertebrates and Drosophila; vertebrates, Drosophila, and nematodes; or mouse. This database is limited to predictions of miRNA listed in the drop-down menus.

1. Clicking on the buttons leads to an interface where multiple options can be explored:

   (a) Choose the species (from the drop-down menu; Fig. 4A)

   (b) Choose the dataset to be searched (from the drop-down menu; Fig. 4B)

   (c) Choose the miRNA to be investigated (listed in the drop-down menu; Fig. 4C)

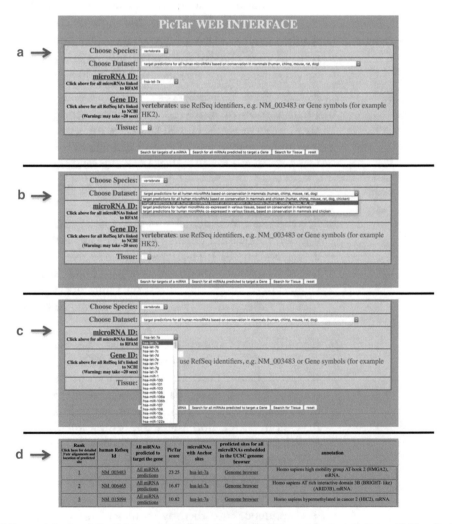

Fig. 4 PicTar: vertebrates (http://pictar.mdc-berlin.de/cgi-bin/PicTar_vertebrate.cgi). Home PicTar site including additional searchable model organisms (http://pictar.mdc-berlin.de/)

2. At this point the "Search for targets of a miRNA" button at the bottom of the page can be used to return predictions in a table below this interface (Fig. 4D). Information displayed includes:

   (a) *Rank*: numbered ranks are links to detailed 3′ UTR alignments and location of predicted site.

   (b) *Species-specific RefSeq Id*: a link to the NCBI database entry of the predicted targeted transcript/gene.

   (c) *All miRNAs predicted to target the gene*: a link to a new PicTar interface page where all miRNA predicted to target this transcript/gene are displayed; including alignments of the target sequence and NCBI entries for each.

   (d) *PicTar score*: the probability that the UTR of the target gene/transcript will be targeted by the chosen miRNA.

   (e) *miRNAs with anchor sites: predicted sites for all miRNAs embedded in the UCSC genome browser*: links to the UCSC (University of California, Santa Cruz) displaying the genomic location of the miRNA.

   (f) *Annotation*: species and name of the transcript predicted to be targeted.

3.4 microRNA.org (www.microrna.org/)

This site provides predicted targets of the inputted microRNA and scores for downregulation of the targets. It also includes searchable miRNA expression patterns from experimental data. Species included are *Homo sapiens, Mus musculus, Rattus norvegicus, Drosophila melanogaster*, and *Caenorhabditis elegans*.

Clicking on the three main tabs along the top of the microRNA. org page allows a number of different searches to be performed:

1. *miRNA tab*:

   (a) Enter search miRNA (a list can be entered with each miRNA separated by a colon) using the correct nomenclature: hsa-mir-#### in the box provided (Fig. 5A).

   (b) Choose the species (from the drop-down menu; Fig. 5B).

   (c) Click on the Go button.

The information displayed includes:

   (a) *miRNA*: identified will be listed in order.

   (b) *Genes Targeted*: The number of predicted genes targeted will be displayed for each miRNA.

   (c) *Links*: Links to

   • *View targets*: displays a list of transcripts predicted to be targeted by the miRNA. Includes the PubMed reference and a link to the alignment details.

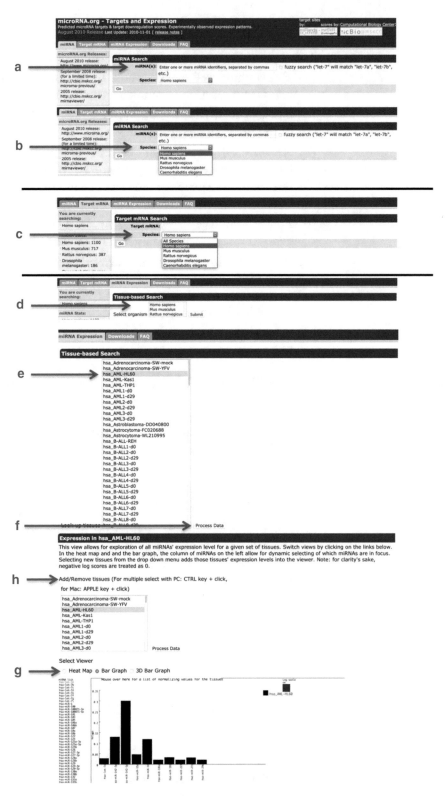

Fig. 5 microRNA.org—Targets and expression. Predicted microRNA targets and target downregulation scores. Experimentally observed expression patterns. (http://www.microrna.org/microrna/home.do)

- *View expression profile*: Displays any tissues specific expression data (if known).

- *View in miRBase*: links to the miRBase entry as described in 3.2 point 4.

- *View in miRò*: Opens a link to the miRò (The miR ontology database). Follow the miRNA link to display general miRNA information. A link to the related miR-Base entry as described in 3.2 point 4.

2 *Target mRNA tab*:

(a) Choose the species (from the drop-down menu; Fig. 5C).

(b) Click on the Go button.

The predicted miRNA transcripts, which target the mRNA of choice, will be listed. Includes the PubMed reference and a link to the alignment details.

3. *miRNA (tissue) expression search*:

(a) Choose the species from the drop-down menu (either *Homo sapiens, Mus musculus* or *Rattus norvegicus*) (Fig. 5D).

(b) Click the submit button.

(c) A new page will load where the possible tissue choices are displayed (multiple tissues can be chosen by holding down the + shift or + ctl key) (Fig. 5E).

(d) Click the Process Data button (Fig. 5F).

(e) The page will load providing the option to view either the expression data as a: Heat Map, Bar Graph, or 3D Bar Graph (Fig. 5G) (requires that Java be activated in your browser). Tissues can be added or removed using the + shift or + ctl keys (Fig. 5H).

The downloads tab provides access to the downloadable target site predictions from the indicated species (as: Good mirSVR score, Conserved miRNA; Good mirSVR score, Non-conserved miRNA; Non-good mirSVR score, Conserved miRNA and Non-good mirSVR score, Non-conserved miRNA).

References

1. Maragkakis M, Alexiou P, Papadopoulos GL, Reczko M, Dalamagas T, Giannopoulos G et al (2009) Accurate microRNA target prediction correlates with protein repression levels. BMC Bioinformatics 10:295

2. Grün D, Wang Y-L, Langenberger D, Gunsalus KC, Rajewsky N (2005) microRNA target predictions across seven Drosophila species and comparison to mammalian targets. PLoS Comput Biol 1(1):e13

3. Fernández-Suárez XM, Rigden DJ, Galperin MY (2014) The 2014 Nucleic Acids Research Database Issue and an updated NAR online molecular biology database collection. Nucleic Acids Res 42(Database issue):D1–D6

4. Vlachos IS, Kostoulas N, Vergoulis T, Georgakilas G, Reczko M, Maragkakis M et al (2012) DIANA miRPath v.2.0: investigating the combinatorial effect of microRNAs in pathways. Nucleic Acids Res 40(Web Server issue):W498–W504

5. Sethupathy P, Corda B, Hatzigeorgiou AG (2006) TarBase: a comprehensive database of experimentally supported animal microRNA targets. RNA 12(2):192–197

6. Megraw M, Sethupathy P, Corda B, Hatzigeorgioum AG (2007) miRGen: a database for the study of animal microRNA genomic organization and function. Nucleic Acids Res 35(Database issue):D149–D155

7. Maragkakis M, Reczko M, Simossis VA, Alexiou P, Papadopoulos GL, Dalamagas T et al (2009) DIANA-microT web server: elucidating microRNA functions through target prediction. Nucleic Acids Res 37(Web Server issue):W273–W276

8. Alexiou P, Maragkakis M, Papadopoulos GL, Simmosis VA, Zhan GL, Hatzigeorgiou AG (2010) The DIANA-mirExTra web server: from gene expression data to microRNA function. PLoS ONE 5(2):e9171

9. Kozomara A, Griffiths-Jones S (2014) miRBase: annotating high confidence microRNAs using deep sequencing data. Nucleic Acids Res 42(Database issue):D68–D73

10. Griffiths-Jones S, Saini HK, van Dongen S, Enright AJ (2008) miRBase: tools for microRNA genomics. Nucleic Acids Res 36(Database issue):D154–D158

11. Kozomara A, Griffiths-Jones S (2011) miRBase: integrating microRNA annotation and deep-sequencing data. Nucleic Acids Res 39(Database issue):D152–D157

12. Griffiths-Jones S, Grocock RJ, Van Dongen S, Bateman A, Enright AJ (2006) miRBase: microRNA sequences, targets and gene nomenclature. Nucleic Acids Res 34(Database issue):D140–D144

13. Krek A, Grün D, Poy MN, Wolf R, Rosenberg L, Epstein EJ et al (2005) Combinatorial microRNA target predictions. Nat Genet 37(5):495–500

14. Betel D, Wilson M, Gabow A, Marks DS, Sander C (2008) The microRNA.org resource: targets and expression. Nucleic Acids Res 36(Database issue):D149–D153

15. John B, Enright AJ, Aravin A, Tuschl T, Sander C, Marks DS (2004) Human MicroRNA targets. PLoS Biol 2(11):e363

16. Betel D, Koppal A, Agius P, Sander C, Leslie C (2010) Comprehensive modeling of microRNA targets predicts functional non-conserved and non-canonical sites. Genome Biol 11(8):R90

17. Vlachos IS, Zagganas K, Paraskevopoulou MD, Georgakilas G, Karagkouni D, Vergoulis T et al (2015) DIANA-miRPath v3.0: deciphering microRNA function with experimental support. Nucleic Acids Res 43(W1):W460–W466

Chapter 19

Visualization and Analysis of MiRNA–Targets Interactions Networks

Luis E. León and Sebastián D. Calligaris

Abstract

MicroRNAs are a class of small, noncoding RNA molecules of 21–25 nucleotides in length that regulate the gene expression by base-pairing with the target mRNAs, mainly leading to down-regulation or repression of the target genes. MicroRNAs are involved in diverse regulatory pathways in normal and pathological conditions. In this context, it is highly important to identify the targets of specific microRNA in order to understand the mechanism of its regulation and consequently its involvement in disease. However, the microRNA target identification is experimentally laborious and time-consuming. The in silico prediction of microRNA targets is an extremely useful approach because you can identify potential mRNA targets, reduce the number of possibilities and then, validate a few microRNA–mRNA interactions in an in vitro experimental model. In this chapter, we describe, in a simple way, bioinformatics guidelines to use miR-Walk database and Cytoscape software for analyzing microRNA–mRNA interactions through their visualization as a network.

Key words miRNA targets, miRNA–mRNA networks, In silico prediction

1 Introduction

MicroRNAs (miRNAs) are a class of small, noncoding RNA molecules of 21–25 nucleotides in length, that regulate gene expression by binding to their complementary target mRNA. MiRNA genes reside in regions of the genome as distinct transcriptional units as well as in clusters of polycistronic units carrying the information of several miRNAs [1, 2]. It has been suggested that approximately half of known miRNA reside in non-protein coding RNAs (intron and exon) or within the intron of protein-coding genes [3].

The miRNA genes are transcribed by RNA polymerase II, generating long primary transcripts (pri-miRNAs) [4]. Subsequently, in the nucleus the RNase III-type enzyme Drosha processes the long primary transcripts (pri-miRNA), yielding a hairpin precursors (pre-miRNA) consisting of approximately 70 nucleotides. These pre-miRNA hairpins are exported to the cytoplasm where

Sweta Rani (ed.), *MicroRNA Profiling: Methods and Protocols*, Methods in Molecular Biology, vol. 1509,
DOI 10.1007/978-1-4939-6524-3_19, © Springer Science+Business Media New York 2017

they are further processed into a 21–25 nucleotide miRNA duplex structures by the RNase III protein Dicer [5]. The less stable of the two strands in the duplex is incorporated into a multiple-protein nuclease complex, the RNA-induced silencing complex (RISC), which regulates protein expression [6]. The miRNAs binds mainly to the 3′ UTR region of the mRNA target. However, it has also been described that miRNAs binds to the coding sequence and 5′ UTR [7, 8]. Once incorporated into RISC, the miRNA regulates the target genes by degrading the mRNA through direct cleavage or by inhibiting protein synthesis [6].

By this mechanism, miRNAs play pivotal roles in multiple processes including normal development, response to internal and external stimuli, and diverse pathologies like cancer, cardiovascular disease, type II diabetes, and neurodegeneration [9–13]. It is important to note that the biological relevance of miRNAs is in their interaction with their target genes and miRNAs are known to interact with multiple mRNAs. On the other hand, an mRNA could be regulated by multiple miRNAs, making it difficult to correctly interpret miRNA–mRNA regulatory network. Moreover, it has been suggested that one-third of human genes is regulated by miRNAs [14]. A good tool to visualize and interpret the whole picture of miRNA regulatory network is the use of graph theory. Graph theory is the study of graphs, which are structures used to model pairwise relations between objects (in our case miRNA–mRNA interactions). In this context, a graph is composed of nodes and edges connect together to build networks. Using network analysis on these graphs, it is possible to identify important nodes or hubs that regulate many other nodes, which in biological terms could be a master regulator. In this chapter, we generate a list of interactions between miRNA-targets and create a network with these interactions and perform an analysis to identify potentially biological relevant miRNAs. To do this, we used miRWalk database and Cytoscape software, which are freely available tools. The example includes a list of human miRNA as starting point; however, the protocol should be applicable to other organisms. In summary, the main aim of this chapter is to provide a detailed protocol to integrate, visualize, and analyze interactions between miRNA and mRNA in a gene network for inexpert users of bioinformatics tools.

2   Materials

1. Computer requirements depend on the amount of data to be analyzed, a minimum of 4 GB of RAM and 10 GB of free space are recommended.

2. The method described here can be applied in any Operative System (Windows, Mac, or Linux).

3. Microsoft Excel or any software to visualize spread-sheets files.

4. The Cytoscape software from www.cytoscape.org. This tutorial was done using Cytoscape 3.2.1.

---

3 Methods

Your starting list could be a set of miRNAs differentially expressed, identified by array or sequencing techniques, or simply, could be a list of selected miRNAs based on scientific literature searching or published miRNAs data. For our purpose, we used a list of 17 differentially expressed miRNAs identified by Next Generation RNA sequencing (miR-132-5p, miR-19a-3p, miR-19b-3p, miR-485-5p, miR-127-3p, miR-128, miR-409-3p, miR-433, let-7 g-3p, miR-370, miR-431-3p, miR-873-3p, miR-136-3p, miR-212-3p, miR-10a-5p, miR-1224-5p, and miR-4448) corresponding to the comparison of cerebrospinal fluid (CSF) samples between healthy and Parkinson's disease patients [15].

3.1 Identify miRNA Validated Targets Using miRWalk Database

There are a great number of tools and databases for miRNA target prediction available. We summarize a few of them in Table 1. Any of these tools can be used to generate the list of miRNA-target pair. However, in order to generate a list of the miRNA–mRNA pair (that we call interactions) and perform a posterior analysis of these interactions, we used miRWalk database [16] and Cytoscape [17] respectively. We chose miRWalk because it contains information about predicted and experimentally validated interaction. Moreover, for predictions, miRWalk integrates multiple algorithms (DIANA-microTv4.0, DIANA-microT-CDS, miRanda-rel2010, mirBridge, miRDB4.0, miRmap, miRNAMap, doRiNA, PicTar2, PITA, RNA22v2, RNAhybrid2.1, and Targetscan6.2), making easy to get a list of interactions predicted by many different tools (*see* **Note 1**).

1. Go to miRWalk web page http://www.umm.uni-heidelberg.de/apps/zmf/mirwalk/index.html. The first look is to identify miRNA targets that previously have been validated by experimental approaches.

   Select the "Validated Target Module" and choose miRNA-gene targets. Select human as species (human, mouse, and rat are available) and then, click on "Database". When you select the database automatically the input identifier format is displayed. In our example, we selected miRBase and miRNA as the database and input identifier respectively. The correct format of the identifiers is displayed in parenthesis. Paste or write your list of miRNAs in the text box. Take care to use the correct nomenclature.

Table 1
Tools to identify miRNA–target interaction

Tool	Type interaction	Website	Version	References
DIANA-TarBase	Validated	http://diana.imis.athena-innovation.gr/DianaTools/index.php?r=tarbase/index	Web	[25, 26]
TargetScan	Predicted	http://www.targetscan.org/	Web	[23]
miRanda	Predicted	http://www.microrna.org/microrna/home.do	Web/standalone	[24]
DIANA-Micro-T-CDS	Predicted	http://diana.imis.athena-innovation.gr/DianaTools/index.php?r=microT_CDS/index	Web	[25, 26]
RNA22	Predicted	https://cm.jefferson.edu/rna22/	Web	[27]
RNAhybrid	Predicted	https://bibiserv2.cebitec.uni-bielefeld.de/rnahybrid	Web/standalone	[28]
TargetMiner	Predicted	http://www.isical.ac.in/~bioinfo_miu/targetminer20.htm	Web/Standalone	[29]

2. Select information related with pre-miRNA and/or mature miRNA according to your study. We performed the analysis with default options. Finally, press the "Search" button.

3. In the results page, go to "Validated miRNA-target interactions" and click the link "miRNA-target interactions". Click on "Download table" and open it in the Microsoft Excel application. Open the file from Excel option, *File → Open* and select the saved table file and follow the instructions of Subheading 3.3.1.

3.2 Identify miRNA Predicted Targets Using miRWalk Database

1. Go to miRWalk web page and now select "Predicted Target Module", "miRNA-gene Targets" in the scroll menu. For database selection, repeat the steps as described in Subheading 3.1. Paste or write your list of miRNAs in the text box (*see* **Note 2**).

2. In "Putative target gene list", you can select and combine the information of binding sites resulting from the miRNA-target prediction programs available in miRWalk. Also, you can select the region that could be tested for interaction with the miRNA; these include 5′ UTR, 3′ UTR, and CDS. Finally, click "search" button. For our analysis, we selected TargetScan, miRanda, RNA22, and miRWalk, and all others parameters were used with default parameters.

3. In "Putative target gene table" click on "3′UTR" under section "Putative target genes predicted by chosen algorithms within mRNA selected regions". Download the complete table. Column 1 contains miRNA name and, the columns 2, 3, and 4 contain gene names, EntrezID, and RefSeqID identifiers for their target mRNAs, respectively. The next columns have the name of the selected algorithms as a header. If the prediction of interactions is positive, a value of 1 is given. The last column has "SUM" as a header, which is the result of the sum of all the algorithms that predict the interaction between miRNA and the specific gene. Usually, it is better if many different algorithms predict the same interaction, so higher values in SUM are very suggestive (but not definitive) of miRNA–mRNA interactions. We recommend selecting only interactions predicted by all algorithms.

3.3 Visualization and Analysis of Interaction miRNA–mRNA Data

To visualize and analyze the data of interaction (validated or predicted) miRNA-target regulatory networks we used Cytoscape. To do this, open Cytoscape, and click on *File → Import → Network → File*. When clicked on file, a new window is displayed. In the *interaction definition* panel choose miRNA column as source node and gene column as Target interaction. Click on "OK". The network is displayed in the main window. To visualize names of nodes, click on *View → Show Graphic Details*. In the next step, we used the validated interaction network obtained in Subheading 3.1.

3.3.1 Importing Gene Interaction Network Data into Cytoscape

3.3.2 Adding Node Attributes into Cytoscape

Interaction networks are useful as models. However, they are most powerful when integrated with additional information. Cytoscape allows the addition of information into node or edge as attributes. Node attributes can include among other gene names, protein name, molecular function (e.g., kinase, transporter or phosphatase) or confidence *p*-values. In a text editor or Excel spread-sheet, create a table with the format of a node attribute. A node attribute file begins with the name of the attribute on the first line (cannot have spaces). Each following line contains the name of the node (e.g., miRNA name); meanwhile, the second column contains the value of that attribute. In our case, to simplify, we separated the attributes as molecule type (mRNA or targets are the attributes) as can be seen in Table 2.

Import the attributes by clicking *File → Import → Table → File* and select the file containing the node attributes. A new window is displayed. In importing type, you can select import data as a node, edge or network attribute. Click "OK" for the attribute association with the respective nodes. With the same procedure, it is possible to add the Edge attributes; for example, gene expression change direction (e.g., activation or repression). The information of attributes is used in the next section to change the visualization of the network.

Table 2
Example of node/attributes table

Node_name	Attribute
miR-132-5p	miRNA
miR-19a-3p	miRNA
miR-19b-3p	miRNA
PDGR1	Target
EPC1	Target

3.3.3 Styles and Layout of Network Visualization

Cytoscape includes pre-configured network styles that could be loaded from Control panel. Moreover, also allows customization of network visualization that is facilitated by using attributes. The custom visualization includes node and edge shape, color, and size, among others. For network style modification, use the Control Panel, select the "Style" tab and click on the desired characteristic to change (e.g., fill color). Different options are displayed; then, select "Column" and select the attribute to be shown, in our case "type". Under "Mapping type" select "Discrete Mapping". "Discrete Mapping" can map different types of molecules for colors or shapes, for example, a black rectangle for miRNA and a white circle for mRNA genes (Fig. 1).

Node and edge position adjusting is possible by changing the network layout. The Layout menu has an array of features for organizing the network visually according to one of the several algorithms, aligning and rotating groups of nodes and adjusting the size of the network. As option are available Circular, Hierarchical, Organic, Grid and Force Directed Layouts among others. In this pipeline, we choose Force Directed Layout, which is based in "force-directed" paradigm. The main advantage of this layout is their speed and also that with the right parameters can provide a pleasing layout. Force-directed graph drawing algorithms assign forces among the set of edges and the set of nodes of a graph drawing. Typically, spring-like attractive forces are used to attract pairs of endpoints of the graph's edges towards each other, while simultaneously repulsive forces are used to separate all pairs of nodes. In equilibrium states, the edges tend to have a uniform length, and nodes that are not connected by an edge tend to be drawn further apart. Resulting layouts often expose the inherent symmetric and clustered structure of a graph; they show a well-balanced distribution of nodes and have few edge crossings (*see* **Note 3**).

To apply this algorithm to the network, select *Layout → Prefuse Force Directed Layout*. This layout is useful to distinguish highly connected regions of the graph from sparse ones. However, you can create networks that visually are easy to interpret, and can

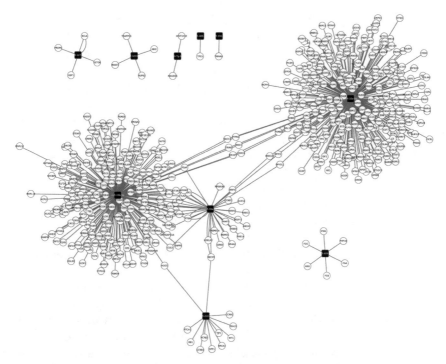

Fig. 1 Gene miRNA regulatory networks. The *black rectangles* are miRNAs and the *white circles* are mRNA targets. The edge connecting two nodes are indicative of regulation. The graph is generated in Cytoscape 3.2 and drawing using the Force Directed Layout

easily identify hub nodes. On the other hand, you could have complex networks that require mathematical calculations to identify important nodes. In the last case, you need to employ a different approach. To do this we analyze the network topology.

3.3.4 Network Topology

Networks generated by following the miRNA–mRNA predictions as described in Subheading 3.2 generally have a large number of miRNA–mRNA interactions. In these particular situations, it is relevant to reduce the number of interactions. A small number of interactions could be biologically important or related to the process in the study. Network topology analysis is a powerful way to prioritize nodes that can be important for gene network function.

Cytoscape includes built-in tools that can give us basic network statistics, such as node degree (number of edges incidents to the node), betweenness centrality (indicator of a node's centrality in a network), and cluster coefficient (measure of the degree to which nodes in a graph tend to cluster together), among others. Also, the full potential of Cytoscape can be used, by using different apps that can be downloaded and loaded into your desktop session that performs network statistics and others interesting analysis. The web page of Cytoscape has an App Store (http:// apps.Cytoscape. org/). The App Store is a repository of multiple kinds of plugins that allow increasing the analysis capabilities of Cytoscape. These plugins can be downloaded and installed, via web page or from the *Apps→ Apps Manager* option from Cytoscape. To illustrate the potential analysis of apps, we employed the CentiScaPe plugin available for Cytoscape App to calculate network statistics. We chose CentiScaPe because it is capable of computing multiple parameters for network analyzer [18]. These parameters allow identifying significant nodes in a complex network, generating numerical and graphical output making it easy to find key nodes in large networks.

To open the CentiScaPe tool, click on *Apps→ CentiScaPe*. A new panel is open showing all the parameters available. You must select the centrality value you want to calculate. Interestingly, this plugin gives a description of the parameter to calculate, in mathematical and biological terms. To see the description click the "?" button next to parameter name.

Since our network connections are based on directed connections, we chose the "Directed Networks" option. Then click "Start" to calculate. The "Results Panel" summarizes the network analysis results. Once calculated, network statistics can be used as attributes and added as visual cues using the "Control Panel" as we described above. For example, we can visualize node degree by making node size proportional to this statistic. "Node degree" indicates the number of connections that a node have, this means how many edges are attached to a node in the network. The most connected nodes or hubs are important for network structure and often regarded as key for biological network function. This example shows how a simple network analysis can be a powerful tool to identify key regulatory miRNA and their putative targets (*see* **Note 4**).

3.3.5 Cluster Analysis of Networks

Usually in biological networks, the nodes that work together, i.e., play a role in the same pathway, are highly interconnected. These interconnected nodes or cluster potentially could be an important cellular module. These nodes can be identified by visual exploration of the network. However, in a complex network, identifying these clusters is more difficult. To make it there are many plugins available from Cytoscape Apps (*see* **Note 5**). In our example, we employed ClusterViz plugin. We used ClusterViz for validated interaction Network and the EAGLE algorithm with default options. This analysis results in five major sub-networks containing most of the nodes and other smaller clusters (Fig. 2). In this section, you can select the major modules and create sub-networks, as you prefer.

3.4 Gene Ontology Overrepresentation Analysis

Gene ontology (GO) enrichment analysis is possible over the whole network or sub-selected network. In this part, we used the plugin BiNGO [19]. BiNGO is a Cytoscape plugin that identifies the GO categories that are statistically overrepresented in a set of genes or

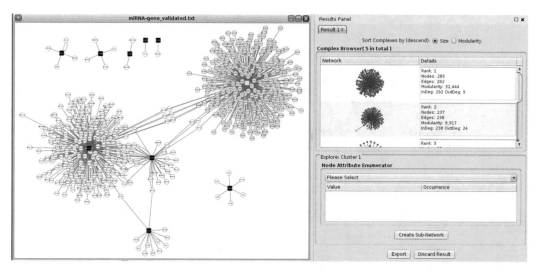

Fig. 2 A screenshot of Cytoscape showing the results of clustering using ClusViz. In the *left side* of the picture is the whole network (same as Fig. 1). The *right side* of the figure shows the resulting windows of ClusViz. In this section, the sub-networks are sorted by rank. The sub-selected network is shown as *yellow nodes* in the whole network

a sub-graph of a biological network. BiNGO maps the predominant functional themes of a given gene set on the GO hierarchy and outputs this mapping as a Cytoscape graph. Gene sets can either be selected or computed from a Cytoscape network (as sub-graphs) or compiled from sources other than Cytoscape (e.g., a list of genes regulated by miRNAs). The main advantage of BiNGO over other GO tools is the fact that it can be used directly and interactively on molecular interaction graphs.

Select the nodes of the network that you want to analyze or the whole network. We used the rank1 module obtained by ClusViz. After installing BiNGO from Cytoscape App store, go to "Apps", and click on BiNGO. In the new window, put a name in "Cluster name", select or deselect the options according to your biological question. We used Binomial as statistical test followed by a multiple hypothesis corrections by false discovery rate ($p = 0.05$). In ontology file we use "GO_Biological_Process" and we selected *Homo sapiens*, then we clicked on "Start BiNGO".

As a result, you get a graph representing the gene ontology terms overrepresented in your sample (Fig. 3) and a table with all the data, including p-value, corrected p-value and cluster frequency. As we can see, in our example cellular metabolic process are overrepresented in module 1 obtained with ClusViz. The cellular metabolic process is a very general gene ontology term. Proteostasis, oxidative stress, mitochondrial dysfunction, excitotoxicity, and neuroinflammation have all been associated with Parkinson disease [20–22], and most of them have a component of the cellular metabolic process. This simple, but integrative bioinformatics approach

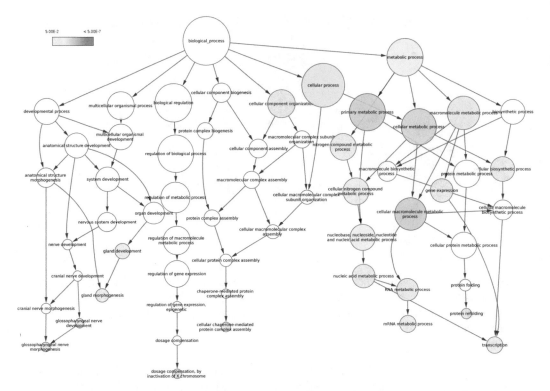

Fig. 3 Overrepresented Gene Ontology categories for Biological Process in sub-network rank1. Given that gene ontology categories are hierarchical, we employed the hierarchical layout for the graph. The nodes are *colored* according to their significant *p*-value

allowed us to identify the modular structure of the miRNA target network in CSF of Parkinson patients and sub-select a miRNA-related with deregulated biological pathways (*see* **Note 6**). The idea behind this whole pipeline is to prioritize one or few miRNA from the "big list" to perform functional studies for their interaction validation.

4   Notes

1. This protocol, for simplicity, used miRWalk as a source of miRNA–mRNA interaction data. However, any other tools or web page that generates an output list of miRNAs and its targets could be used in the network analysis and visualization. This means that this protocol can be used for any organism with available interaction data. Moreover, the network analysis data could be applied to any network, including protein–protein interaction network.

2. miRWalk database, limits the search to 20 miRNA when you choose the prediction methods. So if the list of miRNA you want to check is larger than 20, you can analyze them separately

and then merge the tables. However, if your list of miRNA is extremely large, i.e., hundreds of miRNAs, the gene network generated contain a great number of nodes, making it difficult to extract insightful information. So when you have a larger number of miRNAs, you should use validated interactions.

3. When miRNA–target interaction has been validated by more than one paper, you will see in the validated interaction the same pair miRNA-gene multiple times. In order to avoid the problem with the network analysis, keep only one before importing to Cytoscape. In the network, if a pair is repeated in the list, it can be visualized like two nodes with multiples edges connecting them.

4. When you work with Cytoscape, you can save your network at any moment, so you do not need to repeat all the procedure in a new session. To do this, go to *File → Save as* and chose location and name of the file. The extension of Cytoscape files is by default *.cys*.

5. The clustering plugins from Cytoscape app Store are very useful for the analysis of very large networks. Usually, this kind of networks is produced when the list of input miRNAs is large and/or when the prediction interaction algorithm is used.

6. The data, methods, and parameters used at each step are for demonstration purposes and are not the only way or as a general rule to carry out data analyses. Changes in methods and parameters can have a significant impact on your final results. Considering this, any change should be carefully evaluated and decided upon depending on your biological question, scientific aims, and experimental design.

Acknowledgements

This work was supported by Proyecto Mineduc-UDD PMI 1204 "De la ciencia a la innovación en salud: adopción en la actividad clínica, nacional e internacional, de nuevos productos, procesos y prácticas de clase mundial, basados en investigación científica de la UDD y de terceros."

References

1. Lau NC, Lim LP, Weinstein EG, Bartel DP (2001) An abundant class of tiny RNAs with probable regulatory roles in Caenorhabditis elegans. Science 294:858–862

2. Lee Y, Jeon K, Lee J-T, Kim S, Kim VN (2002) MicroRNA maturation: stepwise processing and subcellular localization. EMBO J 21:4663–4670

3. Rodriguez A, Griffiths-Jones S, Ashurst JL, Bradley A (2004) Identification of mammalian microRNA host genes and transcription units. Genome Res 14:1902–1910

4. Kim VN (2005) MicroRNA biogenesis: coordinated cropping and dicing. Nat Rev Mol Cell Biol 6:376–385

5. Sontheimer EJ (2005) Assembly and function of RNA silencing complexes. Nat Rev Mol Cell Biol 6:127–138

6. Iwakawa H-O, Tomari Y (2015) The functions of MicroRNAs: mRNA decay and translational repression. Trends Cell Biol 25:651–665

7. Liu G, Zhang R, Xu J, Wu C-I, Lu X (2015) Functional conservation of both CDS- and 3′-UTR-located microRNA binding sites between species. Mol Biol Evol 32:623–628

8. Zhou H, Rigoutsos I (2014) MiR-103a-3p targets the 5′ UTR of GPRC5A in pancreatic cells. RNA 20:1431–1439

9. Ardekani AM, Naeini MM (2010) The role of MicroRNAs in human diseases. Avicenna J Med Biotechnol 2:161–179

10. Ivey KN, Srivastava D (2015) microRNAs as developmental regulators. Cold Spring Harb Perspect Biol 7:a008144

11. Abente EJ, Subramanian M, Ramachandran V, Najafi-Shoushtari SH (2015) MicroRNAs in obesity-associated disorders. Arch Biochem Biophys. doi:10.1016/j.abb.2015.09.018

12. Femminella GD, Ferrara N, Rengo G (2015) The emerging role of microRNAs in Alzheimer's disease. Front Physiol 6:40

13. Jansson MD, Lund AH (2012) MicroRNA and cancer. Mol Oncol 6:590–610

14. Lim LP, Glasner ME, Yekta S, Burge CB, Bartel DP (2003) Vertebrate microRNA genes. Science 299:1540

15. Burgos K, Malenica I, Metpally R, Courtright A, Rakela B, Beach T, Shill H, Adler C, Sabbagh M, Villa S et al (2014) Profiles of extracellular miRNA in cerebrospinal fluid and serum from patients with Alzheimer's and Parkinson's diseases correlate with disease status and features of pathology. PLoS One 9, e94839

16. Dweep H, Sticht C, Pandey P, Gretz N (2011) miRWalk–database: prediction of possible miRNA binding sites by 'walking' the genes of three genomes. J Biomed Inform 44:839–847

17. Shannon P, Markiel A, Ozier O, Baliga NS, Wang JT, Ramage D, Amin N, Schwikowski B, Ideker T (2003) Cytoscape: a software environment for integrated models of biomolecular interaction networks. Genome Res 13:2498–2504

18. Scardoni G, Petterlini M, Laudanna C (2009) Analyzing biological network parameters with CentiScaPe. Bioinformatics 25:2857–2859

19. Maere S, Heymans K, Kuiper M (2005) BiNGO: a Cytoscape plugin to assess overrepresentation of gene ontology categories in biological networks. Bioinformatics 21:3448–3449

20. Hirsch EC, Hunot S (2009) Neuroinflammation in Parkinson's disease: a target for neuroprotection? Lancet Neurol 8:382–397

21. He F, Balling R (2013) The role of regulatory T cells in neurodegenerative diseases. Wiley Interdiscip Rev Syst Biol Med 5:153–180

22. Schwartz M, Kipnis J, Rivest S, Prat A (2013) How do immune cells support and shape the brain in health, disease, and aging? J Neurosci 33:17587–17596

23. Agarwal V, Bell GW, Nam J-W, Bartel DP (2015) Predicting effective microRNA target sites in mammalian mRNAs. Elife 4

24. John B, Enright AJ, Aravin A, Tuschl T, Sander C, Marks DS (2004) Human MicroRNA targets. PLoS Biol 2:e363

25. Maragkakis M, Alexiou P, Papadopoulos GL, Reczko M, Dalamagas T, Giannopoulos G, Goumas G, Koukis E, Kourtis K, Simossis VA et al (2009) Accurate microRNA target prediction correlates with protein repression levels. BMC Bioinformatics 10:295

26. Maragkakis M, Reczko M, Simossis VA, Alexiou P, Papadopoulos GL, Dalamagas T, Giannopoulos G, Goumas G, Koukis E, Kourtis K et al (2009) DIANA-microT web server: elucidating microRNA functions through target prediction. Nucleic Acids Res 37:W273–W276

27. Miranda KC, Huynh T, Tay Y, Ang Y-S, Tam W-L, Thomson AM, Lim B, Rigoutsos I (2006) A pattern-based method for the identification of MicroRNA binding sites and their corresponding heteroduplexes. Cell 126:1203–1217

28. Kruger J, Rehmsmeier M (2006) RNAhybrid: microRNA target prediction easy, fast and flexible. Nucleic Acids Res 34:W451–W454

29. Bandyopadhyay S, Mitra R (2009) TargetMiner: microRNA target prediction with systematic identification of tissue-specific negative examples. Bioinformatics 25:2625–2631

Chapter 20

Guidelines on Designing MicroRNA Sponges: From Construction to Stable Cell Line

Manoela Marques Ortega and Hakim Bouamar

Abstract

Single microRNA (miRNA) can be inhibited using antagomiR which efficiently knockdown a specific miRNA. However, the effect is transient and often results in subtle phenotype. Here we report a guideline on designing miRNA sponge inhibiting a miRNA family. As a model system, we targeted miR-30 family, known as tumor suppressor miRNAs in multiple tumors. To achieve an efficient knockdown, we generated perfect and bulged-matched miRNA binding sites (MBS) and introduced multiple copies of MBS. The protocol here demonstrates the miRNA sponge as a useful tool to examine the functional impact of inhibition miRNAs.

Key words microRNAs (miRNA) sponges, Vectors construction, miR-30a inhibition

1 Introduction

microRNAs (miRNA) are small endogenous RNAs that can inhibit protein expressions of target mRNAs, by interacting mainly to its 3′ untranslated region (UTR) and thus degrade mRNAs or inhibit translation [1, 2]. The involvement of miRNAs in cancer includes the regulation of key cancer-related pathways, such as cell cycle control and the DNA damage response [3–12]. A miRNA sponge, unlike the antagomiR, is a complementary synthetic RNA to the target miRNAs [13–15]. miRNA sponge is a DNA construct that produces artificially designed miRNA binding sites (MBS) in the 3′ UTR region of a nontoxic gene such as green fluorescence protein (GFP) or luciferase. The expression of artificial RNA with specific and multiple MBS can absorb endogenous miRNA depleting the target miRNA in cells. Although antagomiR has advantages including ease of synthesis and diverse chemical modification to improve its stability [16, 17], miRNA sponge can achieve stable inhibition as well as inducible tissue specific inhibition of target miRNAs in vitro/vivo [18, 19].

Sweta Rani (ed.), *MicroRNA Profiling: Methods and Protocols*, Methods in Molecular Biology, vol. 1509,
DOI 10.1007/978-1-4939-6524-3_20, © Springer Science+Business Media New York 2017

2 Materials

As a model system, we targeted miR-30 family, tumor suppressor miRNAs in diffuse large B cell lymphoma (DLBCL) [10]. The microRNA sponge is designed in such a way that it presents 4-nt spacers (Fig. 1, blue), called also bulge, as it has been shown that it prevents cleavage by RISC proteins [20]. The rest of the sequence of miRNA sponge is complementary to the miRNA of interest and flanked by the restriction site SanDI (discussed in Subheading 2.1) for directional subcloning into pEGFP-C3-vector (Clontech, Palo Alto, USA). Although the sponge construction was based on the miR-30a seed and mature sequence, it is expect to be recognized as target by multiple miRNAs that share the same seed sequence. Thus, miR-30 family members are also able to achieve stable inhibition of target miRNA in vitro (Fig. 1).

2.1 Construction of miRNA-30a Sponge

1. First, a linker consisting of SanDI (for directional multidimerization) flanked by BglII/EcoRI sites is digested. A stop codon added in frame immediately following BglII restriction site (Fig. 2). SanDI recognizes the 7 base pair (bp) interrupted palindrome 5′-GG/GWCCC-3′ (W = A or T) and cleaves double-stranded DNA after the second G in the sequence, producing 3-nt long 5′ protruding ends [21] (Fig. 3).

2. The sequences for SanDI oligonucleotide are as follows: Upper strand: 5′-CAG__GAATTC__atattc*GGGTCCC*atatt**TCACA**__GATCT__cgt-3′; lower strand: 5′-ACG__AGATCT__G**TGA**aatat*GGG ACCC*gaatat__GAATTCC__TG-3′ (underlined: restriction enzyme sites; lower case: spacer; bold: stop codon; italic: SanDI sequence).

bulge

sponge miRNA-30a	TGTAAACA—AATCGACTGGAAG
miRNA-30a	UGUAAACAUCCUCGACUGGAAG
miRNA-30b	UGUAAACAUCCUACACUCAGCU
miRNA-30c	UGUAAACAUCCUACACUCUCAGC
miRNA-30d	UGUAAACAUCCCCGACUGGAAG
miRNA-30e	UGUAAACAUCCUUGACUGGAAG

Fig. 1 Sponge construction is based on the miRNA-30a seed (*red*) and mature (*black*) sequences. It is expected that sponge based on the sequence of miR-30a to be recognized as targets by miRNA-30 family members (b–e). *Highlighted yellow* nucleotides within miRNA sequences are the ones that do not match sponge (miR-30a is used as reference with 100 % match)

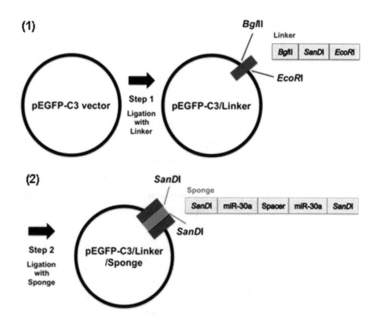

Fig. 2 SanDI linker was added at each end the sponge monomer for directional cloning. Two-steps for miRNA sponge construction: (*1*) linker was inserted through BglII/EcoRI sites and (*2*) sponge monomer was directionally ligated into the SanDI site (adapted from Jung et al., 2015) [22]

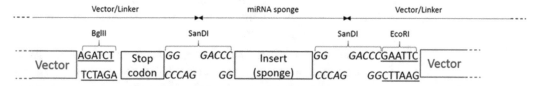

Fig. 3 Sponge constructions include a linker consisting of SanDI flanked by BglII/EcoRI sites and a stop codon added in frame immediately following BglII restriction site

3. After that, an oligonucleotide pair harboring MBS of miR-30a (TGTAAACA) with spacers (ATATTC) was designed and SanDI linker was added at each end. This monomer unit was ligated to the pEGFP-C3/SanDI linker vector by SanDI site. This ligation generated monomer but also tandem-repeated miRNA binding sites, by changing vector to insert ratio. The sponge sequences included bulged sites (--AA) located just after the seed sequence (nucleotides 9–12) promoting a mispairing and thus forming more stable interactions with the miRNA.

4. The sponge oligonucleotides are designed as follows. Upper strand: 5'-CGGATC*GGGA*CCC<u>CTTCCAGTCGATT</u> --TG <u>TTTACA</u>gaatat<u>CTTCCAGTCGATT</u> --TG <u>TTTACA</u>*GGGA* *CCC*CGGATC-3'; lower strand: 5'-GATCCG*GGGTCCC*<u>TGT</u> <u>AAACA</u> --AA   TCGACTGGAAGatattc<u>TGTAAACA</u> --AA TCGACTGGAAG*GGGTCCC*GATCCG-3'   (underlined: sponge miRNA-30a; lower case: spacer; italic: SanDI sequence).

5. A control sponge, scrambled sequence that does not match any human miRNA, was similarly designed and cloned using the siRNA Wizard software (http://www.sirnawizard.com/scrambled.php). This tool generates a negative control for siRNA. It accepts a short DNA sequence, and outputs a scrambled sequence. The scrambled sequence will have the same nucleotide composition as the input sequence and it will have passed siRNA filtering for the standard search. Moreover, it will have no match with any mRNA of the selected organism database, and no known miRNA seed recognition sequence.

6. The control sponge oligonucleotides are designed as follows: Upper strand: 5′-CGGATC*GGGACCCC*CTTCCAGTCGATT --TGTTTACA gaatat CTTCCAGTCGATT --TGTTTACA *GGGACCCC*GGATC-3′; lower strand: 5′-GATCCG*GGG TCCC*TGTAAACA --AA TCGACTGGAAG atattc TGTA AACA--AA TCGACTGGAAG GGGTCCCGATCCG-3′ (underlined: scrambled sequence; lower case: spacer; italic: SanDI sequence).

2.2 Cloning of SanDI: pEGFP-C3/Linker

Prepare all solutions using ultrapure deionized water.

1. TE buffer: 10 mM Tris–HCl, pH 7.5; 50 mM NaCl; 1 mM EDTA. Add 0.5 mL of 1 M Tris–HCl pH 7.5 and 0.5 mL of 5 M NaCl and 0.1 mL of 0.5 M EDTA in a 50 mL Falcon tube. Bring the volume up to 50 mL with water. Mix and stock at room temperature.

2. Annealing reaction: first, resuspend forward and reverse SanDI oligonucleotides to get a final concentration of 200 μM each in TE buffer. Second, dilute 200 μM forward to final concentration of 20 μM with TE buffer. Repeat the same using the reverse oligonucleotide. Finally, mix 1 μL of 20 μM forward plus 249 μL TE buffer to get 80 nM. Repeat above steps using reverse oligonucleotide. Mix 25 μL of 80 nM forward plus 25 μL of 80 nM reverse oligonucleotides in a 250 μL microcentrifuge tube (final concentration each is 40 nM). Bring the volume up to 200 μL with water.

3. Heat the mixed oligonucleotides to allow the duplex oligo to form (*see* **Note 1**).

4. BglII and EcoRI digestion (duplex oligo): 90 μL of duplex, 12 μL EcoRI 10× buffer, 12 μL 10× BSA [1 μL of 100× BSA (NEB, USA) plus 9 μL water], 2 μL of each BglII and EcoRI restriction enzymes. Bring the volume up to 120 μL with water. Digest at 37 °C for 2–3 h.

5. BglII and EcoRI digestion (pEGFP-C3vector): 1 μg vector, 2 μL EcoRI 10× buffer, 2 μL 10× BSA, 1 μL of each BglII and EcoRI restriction enzymes. Bring the volume up to 20 μL with water. Digest at 37 °C for 2–3 h.

6. Run in 4 lanes in a 2% agarose gel [2 g agarose in 100 mL Tris/Borate/EDTA (TBE) buffer and 1 μL ethidium bromide (EtBr)]: (1) the linearized pEGFP-C3 vector, (2) digested duplex, (3) 50 μL of 80 nM SanDI oligonucleotide forward, and (4) 50 μL of 80 nM SanDI oligonucleotide reverse. Lanes 3–4: are used as controls.

7. T4 ligation reaction (ratio 1:2): 2 μL 10× T4 DNA ligase buffer, 10 ng pEGFP-C3, 0.1 ng duplex oligos, 1 μL T4 ligase. Bring the volume up to 20 μL with water.

8. Transformation of competent *Escherichia coli* (*E. coli*) DH5α cells can be performed using 2, 5, and 10 μL of ligation reaction by heat shock method (*see* **Note 2**).

9. Transformed bacteria are streaked into Lennox Broth medium (LB) agar (*see* **Note 4**) plate supplemented with 50–100 μg/mL kanamycin antibiotics and incubated at 37 °C overnight (*see* **Note 3**).

10. Pick 3–5 single colonies from each plate using a pipette tip and drop it into 5 mL LB medium supplemented with 50–100 μg/mL kanamycin antibiotic (*see* **Note 5**). Incubate at 37 °C, 5 × *g* shaking overnight.

11. Prepare minipreps (Qiagen, USA) from each colony and screen the plasmids by digesting with SanDI and/or BglII/EcoRI.

2.3 Cloning of miR30a and Scrambled Sponges

1. Annealing reactions: first, resuspend in TE buffer forward and reverse miR-30a sponge and scrambled oligonucleotides to get a final concentration of 200 μM each. Second, dilute 200 μM forward to final concentration of 20 μM with TE buffer. Third, mix 1 μL of 20 μM forward plus 249 μL TE buffer to get 80nM. Repeat the same using the reverse oligonucleotides. Finally, mix 25 μL of 80 nM forward plus 25 μL of 80nM reverse oligonucleotides in a 250 μL Eppendorf tube (final concentration each: 40 nM). Bring the volume up to 200 μL with water.

2. Annealing protocol: see **step 3** of Subheading 2.2.

3. SanDI digestion (duplex oligo): 15 μL annealing reactions (miR-30a sponge or scrambled), 2 μL 10× restriction buffer, 2 μL 10 % BSA, 1 μL SanDI restriction enzyme. Bring the volume up to 10 μL with water.

4. SanDI digestion (pEGFP-C3/Linker as shown in Fig. 3 and prepared in Subheading 2.2): 1 μg vector, 2 μL 10× restriction buffer, 2 μL 10× BSA, 1 μL SanDI enzyme. Bring the volume up to 10 μL with water.

5. T4 ligation: 38 μL miR-30a sponge or scrambled annealing reactions (prepared in **step 3** of Subheading 2.3), 2 μL T4 ligase, 4.44 μL T4 10× DNA Ligase buffer.

6. See **steps 8–10** of Subheading 2.2. Follow **step 11** of Subheading 2.2 but digest only with BglII/EcoRI.

7. T4 ligation (*see* **Note 6**):

   - **miR-30a (200–300 bp) T4 ligation (1:10)**: 1 μL (15.4 ng) pEGFP-C3+SandI, 10 μL miR-30a sponge annealing reaction (120 ng), 1 μL T4 ligase, 2.5 μL 10× T4 buffer, 5.5 μL water.

   - **miR-30a (200–300 bp) T4 ligation (1:100)**: 1 μL 1:10 dilution peGFP-C3+SandI (1.55 ng), 10 μL miR-30a annealing reaction (120 ng), 1 μL T4 ligase, 2 μL T4 buffer, 6 μL water.

   - **miR-30a (300–500 bp) T4 ligation (1:10)**: 1 μL (15.4 ng) pEGFP-C3+SandI, 1.2 μL miR-30a annealing reaction (13.1 ng), 1 μL T4 ligase, 2 μL 10X T4 buffer, 14.8 μL water.

   - **miR-30a (300–500 bp) T4 ligation (1:100)**: 1 μL pEGFP-C3+SandI (15.4 ng), 12 μL miR-30a annealing reaction (131 ng), 1 μL T4 ligase, 2 μL T4 buffer, 4 μL water.

   - **Scrambled (200–300 bp) T4 ligation (1:10)**: 1 μL (15.4 ng) pEGFP-C3+SandI, 2.4 μL 1:10 dilution scrambled annealing reaction (8.2 ng), 1 μL T4 ligase, 2 μL T4 buffer, 13.6 μL water.

   - **Scrambled (200–300 bp) T4 ligation (1:100)**: 1 μL pEGFP-C3+SandI (15.4 ng), 2.4 μL scrambled annealing reaction (8.2 ng), 1 μL T4 ligase, 2 μL T4 buffer, 13.6 μL water.

   - **Scrambled (300–500 bp) T4 ligation (1:10)**: 1 μL (15.4 ng) pEGFP-C3+SandI, 1 μL scrambled annealing reaction (13 ng), 1 μL T4 ligase, 2 μL T4 buffer, 15 μL water.

   - **Scrambled (300–500 bp) T4 ligation (1:100)**: 1 μL pEGFP-C3+SandI (15.4 ng), 10 μL scrambled annealing reaction (130 ng), 1 μL T4 ligase, 2 μL T4 buffer, 6 μL water.

8. Oligonucleotides used for polymerase chain reaction (PCR) and sequencing are as follows: Upper strand: 5′- GAT CAC ATG GTC CTG CTG GA -3′; lower strand: 5′-TGT TTC AGG TTC AGG GGG AG -3′.

3 Methods

Carry out all procedures on ice unless otherwise specified.

3.1 Cloning of SanDI

1. Prepare 200 μL of annealing reaction using forward and reverse SanDI oligonucleotides (*see* **Note 7**). Heat at 94 °C for 10 min (*see* **Note 1**).

2. Perform BglII and EcoRI digestion using annealing reaction above and pEGFP-C3 vector at 37 °C for 2–3 h (*see* **Note 8**).

3. Add 1 μL alkaline phosphatase, Calf Intestinal (CIP) enzyme, to the pEGFP-C3 digested vector and incubate for 1 h at 37 °C. After, incubate 15–60 min at 65 °C.

4. Run in a 2% agarose gel the duplex oligos and linearized pEGFP-C3 from **step 2** and of Subheading 3.1 and respectively. Add in the same gel 1 μg of non-digested pEGFP-C3-vector as control.

5. Cut the pEGFP-C3 linearized vector out of the agarose gel and perform the gel purification using gel purification kit.

6. Perform T4 ligation enzyme using 10 ng pEGFP-C3-vector plus 0.1 ng annealed reaction overnight at 16 °C.

7. Transform the competent cells by heat shock method.

8. The transformed cells are streaked into LB medium agar plate with 50 μg/mL kanamycin and incubate overnight at 37 °C.

9. Pick 3–5 single kanamycin resistant colonies from each LB medium agar plate into 5 mL LB medium + antibiotic. Incubate overnight at 37 °C in a shaker incubator at $5 \times g$.

10. Harvest DNA using mini-prep kit (*see* **Note 9**).

11. The clones can be screened by two different ways: (1) EcoRI + BglII and/or SanDI digestion or (2) sequencing (Fig. 4).

3.2 Cloning of miR30a and Scrambled Sponges

1. miR-30a sponge forward and reverse and scrambled forward and reverse are dissolved in TE buffer to obtain a final concentration of 200 μM.

2. Prepare 200 μL of annealing reaction using miR-30a forward and reverse oligonucleotides and scrambled forward and reverse oligonucleotides (*see* **Note 7**). Heat at 94 °C for 10 min (*see* **Note 1**).

3. Perform PCR purification using a purification kit (*see* **Note 10**).

4. Digest overnight at 37 °C the annealing reaction (miR-30a and scrambled) and pEGFP-C3 + SandI vector by using SandI restriction enzyme (*see* **Note 11**).

5. Add in the pEGFP-C3 + SandI vector reaction, 2 μL CIP plus 2 μL buffer 3 and incubate for 1 h at 37 °C. Then, incubate reactions at 65 °C for 1 h.

6. Run above reaction in a 1% agarose gel [1 g agarose in 100 mL TBE buffer and 1 μL EtBr] and extract the digested band from gel.

7. Perform gel purification using Gel Purification kit.

8. Perform T4 ligation only using annealing reactions (miR-30a and scrambled) overnight at 16 °C (annealing reactions concatemerization).

9. Run concatemerized annealing reactions in a 2% agarose gel. A DNA smear ranging from 200 to 500 bp should be observed

GCTCAGAGCGCGATCCTGGTCCTGCTGGAGTTCGTGACCGCCGCC

GGGATCACTCTCGGCATGGACGAGCTGTACAAG**TACTCAGATCT**G

TGAAATAT<u>GGGACCC</u>GAATAT**GAATTC**TGCAGTCGACGGTACCGC

GGGCCCGGGATCCACCGGATCTAGATAACTGATCATAATCAGCCA

TACCACATTTGTAGAGGTTTTACTTGCTTTAAAAAACCTCCCACAC

CTCCCCCTGAACCTGAAACATAAAATGAATGCAATTGTTGTTGTT

AACTTGTTTATTGCAGCTTATAATGGTTACAAATAAAGCAATAGC

ATCACAAATTTCACAAATAAAGCATTTTTTTCACTGCATTCTAGTT

GTGGTTTGTCCAAACTCATCAATGTATCTTAACGCGTAAATTGTA

AGCGTTAATATTTTGTTAAAATTCGCGTTAAATTTTTGTTAAATCA

GCTCATTTTTTAACCAATAGGCCGAAATCGGCAAAATCCCTTATA

AATCAAAAGAATAGACCGAGATAGGGTTGAGTGTTGTTCCAGTTT

GGAACAAGAGTCCACTATTAAAGAACGTGGACTCCAACGTCAAA

GGGCGAAAAACCGTCTATCAGGGCGATGGCCCACTACGTGAACC

ATCACCCTAATCAAGTTTTTTGGGGTCGAGGTGCCGTAAAGCACT

AAATCGGAACCCTAAAGGGAGCCCCCGATTTAGAGCTTGACGGG

GAAAGCCGGCGAACGTGGCGAGAAAGGAAGGGAAGAAAGCGAA

AGGAGCGGGCGCTAGGGCGCTGGCAAGTGTAGCGGTCACGCTGC

GCGTAACCACCACACCCGCCGCGCTTAATGCGCCGCTACAGGGCG

CGTCAGGTGGCACTTTTCGGGGAAATGTGCGCGGAACCCCTATTT

GTTTATTTTTCTAAATACATTCAAATATGTATCCGCTCATGAGACA

ATAACCCTGATAAATGCTTCAATAATATTGAAAAAGGAAGAGTCC

TGAGGCGGAAAGAACCAGCTGTGGAAATGTGTGTCAGTTAGGGT

GTGAAAGTCCCCAGGCTCCCCAGCAGGCAGAAGTATGCAAGCAT

Fig. 4 Result of sequencing of peGFP-C3 + SandI positive colony showing a perfect cloning of oligonucleotide SanDI (in *blue*). The *red* sequences represent BglII and EcoRI restriction sites. *Green* sequence refers to GFP sequence from pEGFP-C3 plasmid

in the gel (the DNA size is dependent on the efficiency of the ligation). Cut the smear out of the gel in two pieces as follow: 200–300 bp and 300–500 bp.

10. Perform gel purification using Gel Purification Qiagen kit.

11. Perform the T4 ligation reaction using 200–300 bp and 300–500 bp annealing reactions (miR-30a and scrambled) plus pEGFP-C3 + SandI vector in a 1:10 and 1:100 (vector–insert) ratio.

12. Transformation of DH5α competent cells is performed by heat shock method (*see* **Note 2**).

13. The transformed competent cells are streaked into LB medium agar plate with 50 μg/mL kanamycin and incubate overnight at 37 °C.

14. Resuspend each colony in 50 μL LB medium with kanamycin in a 96-well plate (*see* **Note 12**). Perform a PCR for screening the colonies (*see* **Note 13**).

15. Positive colonies are grown in 5 mL LB medium + antibiotic at 37 °C, 5 ×*g* shaking overnight.

16. Harvest DNA using Mini-prep kit (*see* **Note 9**).

17. Two different tests can be performed for positive selection colonies: EcoRI + BglII digestion (Fig. 5) and sequencing (Fig. 6) using the pEGFP-C3 forward sequencing primer.

18. After sequencing confirmation, perform Max-prep using Max-prep kit.

3.3 Generation of Stable Genetic Models of miR-30a

1. A panel of four cell lines—two DLBCL (SU-DHL7 and OCI-Ly18) and two T-ALL (KOPT-K1 and DND-41)—are

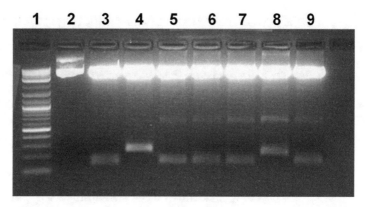

Fig. 5 2 % agarose gel showing scrambled and miR-30 colonies after BglII and EcoRI digestion. A perfect matched and bulged-matched miRNA binding sites were generated, ranging from two (scrambled: 3, 5, 6; miR30a: 7, 9) and six (scrambled: 4; miR30a:8) MBS in the miRNA sponges. *1*: Marker DNA ladder 100 bp; *2*: no digested miR-30 sponge as control

GCCCCAGAAGCGCGATCCTGGTCCTGCTGGAGTTCGTGACCGCCGCCGGGA

TCACTCTCGGCATGGACGAGCTGTACAAGTACTCAGATCT**GTG**AAATATGG

GACCCGTACCTGTTTACGTTCTAACTGAATATGTACCTGTTTACGTTCTAACT

GGGACCCGTACCTGTTTACGTTCTAACTGAATATGTACCTGTTTACGTTCTA

ACTGAATATGTACCTGTTTACGTTCTAACTGGGACCCGTACCTGTTTACGTTC

TAACTGAATATGAATTCTGCAGTCGACGGTACCGCGGGCCCGGGATCCACC

GGATCTAGATAACTGATCATAATCAGCCATACCACATTTGTAGAGGTTTTAC

TTGCTTTAAAAAACCTCCCACACCTCCCCCTGAACCTGAAACATAAAATGAA

TGCAATTGTTGTTGTTAACTTGTTTATTGCAGCTTATAATGGTTACAAATAAA

GCAATAGCATCACAAATTTCACAAATAAAGCATTTTTTTCACTGCATTCTAG

TTGTGGTTTGTCCAAACTCATCAATGTATCTTAACGCGTAAATTGTAAGCGT

TAATATTTTGTTAAAATTCGCGTTAAATTTTTGTTAAATCAGCTCATTTTTTA

ACCAATAGGCCGAAATCGGCAAAATCCCTTATAAATCAAAAGAATAGACCG

AGATAGGGTTGAGTGTTGTTCCAGTTTGGAACAAGAGTCCACTATTAAAGA

ACGTGGACTCCAACGTCAAAGGGCGAAAAACCGTCTATCAGGGCGATGGCC

CACTACGTGAACCATCACCCTAATCAAGTTTTTTGGGGTCGAGGTGCCGTAA

AGCACTAAATCGGAACCCTAAAGGGAGCCCCCGATTTAGAGCTTGACGGGG

AAAGCCGGCGAACGTGGCGAGAAAGGAAGGTAAGAAAGCGAAAGGAGCG

GGCGCTAGGGCGCTGGCAAGTGTAGCGGTCACGCTGCGCGTAACCACCACA

CCCGCCCGCGCTTAATGCGCGGCTACAGGCGCGTTCAGGGGCACTTTTCGGG

AAATGTGCGCGGAACCCCCTAATTGTTTATTTTTCTAAATACCATTCCAACA

TGGTATCCGCCTCATGAGCACAATAACTCTGTATAACTGCCTT

Fig. 6 Sequencing of scrambled positive colony showing miRNA binding sites sequences (*pink*) cloned into peGFP-C3 + SandI vector, 7-bp interrupted palindrome 5′-GG/GWCCC-3′ (W = A or T) (*blue*), and spacer (*green*). *Red* sequences represent BglII and EcoRI restriction sites, respectively. *Bold*: stop codon

generated with stable expression of sponge constructs directed at miR-30a or a scrambled sequence.

2. Cell lines are generated by electroporation and then selected by G418 antibiotic. Finally, GFP expressing cells can be sorted by flow cytometry (*see* **Note 14**).

4   Notes

1. Heat at 94 °C for 10 min in a thermocycler. Cool down slowly (5 °C/5 min). Then, keep the duplex oligos on ice or at –20 °C as stocks.

2. DH5α transformation using the heat shock method consists of inserting a ligation product into bacteria. After 30 min incubation in ice, a mixture of chemically competent bacteria and DNA insert is placed at 42 °C for 45 s (heat shock) and then placed back on ice for 2 min. SOC medium is added and the transformed cells are incubated at 37 °C for 1 h with agitation $5 \times g$. The transformed DH5α cells are then streaked on LB medium agar plate supplemented with kanamycin antibiotic and incubated at 37 °C overnight.

3. LB medium: Dissolve 10 g tryptone, 5 g yeast extract, and 10 g NaCl in 950 mL deionized water. Adjust the pH of the medium to 7.0 using 1 N NaOH and bring volume up to 1 L. Autoclave on liquid cycle for 20 min. Allow solution to cool to 55 °C, and add antibiotic if needed [1 mL of stock solution (*see* **Note 5**) per liter of LB medium]. Store the medium at +4 °C.

4. LB medium agar: to the LB medium described above, add 15 g/L agar before autoclaving. After autoclaving, cool to approximately 55 °C, add antibiotic, and pour into Petri dishes. Let agar harden, then invert and store at +4 °C in the dark.

5. Stock solution of kanamycin (50 mg/mL): weigh 500 mg kanamycin in 10 mL sterile water. Filter the solution using 0.2 μm filter and store aliquots at –20 °C. For competent cells selection, the antibiotic must be used at a final concentration of 50 μg/mL.

6. DNA concentration after gel purification. *The following numbers are given just for a better understanding of the method.*

   - peGFP-C3MSCV + SandI vector concentration: 15.4 ng/μL
   - miR-30a (200–300 bp) annealing reaction: 12.0 ng/μL.
   - miR-30a (300–500 bp) annealing reaction: 11.2 ng/μL.
   - scrambled (200–300 bp) annealing reaction: 34.1 ng/μL.
   - scrambled (300–500 bp) annealing reaction: 13.0 ng/μL.

7. Divide the 200 μL of annealing reaction in eight PCR tubes with 25 μL each.

8. Perform BglII and EcoRI digestion in a water bath.

9. Store about 500 μL transformed bacteria at 4 °C. After confirming by sequencing, colonies can be grown in 250–500 mL LB medium with 50 μg/mL kanamycin and DNA can be extracted by using max-prep DNA extraction kit.

10. Resuspend the annealing reaction in 30–40 μL final volume.

11. Keep annealing reactions (miR-30a and scrambled) at –20 °C.

12. Note that few colonies will be observed per plate (2–3 per plate).

13. PCR reaction per sample: 2.5 μL buffer Taq polymerase 10×, 0.5 μL dNTP 100 mM, 0.5 μL primers forward + reverse (5 μM of each SanDI), 0.5 μL Taq polymerase, 20.5 μL water, 1 μL each colony (dissolved in 50 μL LB medium).

14. Electroporation was performed using a Bio-Rad Gene Pulser MX Cell (Bio-Rad Laboratories) with parameters set at 250 V, 975 μF, and ∞ resistance. The transfected cells are kept on ice for 10 min and then cultured in Dulbecco's modified Eagle medium with 20 % fetal bovine serum for 24–48 h before G418 selection.

Acknowledgement

We thank Dr. Ricardo CT Aguiar from The University of Texas Health Science Center at San Antonio, USA, for the valuable advices during the sponge constructions.

References

1. Eulalio A, Huntzinger E, Izaurralde E (2008) Getting to the root of miRNA-mediated gene silencing. Cell 132:9–14

2. Georges M, Coppieters W, Charlier C (2007) Polymorphic miRNA-mediated gene regulation: contribution to phenotypic variation and disease. Curr Opin Genet Dev 17:166–176

3. Rai D, Karanti S, Junk I, Dahia P, Aguiar RC (2008) Coordinated expression of microRNA-155 and predicted target genes in DLBCL. Cancer Genet Cytogenet 181:8–15

4. Chaubey A, Karanti S, Rai D, Oh T, Adhvaryu SG, Aguiar RC (2009) MicroRNAs and deletion of the derivative chromosome 9 in chronic myeloid leukemia. Leukemia 23:186–188

5. Jung I, Aguiar RC (2009) MicroRNA-155 expression and outcome in diffuse large B-cell lymphoma. Br J Haematol 144:138–140

6. Li C, Kim SW, Rai D, Bolla A, Kinney M, Robetorye R, Aguiar RC (2009) Copy number abnormalities, MYC activity and the fingerprint of normal B-cells define the microRNA profile of DLBCL. Blood 113:6681–6690

7. Rai D, Kim SW, McKeller MR, Dahia PLM, Aguiar RC (2010) Targeting of SMAD5 links microRNA-155 to the TGFβ pathway and lymphomagenesis. Proc Natl Acad Sci U S A 107:3111–3116

8. Kim SW, Ramasamy K, Bouamar H, Lin AP, Jiang D, Aguiar RC (2012) MicroRNAs miR-125a and miR-125b constitutively activate the NF-kB pathway by targeting the tumor necrosis factor alpha-induced protein 3 (TNFAIP3, A20). Proc Natl Acad Sci USA 109: 7865–7870

9. Jiang D, Aguiar RC (2014) MicroRNA-155 controls RB phosphorylation in normal and malignant B lymphocytes via the non-canonical TGFB1-SMAD5 signaling module. Blood 123:86–93

10. Ortega M, Bhatnagar H, Lin AP, Wang L, Aster JC, Sill H, Aguiar RC (2015) A microRNA-mediated regulatory loop modulates NOTCH and MYC oncogenic signals in B- and T-cell malignancies. Leukemia 29:968–976

11. Jeong D, Kim J, Nam J, Sun H, Lee YH, Lee TJ, Aguiar RC, Kim SW (2015) MicroRNA-124 links p53 to the NF-kB pathway in B cell lymphomas. Leukemia 29:1868–1874

12. Bouamar H, Jiang D, Wang L, Lin AP, Ortega M, Aguiar RC (2015) MicroRNA-155 control of p53 activity is context dependent and mediated by Aicda and Socs1. Mol Cell Biol 35:1329–1340

13. Ebert MS, Neilson JR, Sharp PA (2007) MicroRNA sponges: competitive inhibitors of

small RNAs in mammalian cells. Nat Methods 4:721–726

14. Piva R, Spandidos DA, Gambari R (2013) From microRNA functions to microRNA therapeutics: novel targets and novel drugs in breast cancer research and treatment (Review). Int J Oncol 43:985–994

15. Esau CC (2008) Inhibition of microRNA with antisense oligonucleotides. Methods 44:55–60

16. Takahashi M, Yamada N, Hatakeyama H, Murata M, Sato Y, Minakawa N, Harashima H, Matsuda A (2013) In vitro optimization of 2′-OMe-4′-thioribonucleoside-modified anti-microRNA oligonucleotides and its targeting delivery to mouse liver using a liposomal nanoparticle. Nucleic Acids Res 41:10659–10667

17. Lennox KA, Owczarzy R, Thomas DM, Walder JA, Behlke MA (2013) Improved performance of anti-miRNA oligonucleotides using a novel non-nucleotide modifier. Mol Ther Nucleic Acids 2:e117

18. Wu SQ, Xu ZZ, Lin J, Zhan R (2012) Construction of miRNA sponge targeting miR-20a and stable expression in Jurkat leukemia cell line. J Exp Hematol 20:1056–1062

19. Chen L, Zhang K, Shi Z, Zhang A, Jia Z, Wang G, Pu P, Kang C, Han L (2014) A lentivirus-mediated miR-23b sponge diminishes the malignant phenotype of glioma cells in vitro and in vivo. Oncol Rep 31:1573–1580

20. Kluiver J, Slezak-Prochazka I, Smigielska-Czepiel K, Halsema N, Kroesen BJ, van den Berg A (2012) Generation of miRNA sponge constructs. Methods 58:113–117

21. Simcox TG, Fabian L, Kretz K, Hedden V, Simcox ME (1995) SanDI, a new type-II restriction endonuclease that recognizes 5′-GG/GWCCC-3′. Gene 155:129–130

22. Jung J, Yeom C, Choi YS, Kim S, Lee E, Park MJ, Kang SW, Kim SB, Chang S (2015) Simultaneous inhibition of multiple oncogenic miRNAs by a multi-potent microRNA sponge. Oncotarget 6:20370–20387

Chapter 21

Customization of Artificial MicroRNA Design

Tien Van Vu and Vinh Nang Do

Abstract

RNAi approaches, including microRNA (miRNA) regulatory pathway, offer great tools for functional characterization of unknown genes. Moreover, the applications of artificial microRNA (amiRNA) in the field of plant transgenesis have also been advanced to engineer pathogen-resistant or trait-improved transgenic plants. Until now, despite the high potency of amiRNA approach, no commercial plant cultivar expressing amiRNAs with improved traits has been released yet. Beside the issues of biosafety policies, the specificity and efficacy of amiRNAs are of major concerns. Sufficient cares should be taken for the specificity and efficacy of amiRNAs due to their potential off-target effects and other issues relating to in vivo expression of pre-amiRNAs. For these reasons, the proper design of amiRNAs with the lowest off-target possibility is very important for successful applications of the approach in plant. Therefore, there are many studies with the aim to improve the amiRNA design and amiRNA expressing backbones for obtaining better specificity and efficacy. However, the requirement for an efficient reference for the design is still needed. In the present chapter, we attempt to summarize and discuss all the major concerns relating to amiRNA design with the hope to provide a significant guideline for this approach.

Key words Artificial microRNA, amiRNA design, PTGS, RNAi, microRNA

1 Introduction

There are many types of identified small RNAs acting in various RNA interference (RNAi) pathways including the major class, microRNA (miRNA). Quickly after the identification of miRNAs, synthetic miRNAs (the so-called artificial microRNAs or amiRNAs) were designed to efficiently degrade cognate mRNAs [1–3], thus introducing a highly potential technology to gene functional characterization. Furthermore, it was shown that amiRNAs targeted cognate mRNAs equally or even more efficiently than siRNAs did [1, 3]. Artificial miRNAs were proven to be a highly potential approach not only for functional characterization of genes but also for efficient silencing of exotic genes or undesirable genes [4].

AmiRNA approach has been applied successfully to not only animals but also plants. The most important aspect of amiRNA application is the generation of mature amiRNA based on targeted

Sweta Rani (ed.), *MicroRNA Profiling: Methods and Protocols*, Methods in Molecular Biology, vol. 1509,
DOI 10.1007/978-1-4939-6524-3_21, © Springer Science+Business Media New York 2017

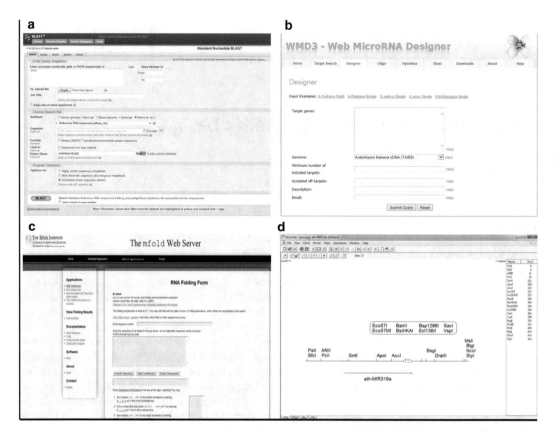

Fig. 1 Interface of some bioinformatics programs used in amiRNA design. (**a**). BLASTN (http://blast.ncbi.nlm.nih. gov/Blast.cgi?PROGRAM=blastn&PAGE_TYPE=BlastSearch&LINK_LOC=blasthome); (**b**) WMD3-Web MicroRNA Designer (http://wmd3.weigelworld.org/cgi-bin/webapp.cgi?page=Designer;project=stdwmd); (**c**). MFOLD (http://unafold.rna.albany.edu/?q=mfold/rna-folding-form) and (**d**) SECentral (Clone Manager Professional, http://www.scied.com/pr_cmpro.htm)

sequence and the integration of the designed sequence into an appropriate stem-loop backbone in such a way that the newly formed precursor (namely, amiRNA expressing precursor or pre-amiRNA, which helps processed the amiRNAs in vivo) properly matches the characteristics of the natural precursor used [5]. For designing amiRNAs to target known sequences in animal, researchers have used many approaches, which showed significant levels of mature amiRNA accumulation. Even in some approaches, they inserted siRNA sequences in the place of mature miRNAs of the respectively natural pre-amiRNAs [1, 2]. In plants, Schwab and coworkers [5] conducted research on amiRNAs in *Arabidopsis* using *ath*-MIR319a as a stem-loop backbone for targeting diverse range of functional genes. The idea of their research was to design amiRNA sequences based on the properties of plant's natural miR-NAs and integrate these into the backbone so as to mimic the natural precursor. This is to ensure that the amiRNA and the subsequently selected precursor will be preferable substrate for DCL1.

On the other hand, it is also good for directing the selection of guide strand used in miRISC. The guide strand selection depends on energy balance between 3′ and 5′ regions calculating by the number of hydroxyl bond between nucleotides in the double-stranded miRNA/amiRNA. Moreover, the recruitment of the designed miRNA by AGO complex could be control using prioritized nucleotide at the 5′ terminal of the amiRNA [6]. The other concerns are to ensure: lowest or zero possibility of off-target effects; in silico folded conformation of pre-amiRNA perfectly matches that of the natural one; and efficient expression of the amiRNA in selected plants by appropriate pre-miRNAs.

However, it is impossible to design an amiRNA, and subsequently pre-amiRNAs, which fully mimic natural ones, due to sequence differences. In addition, the expression of amiRNAs in plants sometimes induced side-effects (off-target effects) that were more or less impact on plant depending on the levels of similarity between amiRNA/pre-amiRNA and the correspondingly natural backbone. Further, there is no detailed guideline for the design of amiRNA in plant. With these views, we attempt to summarize and comment on the amiRNA/pre-amiRNA design to offer a useful guideline for more efficient applications of amiRNA approach in plants.

2 Materials

2.1 Databases

In this method some of the following databases are used: GenBank, Mirbase, EMBL, and PGDB.

2.2 Bioinformatics Programs

In this method we mostly use bioinformatics software to design amiRNAs, to assemble them into appropriate precursors and to predict secondary structures have the designed precursor and natural one, as well. Some of the programs are BLASTN, WMD3 (Web MicroRNA Designer), MFOLD, and SECentral (Fig. 1).

3 Methods

This method applies to the design of 21-nt amiRNA to act in posttranscriptional gene silencing (PTGS) pathway in plant.

3.1 Identification of Silencing Scenario

There are two main scenarios for targeting a gene by amiRNA: (1) Knockout, in PTGS pathway this means all the mRNA of the targeted gene should be cleaved and degraded; and (2) Knockdown, this means suppression of targeted gene expression (*see* **Note 1**)

3.2 Identification of Targeted Sequence(s)

1. Retrieval of targeted genes. For 21 nt-amiRNA designs for PTGS, targeted sites should be from Open Reading Frames (ORFs) of the genes (*see* **Notes 1** and **2**).

2. Using Clone Manager module of SECentral software to search for ORFs of the targeted genes.

3. Using NCBI BLASTN to search for conservative regions among the targeted ORFs (targeted ORFs from the same gene family or from organisms in one species). The conservative fragments will be used to design amiRNAs.

3.3 Design of 21 nt-amiRNA Sequence(s)

1. Submission of the conservative fragments to WMD3 website to design amiRNAs using corresponding PGDB database of the amiRNA-expressing plant as reference for excluding off-targets.

2. Analyses of WMD3 results and selection of amiRNAs based on their features for further research. A Uracil should be positioned at 5′ end of the amiRNA. One mismatch is introduced to position 18–20 of each amiRNA to prevent any potential production of phased-siRNAs (*see* **Notes 1–3**). The selected and modified amiRNAs should be used to search for any off-target in human genome database or human expressed sequence tags (ESTs) database for safety purpose (if needed in the future).

3.4 Precursor Selection

Appropriate precursor sequences are retrieved and selected from miRBase database for expressing amiRNAs in plants. Precursors to be selected should naturally exist and experimentally express in plants. Single, dual, triplex or multiplex amiRNA expressing precursor may be used for different purposes (*see* **Notes 4** and **5**).

3.5 Pre-amiRNA Assembly

1. Identification and design of amiRNA*s for building pre-amiRNAs. amiRNA*s for assembling to *ath*-MIR319a are designed by WMD3. amiRNA*s for assembling to other precursors are designed according to the features of miRNA*s on the natural backbones (*see* **Note 6**).

2. Replacement of the natural sequences of miRNA and miRNA* on the selected precursors by the designed amiRNAs and amiRNA*s in the same order to form pre-amiRNAs.

3. *In silico* validation of the assembled precursor by using MFOLD software to predict their secondary structure. Secondary structure of the assembled precursor should be exactly same as their natural donors (*see* **Note 7**).

3.6 Pre-amiRNA Synthesis

The in silico validated precursor sequences are sent directly to commercial company for chemical syntheses. The next stage will be cloning of the synthesized precursors into binary vectors (pBI121 or pCAMBIA1301) for plant transformation and analysing transgenic plants for amiRNA expression at various generations.

4 Notes

1. As shown by various reports, the silencing modes were driven by the activity of AGO proteins in the RISC complex as well as the levels of base-pairing complementarity between miRNA and targeted RNA sequences. In *Arabidopsis*, only AGO1, AGO2, AGO4, AGO7, and AGO10 proteins were shown to exhibit slicer activity [7–10]. On the other hand, it was shown that few mismatches outside the core region (nucleotide 2–12 from 5′ end) of miRNAs did not significantly alter the slicing activity. In contrast, more than one mismatch in the core region, especially at position 10–11 from 5′ end, would lead to inhibition of slicing activity [5]. To approach cleavage mechanism, the amiRNA should carry a signal (i.e., 5′ U) to be recruited into an endonuclease domain containing AGO protein (mostly AGO1 and its orthologs in plants) and is highly complementary to its targeted sequence, especially in the core region.

2. Sorting of miRNAs into AGO proteins in *Arabidopsis* is directed by their 5' terminal nucleotides, which are selectively anchored by specific pockets in the MID domains of AGO proteins [6, 11, 12]. Biochemical studies indicated that key amino acid residues at the active site (i.e., bases 10 and 11 from 5′ end of guide strand miRNA) and those lining the 5′-phosphate-binding pocket made up of the MID domain are critical for cleavage activity [13]. Bioinformatics analysis revealed that AGO2 and AGO4 preferentially recruit small RNAs with a 5′ terminal adenosine (A, 92 % and 79 % association, respectively), whereas AGO1 harbors miRNAs that favor a 5′ terminal Uracil (U, 86 % association). AGO5 predominantly binds small RNAs that initiate with cytosine (C, 83 % association) [5]. Further analyses showed that most *Arabidopsis* miRNAs have a 5′ terminal U, and these were predominantly associated with AGO1. Moreover, changing the 5′ terminal nucleotide of a miRNA predictably redirected it into a different AGO complex and alters its biological activity [5, 11, 12].

3. Off-target effects are a major concern in RNAi application and amiRNA design as well. The variation in miRNA length may also contribute to off-target effects [14]. For example, miRNAs of 22 nt length were shown to be triggers of phased siRNAs (phasiRNAs) and these small RNAs could silence endogenous genes *in trans* [15, 16]. Off-target effects induced by amiRNAs were shown to seriously affect leaf morphology [17, 18] and to significantly reduce the plant regeneration efficiency [19] in tomato transgenic plants. Therefore, it is important to select amiRNA sequence, which does not contain regions complementary to any functional gene of the plant. The alterations in the 3′ nucleotide of amiRNAs to contain

1–3 mismatches (between amiRNAs and targeted mRNAs) can prevent producing phasiRNA [20]. Another solution is to design multiple amiRNAs and their precursors and then screen for the optimized one, which may produce single amiRNA of interest [21, 22]. To better understanding the production of amiRNA processing in vivo, amiRNAs should be cloned using stem-loop primers [23] and then sequenced to assess the presence of interest amiRNAs in the plant cells.

In the other aspect, rice MIR168a was shown to function in cross-kingdom manner [i.e., the food-derived exogenous miRNA can pass through the mouse gastrointestinal track and enter the circulation and various organs especially the liver where it regulates mouse LDLRAP1 protein expression and physiological condition] [24] and hence in case of amiRNA applications in plants which could be used as food sources for human or animals, off-target effects may need to be taken care by finding complementary sites of amiRNAs in genomes of the cross-kingdoms.

4. The conformation of precursor backbone of miRNA plays important role for precise dicing of DCL1 and the competition of different DCLs for their substrates [25]. The combination of mature miRNA and its precursor may alternate the structure and thus decide the efficacy of dicing [26]. An amiRNA was proven to express at different levels by various backbones in transgenic plants [5, 19]. In most of previous reports, amiR-NAs levels were shown to correlate with gene silencing levels [5, 17–19, 27–31].

5. Polycistronic pre-miRNAs producing more than one mature sequence of miRNA from one transcript were reported in rice [osa-MIR395 family [32]] and Arabidopsis [Ath-MIR859-774a [33]]. Recently, the polycistronic pre-miRNAs were applied for silencing multiple genes in plants [33–35] with significant successes. The approach opens a novel strategy for the application of amiRNA technology in plants omitting the uses of complicate systems for double transformation or tri-transformation of two or three genes and/or multiple pre-amiRNA expression cassettes.

6. Mature miRNA duplex is loaded into AGO protein with the support from DCL and other cytosolic proteins like double-stranded RNA binding protein (DRB1, similar to HYL1), CYP40, SQN, and HSP90. Subsequently, the guide strand is selected upon asymmetric thermostability of the duplex termini [36, 37]. Energy balance of the miRNA duplex is the key determinant of the thermodynamic selection. The strand with lower thermodynamic stability at its 5′ end (fewer number of hydroxyl bond compared to its 3′ end) is selected as guide strand and the opposite strand (passenger strand or star strand)

will be removed along with the release of the AGO1-associated proteins [37]. The passenger strand removal may be assisted by the dissociation of SQN and HSP90 from AGO protein [37].

7. The secondary conformation (i.e., stem structure and loop distribution) of miRNA precursor affects the precision of catalytic activity of DCL1 via facilitating specific binding of proteins (e.g., HYL1, SE, TGH, and DDL) [26, 38–42]. Therefore, it is important to verify in silico whether the secondary structure of pre-amiRNAs is exactly same as the corresponding natural one. Some excellent software was programmed to predict secondary structure of pre-amiRNAs. In our opinion, MFOLD (http://mfold.rit.albany.edu/?q=mfold/RNA-Folding-Form) [43] is the best software for folding pre-miRNAs and pre-amiRNAs with the ease to compare and visually find out any variation in secondary structures of both the precursors. MFOLD can also be used to calculate free binding energy of amiRNA-targeted RNA.

References

1. Zeng Y, Wagner EJ, Cullen BR (2002) Both natural and designed micro RNAs can inhibit the expression of cognate mRNAs when expressed in human cells. Mol Cell 9(6):1327–1333

2. McManus MT, Petersen CP, Haines BB, Chen J, Sharp PA (2002) Gene silencing using microRNA designed hairpins. RNA 8(6):842–850

3. Boden D, Pusch O, Silbermann R, Lee F, Tucker L, Ramratnam B (2004) Enhanced gene silencing of HIV-1 specific siRNA using microRNA designed hairpins. Nucleic Acids Res 32(3):1154–1158

4. Zhou M, Luo H (2013) MicroRNA-mediated gene regulation: potential applications for plant genetic engineering. Plant Mol Biol 83(1-2):59–75. doi:10.1007/s11103-013-0089-1, Epub 2013 Jun 15

5. Schwab R, Ossowski S, Riester M, Warthmann N, Weigel D (2006) Highly specific gene silencing by artificial microRNAs in *Arabidopsis*. Plant Cell 18(5):1121–1133

6. Mi S, Cai T, Hu Y, Chen Y, Hodges E, Ni F, Wu L, Li S, Zhou H, Long C, Chen S, Hannon GJ, Qi Y (2008) Sorting of small RNAs into *Arabidopsis* argonaute complexes is directed by the 5′ terminal nucleotide. Cell 133(1):116–127

7. Baumberger N, Baulcombe DC (2005) Arabidopsis ARGONAUTE1 is an RNA Slicer that selectively recruits microRNAs and short interfering RNAs. Proc Natl Acad Sci U S A 102(33):11928–11933

8. Qi Y, He X, Wang XJ, Kohany O, Jurka J, Hannon GJ (2006) Distinct catalytic and non-catalytic roles of ARGONAUTE4 in RNA-directed DNA methylation. Nature 443(7114):1008–1012, Epub 2006 Sep 24

9. Ji L, Liu X, Yan J, Wang W, Yumul RE, Kim YJ, Dinh TT, Liu J, Cui X, Zheng B, Agarwal M, Liu C, Cao X, Tang G, Chen X (2011) ARGONAUTE10 and ARGONAUTE1 regulate the termination of floral stem cells through two microRNAs in Arabidopsis. PLoS Genet 7(3):e1001358. doi:10.1371/journal.pgen.1001358

10. Carbonell A, Fahlgren N, Garcia-Ruiz H, Gilbert KB, Montgomery TA, Nguyen T, Cuperus JT, Carrington JC (2012) Functional analysis of three Arabidopsis ARGONAUTES using slicer-defective mutants. Plant Cell 24(9):3613–3629. doi:10.1105/tpc.112.099945, Epub 2012 Sep 28

11. Takeda A, Iwasaki S, Watanabe T, Utsumi M, Watanabe Y (2008) The mechanism selecting the guide strand from small RNA duplexes is different among argonaute proteins. Plant Cell Physiol 49(4):493–500. doi:10.1093/pcp/pcn043

12. Montgomery TA, Howell MD, Cuperus JT, Li D, Hansen JE, Alexander AL, Chapman EJ, Fahlgren N, Allen E, Carrington JC (2008) Specificity of ARGONAUTE7-miR390 interaction and dual functionality in TAS3 trans-acting siRNA formation. Cell 133(1):128–141. doi:10.1016/j.cell.2008.02.033, Epub 2008 Mar 13

13. Wang Y, Li Y, Ma Z, Yang W, Ai C (2010) Mechanism of microRNA-target interaction:

molecular dynamics simulations and thermodynamics analysis. PLoS Comput Biol 6(7):e1000866. doi:10.1371/journal.pcbi.1000866

14. Rogers K, Chen X (2013) Biogenesis, turnover, and mode of action of plant microRNAs. Plant Cell 25(7):2383–2399. doi:10.1105/tpc.113.113159, Epub 2013 Jul 23

15. Chen HM, Chen LT, Patel K, Li YH, Baulcombe DC, Wu SH (2010) 22-Nucleotide RNAs trigger secondary siRNA biogenesis in plants. Proc Natl Acad Sci U S A 107(34):15269–15274. doi:10.1073/pnas.1001738107, Epub 2010 Jul 19

16. Cuperus JT, Carbonell A, Fahlgren N, Garcia-Ruiz H, Burke RT, Takeda A, Sullivan CM, Gilbert SD, Montgomery TA, Carrington JC (2010) Unique functionality of 22-nt miRNAs in triggering RDR6-dependent siRNA biogenesis from target transcripts in Arabidopsis. Nat Struct Mol Biol 17(8):997–1003. doi:10.1038/nsmb.1866, Epub 2010 Jun 18

17. Yadava P, Suyal G, Mukherjee SK (2010) *Begomovirus* DNA replication and pathogenicity. Curr Sci 98(3):360–368

18. Yadava P, Mukherjee SK (2012) Artificial microRNA and its applications. In: Bibekanand M, Zhumur G (eds) Regulatory RNAs: basics, methods and applications. Springer, Berlin, Germany, pp 505–521

19. Vu TV, Choudhury NR, Mukherjee SK (2013) Transgenic tomato plants expressing artificial microRNAs for silencing the pre-coat and coat proteins of a begomovirus, tomato leaf curl New Delhi virus, show tolerance to virus infection. Virus Res 172(1-2):35–45. doi:10.1016/j.virusres.2012.12.008, Epub 2012 Dec 28

20. Zhang C, Ng DW, Lu J, Chen ZJ (2012a) Roles of target site location and sequence complementarity in trans-acting siRNA formation in Arabidopsis. Plant J 69(2):217–226. doi:10.1111/j.1365-313X.2011.04783.x, Epub 2011 Oct 25

21. Fellmann C, Hoffmann T, Sridhar V, Hopfgartner B, Muhar M, Roth M, Lai DY, Barbosa IA, Kwon JS, Guan Y, Sinha N, Zuber J (2013) An optimized microRNA backbone for effective single-copy RNAi. Cell Rep 5(6):1704–1713. doi:10.1016/j.celrep.2013.11.020, Epub 2013 Dec 12

22. Carbonell A, Takeda A, Fahlgren N, Johnson SC, Cuperus JT, Carrington JC (2014) New generation of artificial microRNA and synthetic trans-acting small interfering RNA vectors for efficient gene silencing in Arabidopsis. Plant Physiol 165(1):15–29. doi:10.1104/pp.113.234989, Epub 2014 Mar 19

23. Chen C, Ridzon DA, Broomer AJ, Zhou Z, Lee DH, Nguyen JT, Barbisin M, Xu NL, Mahuvakar VR, Andersen MR, Lao KQ, Livak KJ, Guegler KJ (2005) Real-time quantification of microRNAs by stem-loop RT-PCR. Nucleic Acids Res 33(20):e179

24. Zhang L, Hou D, Chen X, Li D, Zhu L, Zhang Y, Li J, Bian Z, Liang X, Cai X, Yin Y, Wang C, Zhang T, Zhu D, Zhang D, Xu J, Chen Q, Ba Y, Liu J, Wang Q, Chen J, Wang J, Wang M, Zhang Q, Zhang J, Zen K, Zhang CY (2012b) Exogenous plant MIR168a specifically targets mammalian LDLRAP1: evidence of cross-kingdom regulation by microRNA. Cell Res 22(1):107–126. doi:10.1038/cr.2011.158, Epub 2011 Sep 20

25. Nagano H, Fukudome A, Hiraguri A, Moriyama H, Fukuhara T (2014) Distinct substrate specificities of Arabidopsis DCL3 and DCL4. Nucleic Acids Res 42(3):1845–1856. doi:10.1093/nar/gkt1077, Epub 2013 Nov 7

26. Kurihara Y, Watanabe Y (2004) *Arabidopsis* micro-RNA biogenesis through Dicer-like 1 protein functions. Proc Natl Acad Sci U S A 101(34):12753–12758

27. Alvarez JP, Pekker I, Godshmidt A, Blum E, Amsellem Z, Eshed Y (2006) Endogenous and synthetic microRNAs stimulate simultaneous, efficient, and localized regulation of multiple targets in diverse species. Plant Cell 18:1134–1151

28. Niu QW, Lin SS, Reyes JL, Chen KC, Wu HW, Yeh SD, Chua NH (2006) Expression of artificial microRNAs in transgenic *Arabidopsis thaliana* confers virus resistance. Nat Biotechnol 24(11):1420–1428

29. Qu J, Ye J, Fang R (2007) Artificial microRNA-mediated virus resistance in plants. J Virol 81(12):6690–6699

30. Warthmann N, Chen H, Ossowski S, Weigel D, Hervé P (2008) Highly specific gene silencing by artificial miRNAs in rice. PLoS One 3(3), e1829

31. Duan CG, Wang CH, Fang RX, Guo HS (2008) Artificial MicroRNAs highly accessible to targets confer efficient virus resistance in plants. J Virol 82(22):11084–11095

32. Guddeti S, Zhang DC, Li AL, Leseberg CH, Kang H, Li XG, Zhai WX, Johns MA, Mao L (2005) Molecular evolution of the rice miR395 gene family. Cell Res 15(8):631–638

33. Merchan F, Boualem A, Crespi M, Frugier F (2009) Plant polycistronic precursors containing non-homologous microRNAs target transcripts encoding functionally related proteins. Genome Biol 10(12):R136. doi:10.1186/gb-2009-10-12-r136, Epub 2009 Dec 1

34. Kung YJ, Lin SS, Huang YL, Chen TC, Harish SS, Chua NH, Yeh SD (2012) Multiple artificial microRNAs targeting conserved motifs of the replicase gene confer robust transgenic resistance to negative-sense single-stranded RNA plant virus. Mol Plant Pathol 13(3):303–317. doi:10.1111/j.1364-3703.2011.00747.x, Epub 2011 Sep 19

35. Fahim M, Larkin PJ (2013) Designing effective amiRNA and multimeric amiRNA against plant viruses. Methods Mol Biol 942:357–377. doi:10.1007/978-1-62703-119-6_19

36. Eamens AL, Smith NA, Curtin SJ, Wang MB, Waterhouse PM (2009) The Arabidopsis thaliana double-stranded RNA binding protein DRB1 directs guide strand selection from microRNA duplexes. RNA 15(12):2219–2235. doi:10.1261/rna.1646909, Epub 2009 Oct 27

37. Iki T, Yoshikawa M, Meshi T, Ishikawa M (2012) Cyclophilin 40 facilitates HSP90-mediated RISC assembly in plants. EMBO J 31(2):267–278. doi:10.1038/emboj.2011.395, Epub 2011 Nov 1

38. Kurihara Y, Takashi Y, Watanabe Y (2006) The interaction between DCL1 and HYL1 is important for efficient and precise processing of pri-miRNA in plant microRNA biogenesis. RNA 12(2):206–212

39. Dong Z, Han MH, Fedoroff N (2008) The RNA-binding proteins HYL1 and SE promote accurate in vitro processing of pri-miRNA by DCL1. Proc Natl Acad Sci U S A 105(29):9970–9975

40. Ren G, Xie M, Dou Y, Zhang S, Zhang C, Yu B (2012) Regulation of miRNA abundance by RNA binding protein TOUGH in Arabidopsis. Proc Natl Acad Sci U S A 109(31):12817–12821. doi:10.1073/pnas.1204915109, Epub 2012 Jul 16

41. Gu S, Jin L, Zhang Y, Huang Y, Zhang F, Valdmanis PN, Kay MA (2012) The loop position of shRNAs and pre-miRNAs is critical for the accuracy of dicer processing in vivo. Cell 151(4):900–911. doi:10.1016/j.cell.2012.09.042

42. Machida S, Yuan YA (2013) Crystal structure of Arabidopsis thaliana Dawdle forkhead-associated domain reveals a conserved phospho-threonine recognition cleft for dicer-like 1 binding. Mol Plant 6(4):1290–1300. doi:10.1093/mp/sst007, Epub 2013 Jan 11

43. Zuker M (2003) Mfold web server for nucleic acid folding and hybridization prediction. Nucleic Acids Res 31(13):3406–3415

INDEX

A

Acid phosphatase assay...............12, 14, 15, 97, 105
Age-related macular degeneration
    angiogenesis assays 98, 110–111
    cytotoxicity assays..........................97–98, 105
    ExoQuick 103
    human retinal pigment epithelial cell line.............96, 102
    miRCURY LNA™ Universal RT microRNA
        PCR.. 96, 99–102
    real-time qPCR 96, 100–101
Artificial microRNA (amiRNA) 235, 237–241

B

Biobanking serum specimens 74, 78
Bioinformatics
    DNA Intelligent Analysis (DIANA)................196–201
    GO (Gene ontology) analysis............................199–201
    KEGG (Kyoto Encyclopaedia of Genes and Genomes)
        analysis.......................................197–199
    microRNA.org............................ 196, 205–207
    miRBase 196, 201–203
    PicTar....................................... 196, 204–205
Breast cancer..................................7, 19, 73, 123–126,
      133–135, 162

C

Cancer biomarkers..7, 162
Cell culture
    cell culture blocks...20
    cell fixing 111
    cell viability.............................. 11, 12, 14, 16
    coating flask...58, 60
    harvesting cells...61
    proliferation 11, 12, 14, 16, 17, 48, 86, 115
    sub-culturing cells..61
    thawing...60–61
Circulating microRNAs 123–136, 161–167
Cluster analysis...216
Colorectal cancer 18, 116
Colorectal fibroblasts................................115–121
Cystic fibrosis
    airway epithelial cells 58, 67
    bronchial brush samples..............................58, 60

primer design...65
TaqMan MicroRNA Arrays............................57
transfection 57, 59, 66–67
Cytoscape 210, 211, 213, 215–217, 219

D

DNA sizing analysis 190

E

Electrophorese...158
Electrophoresis 26, 30, 32–34, 39, 43, 97, 104, 155, 185
Extracellular miRNA carriers................... 161, 162
Extracellular vesicles/exosome
    isolation 5, 43, 44
    ultracentrifugation 38, 40–42, 45

F

Fluorescent gel scanning 190
Formalin-fixed paraffin embedded (FFPE)
    deparaffinisation 19, 21–22
    DNase digestion 19, 22
    Proteinase digestion................................19, 22

G

Gel image analysis 191

H

Hemolysis..................... 72, 78, 111, 126, 133, 134, 136, 146
Homogenization.............................. 26, 28, 35
Human genome database 238

I

Immunoblotting 38–40, 43–45
In silico prediction......................................238, 241
In situ hybridization
    fixing tissue..88
    hybridisation 89, 90
    neurodegenerative disorders...........................86
    sectioning tissue..86
Induced pluripotent stem (iPS) cells
    differentiation................................. 48, 49, 51, 55
    endoderm marker 51, 56
    immunofluorescence 50, 51

Sweta Rani (ed.), *MicroRNA Profiling: Methods and Protocols*, Methods in Molecular Biology, vol. 1509,
DOI 10.1007/978-1-4939-6524-3, © Springer Science+Business Media New York 2017

Induced pluripotent stem (iPS) cells (*cont.*)
    pluripotency 48
    pluripotency markers 50
    RNA isolation 49, 51–52

M

Metabolic syndrome (MetS) 141–149
MicroRNA (miRNA)
    biogenesis 1–7, 86
    cancer 6–7, 11, 17, 116, 117, 120–121,
        123–136, 141, 142, 162, 169, 210, 221
    cardiovascular disease 6, 11, 17, 141, 210
    neurodegenerative diseases 6
    retinal disorder 5–6
    sponges 221–223, 229
    biogenesis 3
    isolation
        miRNeasy Mini Kit 27–28, 30–31,
            35, 73, 133
        miRNeasy serum/plasma kit 74, 78–80
    profiling
        microarray 48, 94, 142, 169–183
        miRCURY LNA™ Universal RT microRNA 96
        miRCURY LNA™ Universal RT microRNA
            PCR 99–102, 170
        miRCURY LNA™ Universal RT miRNA
            qPCR 142, 145
        Next Generation Sequencing 26
        TaqMan low density array 53, 71–83
        TaqMan MicroRNA Arrays 48, 53, 55,
            57, 77, 78
miRNA-mRNA networks 210, 215
miRWalk database 210–213, 218

O

Open Reading Frames (ORFs) 238

P

Plasma 12, 38, 40, 41, 45, 74, 78–80, 83,
    123–126, 128, 130–133, 135, 136, 141–149

R

RNA Integrity Number (RIN) 19, 20, 22, 34, 35, 182
RNA isolation, TriReagent 49–51, 58, 60, 61,
    64, 96, 98, 142, 143, 145, 149
RNA quality analyses
    BioAnalyzer 19, 21, 34, 143, 145, 149, 172, 173
    NanoDrop 21, 33, 173
RNA quantification, NanoDrop 62, 143–145, 149
RNA spike-in 96, 100, 101, 112, 149

S

Secondary metabolites 25–27
Serum 6, 12, 13, 38, 40, 41, 44, 45, 48, 58, 59,
    61, 67, 72–75, 78–81, 83, 87, 94, 96–99, 101–105,
    111, 112, 116, 123–126, 128, 130–136, 142, 145,
    146, 155, 162, 164, 166, 167, 232
Size-exclusion chromatography (SEC) 162

T

Thermal cycler 63, 143, 172, 185, 187, 189, 190
Transmission electron microscopy (TEM) 38–39,
    41–42, 119
Tumor microenvironment (TME) 115, 116

V

Vector construction
    cloning 154, 157–159, 224–226, 238
    gel extraction 155, 158
    ligation 158–159, 223, 225–227, 231
    restriction 152, 154, 158, 222–225, 228
    transformation 159, 225, 229, 231, 238

Printed in the United States
By Bookmasters